D1352506

ENVIRONMENTAL POLICY AND PUBLIC HEALTH

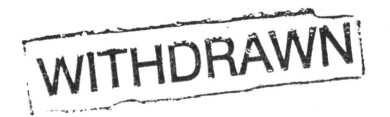
WITHDRAWN

LIVERPOOL JMU LIBRARY

3 1111 01511 9645

ENVIRONMENTAL POLICY AND PUBLIC HEALTH

Air Pollution, Global Climate Change, and Wilderness

WILLIAM N. ROM

FOREWORD BY FRANCES BEINECKE

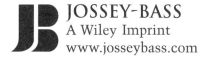

JOSSEY-BASS
A Wiley Imprint
www.josseybass.com

Copyright © 2012 by John Wiley & Sons, Inc. All rights reserved.

Published by Jossey-Bass

A Wiley Imprint

989 Market Street, San Francisco, CA 94103-1741—www.josseybass.com

No part of this publication may be reproduced, stored in a retrieval system, or transmitted in any form or by any means, electronic, mechanical, photocopying, recording, scanning, or otherwise, except as permitted under Section 107 or 108 of the 1976 United States Copyright Act, without either the prior written permission of the publisher, or authorization through payment of the appropriate per-copy fee to the Copyright Clearance Center, Inc., 222 Rosewood Drive, Danvers, MA 01923, 978-750-8400, fax 978-646-8600, or on the Web at www.copyright.com. Requests to the publisher for permission should be addressed to the Permissions Department, John Wiley & Sons, Inc., 111 River Street, Hoboken, NJ 07030, 201-748-6011, fax 201-748-6008, or online at www.wiley.com/go/permissions.

Limit of Liability/Disclaimer of Warranty: While the publisher and author have used their best efforts in preparing this book, they make no representations or warranties with respect to the accuracy or completeness of the contents of this book and specifically disclaim any implied warranties of merchantability or fitness for a particular purpose. No warranty may be created or extended by sales representatives or written sales materials. The advice and strategies contained herein may not be suitable for your situation. You should consult with a professional where appropriate. Neither the publisher nor author shall be liable for any loss of profit or any other commercial damages, including but not limited to special, incidental, consequential, or other damages. Readers should be aware that Internet Web sites offered as citations and/or sources for further information may have changed or disappeared between the time this was written and when it is read.

Jossey-Bass books and products are available through most bookstores. To contact Jossey-Bass directly call our Customer Care Department within the U.S. at 800-956-7739, outside the U.S. at 317-572-3986, or fax 317-572-4002.

Wiley also publishes its books in a variety of electronic formats and by print-on-demand. Not all content that is available in standard print versions of this book may appear or be packaged in all book formats. If you have purchased a version of this book that did not include media that is referenced by or accompanies a standard print version, you may request this media by visiting http://booksupport.wiley.com. For more information about Wiley products, visit us www.wiley.com.

Library of Congress Cataloging-in-Publication Data

Rom, William N.
  Environmental policy and public health : air pollution, global climate change, and wilderness / William N. Rom ; foreword by Frances Beinecke. – 1st ed.
      p. cm. – (Public health/environmental health ; 14)
    Includes bibliographical references and index.
  ISBN 978-0-470-59343-1 (pbk.); 978-1-118-09564-5 (ebk.); 978-1-118-09565-2 (ebk.); 978-1-118-09566-9 (ebk.);
  1. Environmental health–Government policy. 2. Medical policy. I. Title.
  RA566.R66 2012
  362.196$'$98–dc23

                                                                                    2011025363

Printed in the United States of America

FIRST EDITION

PB Printing 10 9 8 7 6 5 4 3 2 1

CONTENTS

FIGURES AND TABLE

*To my wife, Holly, and two children,
Nicole and Meredith, who are documenting and
addressing global climate change as the
mission of the next generation.*

IN THIS VOLUME, Dr. William N. Rom examines environmental challenges that deserve our urgent attention and our best solutions. He explores how the United States has endeavored to reduce the pollution that endangers our public health and the natural systems upon which we depend. He looks at the policies that govern our last remaining wilderness areas. And he discusses global warming, the planetary threat that not only compounds existing pollution and biodiversity problems, but is also emerging as one of the biggest humanitarian crises of our time.

What is especially useful about this book is that Rom examines the interplay between law, science, and advocacy. These three elements have been the building blocks of environmental protection. The Natural Resources Defense Council, where I work, opened its doors in 1970 as the nation's first environmental law firm. John Adams, NRDC's founder, wanted to hold polluters accountable in court, but back then, there was almost no body of environmental law in the United States. You could quickly read through what few statutes existed within an hour. NRDC attorneys, together with other concerned groups, began the work of drafting and passing the Clean Air Act, the Clean Water Act, the Safe Drinking Water Act, the Superfund law, and other bedrock environmental laws.

Legal victories proved effective, but in the 1980s, we began to realize that legal analysis alone could not protect the environment. What is clean water? Lawyers cannot fully answer that question. You need data to measure that, and scientists need to analyze the findings. NRDC brought people on staff to interpret scientific information and to assess what rules would bring us clean air and vibrant forests.

The combination of legal and scientific expertise proved effective, but by the 1990s, when Newt Gingrich's Congress tried to dismantle key environmental protections, we realized that simply proposing good public policies wasn't enough. We had to have the political influence to enact them. At NRDC, we decided to build our membership, because representing a million people—people who tell their representatives that they care about the environment via email, phone, and petitions—is a powerful way to be heard.

Of these three tools for environmental protection—law, science, and advocacy—science holds a place of critical importance. We see this most clearly with the climate crisis. It is scientists who brought this threat to our attention decades ago. For years, politicians and citizens refused to hear the warnings. But in the past five years, the drum beat of climate data has been too deafening to ignore. It reached a crescendo when Vice President Al Gore brought the scientific findings to a mainstream audience with *An Inconvenient Truth* and when the world's leading scientists released the Intergovernmental Panel on Climate Change's fourth report. The report concluded that the warming of the Earth is unequivocal and that most of the observed changes have been caused by humans. For these twin efforts, Al Gore and the IPCC scientists won the Nobel Peace Prize.

Climate science not only outlines the reach of global warming—the amount of Arctic summer sea ice lost each year, the spread of pest infestations such as the white bark pine beetle into northern forests, and the increase in heat-related illnesses. It also conveys the terrible urgency of this crisis. I used to think that we could curb global warming in time so that my grandchildren wouldn't have to face dangerous impacts like punishing droughts and political unrest. Yet we are confronting these very impacts right now, and if we don't act fast, my daughters' generation will really pay the price.

Climate modelers used to say that we could avoid the worst effects if we slashed global warming pollution by 2050, then it was 2040, then 2030. Now a new study has found that sea levels may rise twice as fast as was predicted only two years ago by the IPCC. What has changed since then? Scientists have gained access to more data than the IPCC researchers had on sea temperatures, the role of the Antarctic's ice loss, and the amount of carbon the oceans can absorb.

All of this research points in the same direction: we are running out of time. Back in 2007, Rajendra Pachauri, the head of the IPCC, announced: "If there's no action before 2012, that's too late. What we do in the next two to three years will determine our future." The message is clear: we have to act now.

But as we go forward, we must employ science to shape the policies and laws. Science tells us, for instance, that in order to prevent the worst effects of climate change, we must reduce our global warming pollution by 80 percent by 2050. This is a daunting challenge, but again, science and technology can show the way: Solutions exist today that can achieve these reductions. We can and must shift to low-carbon, clean-energy solutions. As author Bill McKibben says, there is no silver bullet on global warming, but there is silver buckshot.

There are a number of pathways for slashing carbon emissions. NRDC believes the most effective and sustainable are:

- Increasing our energy efficiency
- Improving the fuel economy, and providing environmentally sound alternative fuels for our cars and trucks
- Producing more wind and solar energy
- Using new technologies to capture carbon emissions from coal-fired power plants

Putting these solutions in place will require major shifts in policy and strong national leadership. First and foremost, it will require passing a national law to limit global warming pollution.

We have to be brave and bold in what we do to address global warming, and if we are, we will reap enormous benefits. The process of refashioning our energy sector into something cleaner and more sustainable will generate economic growth across the nation. Shifting to low-carbon fuels will strengthen our national security, and put America in a position of leadership in international climate negotiations.

And confronting global warming will also address the other key areas Rom talks about in this book: pollution and wilderness. Right now, coal-fired power plants are the leading source of carbon dioxide emissions in America, as well as major sources of mercury, sulfur dioxide, nitrogen oxides, and particulate matter in the air. These coal-plant pollutants cause respiratory problems such as asthma and lung disease, and are responsible for 24,000 deaths a year in the United States. Shifting away from coal-fired power and toward cleaner sources of electricity, such as renewable power from wind and solar and greater energy efficiency will dramatically reduce pollution and save lives.

Likewise, turning down the heat on global warming will help us preserve our wilderness landscapes. Scientists predict, for instance, that climate change will intensify three main causes of wildfires: high temperatures, summer dryness, and long-term drought. Fire is a natural part of the forest ecosystem, but overcharged fires can be devastating. Already, from 2000 to 2003, extreme heat and drought combined to kill entire forest expanses of low-elevation forests across 60,000 square miles in the American Southwest, a loss that may be permanent. If we reduce our global warming pollution now, we can help prevent these overly intensified wildfires, as well as the climate-fueled pest infestations and habitat loss that are threatening our wilderness heritage.

Bill Rom has traversed many of the globe's wildest and most iconic landscapes. He has guided canoe trips down remote rivers, and climbed some of the most rugged peaks, including Geladaintong, the 21,700-foot mountain in Tibet that serves as the source of the Yangtze River. But he has also trekked through the halls of Congress, serving as Senator Hillary Rodham Clinton's climate advisor, and has organized international conferences on global warming and public health. And he has been on the front lines of public health as a working doctor in a major urban hospital. With his depth of experience, Rom is an excellent guide through the tangled landscape of environmental law, policy, and science. The issues and case studies he has laid out here will help a new generation of advocates identify the solutions that will best safeguard the Earth, its people, and its wildlife.

Frances Beinecke
President, Natural Resources Defense Council

*E*NVIRONMENTAL POLICY AND *Public Health: Air Pollution, Global Climate Change, and Wilderness* introduces the science and legal framework essential for balancing humans with the environment. This balance is framed by policy choices made by decision makers; how these choices are made has become a field of study called environmental policy. Many of these choices have direct impacts on public health, such as the level of particles or ozone allowed in the ambient air affecting hospital and emergency admissions and mortality, and some indirect such as the preservation of wilderness for our mental health and physical activity. Environmental policy students need to know the principles of American government, including federalism, and learn from this text about the legendary Clean Air Act and its amendments now celebrating their fortieth anniversary. In addition, the student will learn about the Wilderness Act, the Clean Water Act, the National Environmental Policy Act, and many more. With the development of the ozone hole looming over Antarctica during the winter, it is strikingly apparent that humans' anthropogenic pollutants are physically altering the environment of the Earth. This is frightening.

We have enjoyed the lifestyle afforded us by the consumption of fossil fuels with relative abandon. We have warm homes, rapid transit, the fruits of chemical technologies, but these have come at a price documented by the rising CO_2 measurements over the past fifty years from the summit of Mauna Loa in Hawaii. There are now warnings of consequences of anthropogenic climate change in scientific journals, and policy debates on future directions make this volume timely. We can bear the heat waves in the summers and observe the bleaching of corals, the altered weather patterns, the dead evergreens on mountain slopes, the loss of sea ice and glaciers, the warming and expansion of the oceans, but the limits of public forbearance are being reached. Advanced computer models illustrate the challenges facing us in the next few short decades as CO_2 surpasses 450 ppm in the troposphere. Policy decisions affecting our whole economy are upon us. Do we continue to build coal-fired power plants and embrace carbon capture and sequestration, or do we move to natural gas-fired power plans, and how do we achieve this? How are interstate and ocean transmission lines built to harness and transport wind energy? How do we decentralize solar panels to private residences? How do we embrace a built-environment that preserves communities? How do we move from importing oil, especially from the Persian Gulf, to employing alternative sources of energy to protect national security? Most important, what federal government policies will most effectively combat global warming and climate change? How do federal regulatory agencies, namely the Environmental Protection Agency (EPA), protect our environment and enhance economic productivity? EPA protects the public from excessive outdoor air pollution, but as World Trade Center dust invades apartments in New York City, who has jurisdiction over indoor air quality? At what level of priority does human health matter? There are limits, and wilderness best illustrates these limits because it is an ever-shrinking resource. How much do we protect now? Are there alternatives to national parks and wilderness areas that can protect wild lands through conservation easements, and how do we now conserve entire ecosystems and preserve their biodiversity?

To answer these questions, the author has traveled to the most remote regions of the world to observe yak dung biomass fires in Tibetan dwellings and Kun Lun peaks where black carbon settling on the glaciers melts the ice that flows into the Yangtze River. In addition, he has traveled by dogsled to the furthest north Thule Inuit village of Siorapaluk to observe sea ice disappearance, to the bleached corals off Belize and Madagascar, to observe rare and endangered species in the Namibian deserts, and ultimately to the floor of the U.S. Senate to staff the first debate on the McCain-Lieberman bill to combat global warming. As a physician-scientist in environmental medicine and pulmonary diseases, the author has a front-row seat in the development of air pollution science and climate change and represents professional advocacy groups to decision makers at the EPA and other federal agencies. These firsthand experiences are used to illustrate environmental policy in real time. This textbook does have a mission in creating a cadre of well-informed citizens to become the decision makers of the future to protect and enhance the environment by the private sector, federal agencies, nonprofits, and especially by our children!

Acknowledgments

The author wishes to thank the contributing authors for their contributions and their patience with changes wrought by the editing process. I wish to thank the project directors, Kyley Leroy and Katie Schliessman, for their excellent assistance and Sandra Kiselica for editorial assistance. I wish to thank the following reviewers for their many helpful comments: Robert R. Jacobs, Ann Keller, Amy D. Kyle, Michele Morrone, Lee Newman, Daniel Teitelbaum, and Charles D. Treser. I would like to acknowledge the guidance of Andy Pasternack and Seth Schwartz at Jossey Bass.

William N. Rom, MD, MPH, grew up as a guide in the Boundary Waters Canoe Area Wilderness and skied in Aspen, CO, while a student in political science at the University of Colorado. As a medical student at the University of Minnesota, he led the first Earth Day with Sigurd Olson and reminisced on canoe expeditions to the Albany River, Churchill River, and Back River to the Arctic. He is the author of *Canoe Country Wilderness*. While a MPH student at Harvard, he met Dr. Irving Selikoff, the father of environmental medicine, and joined him as a Fellow to study asbestos workers, PBB and PCB-exposed workers, lead-exposed workers, and many others.

Rom was founding director of the Rocky Mountain Center for Occupational and Environmental Health at the University of Utah, where he evaluated coal miners, oil shale workers, and copper smelter workers. At the Pulmonary Branch, National Institutes of Health, he elucidated the mechanisms of asbestosis due to macrophage growth factors. He teaches environmental policy in the Wagner Graduate School of Public Service at NYU. As a Legislative Fellow for Senator Hillary Rodham Clinton, he drafted legislation to protect wilderness, clean the air, and address climate change. He is a member of the Explorer's Club with flag expeditions to Tibet, South Georgia, and Greenland. He directs the NYU Pulmonary Division and the Bellevue Chest Service where he is the Sol and Judith Bergstein Professor. He has trained more than 120 fellows and edits *Environmental and Occupational Medicine*. His research is on early detection of lung cancer, lung fibrosis, and on AIDS and tuberculosis.

Frances Beinecke is president of the Natural Resources Defense Council where she focuses on curbing global warming, developing a clean energy future, reviving the world's oceans, saving endangered wild places, stemming the tide of toxic chemicals, and accelerating the greening of China. As executive director and president she has doubled NRDC's membership to 1.3 million and increased the staff to more than 300. Beinecke received a bachelor's degree from Yale College and a master's degree from the Yale School of Forestry and Environmental Studies. She has received the Rachel Carson Award from the National Audubon Society, the Annual Conservation Award from the Adirondack Council, and the Robert Marshall Award from the Wilderness Society.

Caralee Caplan-Shaw, MD, received her medical degree from McGill University. She completed residency in Internal Medicine and a fellowship in Pulmonary and Critical Care Medicine at Columbia University. She has worked for the Florida Department of Health and provides consultative services to TB patients as a member of Florida's TB Physicians Network. She holds a faculty appointment at NYU, where she attends on the inpatient TB unit and treats patients in the World Trade Center Environmental Health Center and Asthma Clinic at Bellevue Hospital. Her research interests are in environmental lung disease and tuberculosis.

Christopher ("Kim") J. Elliman serves as CEO of the Open Space Institute, a land conservation organization that has protected and/or financed close to 2 million acres and created over 50 new parks or protected areas in the eastern United States. Elliman chairs the Geraldine R. Dodge Foundation and Overhills Foundation, has chaired the Wilderness Society and the Adirondack Council, and has served as vice chairman of the Environmental Defense Fund. He has served on numerous non-profit and philanthropic boards, principally in conservation and cultural institutions. Elliman received his BA from

Yale and now serves on Yale University's Forestry and Environmental Leadership Council.

Kimberly Flynn is a founder and co-coordinator of 9/11 Environmental Action, the community-based organization of Lower Manhattan residents, school parents, and environmental health advocates that formed in April 2002 to ensure that the 9/11-related health needs of the community are met. She currently serves as the community co-chair of the Community Advisory Committee to the World Trade Center Environmental Health Center (WTC EHC), the WTC Center of Excellence that serves affected residents, students, and area workers. She has been engaged in environmental and health advocacy in New York City for more than 20 years.

Craig Hall is the president of WTCRC (World Trade Center Residents Coalition); a downtown residents' grassroots organization founded after 09/11 providing environmental, safety, and rebuilding information. Hall is a World Trade Center Environmental Health Center (WTCEHC) Community Advisory Committee board member, WTC Health Registry Community outreach member, certified NY Battery Park City CERT member, Red Cross First Aider and a founding board member of BPC Cares; a 501C3 charity helping tsunami, earthquake and hurricane victims around the world. He is a family man with three young children and a strongly supporting wife who strives to help others less fortunate.

Catherine McVay Hughes, MBA, is vice chair of Manhattan Community Board 1 and chair of CB1's WTC Redevelopment Committee. She is also an appointed member of the Community Advisory Boards for the WTC Health Registry, WTC EHC, and Gouverneur Healthcare Services. Hughes was appointed by Senator Hillary Clinton as community liaison to the US Environmental Protection Agency WTC Expert Technical Panel. She has testified at NYC Council, NYS, and federal hearings. Hughes holds a degree in engineering from Princeton and an MBA from Wharton. She has lived with her family one block east of the World Trade Center site for 22 years.

Angeliki Kazeros, MD, received her undergraduate degree at New York University and her medical degree from SUNY Downstate Medical School. She completed residency in Internal Medicine at Columbia University and a fellowship in Pulmonary and Critical Care Medicine at Cornell University. She holds a faculty appointment at NYU, where she attends on the inpatient tuberculosis unit, consultation and bronchoscopy service. Kazeros treats patients in the

World Trade Center Environmental Health Center and Asthma clinics at Bellevue Hospital. Her research focus is on noninvasive biomarkers in irritant-induced asthma.

William H. Meadows is president of The Wilderness Society since 1996 and has been active in conservation for over 40 years. He leads a staff of 175 headquartered in Washington, DC and nine regional offices, and acts as key spokesperson and advocate for the Society and its conservation work. Meadows has become a national leader in public land conservation and wilderness preservation, playing an important role in the protection of national forest roadless areas, national parks, wildlife refuges, and national monuments. More than 5 million acres have been added to the National Wilderness Preservation System since Meadows became president of the Wilderness Society.

Sam Parsia, MD, MPH, received his medical degree from Albert Einstein College of Medicine of Yeshiva University and his Master's in Global Public Health from New York University. He completed residency in Internal Medicine at Beth Israel Medical Center in New York, and fellowship in Pulmonary and Critical Care Medicine at New York University. Parsia holds a faculty appointment at NYU, where he treats patients in the World Trade Center Environmental Health Center at Bellevue Hospital and on the Bellevue Chest Service. His research interests are environmental lung disease and global health.

Joan Reibman, MD, is an associate professor of Medicine and Environmental Medicine at New York University. She is the medical director of the NYU/Bellevue Asthma Center, a program initiated to provide state-of-the-art care for asthma for an indigent population, and to serve as a platform for lay and professional education, community outreach and clinical studies. Her research includes epidemiologic and basic science investigations on pollution and asthma and airway immunity, and gene and environment interactions in complex populations. Reibman is also the medical director of the World Trade Center Environmental Health Center, a treatment program for community members with WTC-related illness. Reibman has been the recipient of multiple NIH awards and is the principal investigator for the New York Consortium of the American Lung Association Asthma Clinical Research Centers.

Leonardo Trasande, MD, MPP, is an associate professor of Pediatrics, Environmental Medicine, and Health Policy at New York University. His analysis of the health and economic consequences of mercury pollution played a critical role in preventing the Clear Skies Act from becoming law and provided a major foundation for the multistate lawsuit that overturned EPA's Clean Air Mercury Rule (which relaxed regulations on emissions from coal-fired power plants). Trasande earned a Master's degree in Public Policy from Harvard's Kennedy School of Government, and an MD from Harvard Medical School. He completed a pediatrics residency at Boston Children's Hospital, a Dyson Foundation Legislative Fellowship in the office of Senator Hillary Rodham Clinton, and a fellowship in environmental pediatrics at the Mount Sinai School of Medicine. Trasande is a Fellow of the American Academy of Pediatrics and continues to practice clinically.

ENVIRONMENTAL POLICY AND PUBLIC HEALTH

CHAPTER 1

THE CLEAN AIR ACT AND THE NATIONAL ENVIRONMENTAL POLICY ACT

LEARNING OBJECTIVES

- To understand the history and importance of the Clean Air Act
- To become familiar with the National Ambient Air Quality Standards and how they are created
- To know the requirements of State Implementation Plans
- To understand which air pollutants are hazardous
- To comprehend efforts to protect vital environmental areas and to regulate new sources of pollution

The Clean Air Act is the basic law that frames U.S. environmental policy. This law has seen many versions, beginning in the 1950s with the U.S. Public Health Service (PHS) investigation of the Donora, Pennsylvania, air pollution episode. This investigation found that air pollutants from industrial sources became particularly noxious in a cold air inversion, leading to several dozen deaths directly related to the air pollution. The U.S. PHS investigators related deaths both temporally and etiologically to the air pollution, since most were cardiopulmonary deaths among the elderly. The first air pollution laws primarily funded research for health studies but gradually gave way to federal regulatory efforts that encompassed a unique brand of federalism whereby the states were mandated to carry out the federal regulations in a somewhat cooperative manner. The power to regulate interstate commerce gave the federal government its constitutional mandate, which has been consistently upheld in the courts after industry challenge.

The Clean Air Act

The London Fog and the Donora Fog

The **Clean Air Act (CAA)**, first passed in 1970, is a landmark public law born from public pressure to control smog and air pollution in general. Prior to its enactment, the world experienced some major catastrophic episodes brought about by smog. In particular, the **London Fog** episode in 1952, which killed thousands of people from cardiovascular and pulmonary complications, was due to cold air inversions that increased atmospheric sulfur dioxide, SO_2 and particulate matter (PM). This disaster was preceded by the 1948 Donora, Pennsylvania, air pollution episode (the **Donora Fog**) in which high concentrations of sulfur dioxide, coupled with a temperature inversion and foggy weather, caused twenty people to die due to cardiac and respiratory disease and about half of the town's 12,000 residents to complain of cough, respiratory tract irritation, chest pain, headaches, nausea, and vomiting.[1] The fog was the result of an anticyclone that closed over Donora on the morning of Tuesday, October 26, 1948. Berton Roueché described the event based on eyewitness accounts:

> The weather was raw, cloudy and dead calm, and it stayed that way as the fog piled up all that day and the next. By Thursday, it had stiffened adhesively into a motionless clot of smoke. That afternoon it was just possible to see across the street, and except for the stacks, the mills had vanished. The air began to have a sickening smell, almost a taste. It was the bittersweet reek of sulfur dioxide. Everyone who was out that day remarked on it, but no one was much concerned. The smell of sulfur dioxide, a scratchy gas given off by burning coal

and melting ore, is a normal concomitant of any durable fog in Donora. This time it merely seemed more penetrating than usual.[2]

Early Policy Responses to Air Pollution

The first legislation aimed at controlling air pollution was passed in 1955 as the Air Pollution Control Act (APCA). This was the first federal legislative attempt to control air pollution at its source. It granted $5 million annually for five years for research by the U.S. Public Health Service. The act did little to prevent air pollution, but it made the government aware that the problem existed on the national level. It recognized the dangers facing public health and welfare, agriculture, livestock, and deterioration of property and reserved for Congress the right to control this growing problem. The law, which had been initiated by California's representatives in the Senate and the House, was followed by a number of failed attempts. Air pollution had long been regarded as a local problem, and the federal government was hesitant to interfere with states' rights. As a result, the first APCA was rather narrow in scope and effect.

The First Clean Air Act and Its Amendments

Eight years after passing the APCA, Congress passed the Clean Air Act of 1963.[3] This act dealt with reducing air pollution by setting emissions standards for stationary sources such as power plants and steel mills. It did not take into account mobile sources of air pollution, which had become the largest source of many unhealthy pollutants. Once these standards were set, the government also needed to determine deadlines for companies to comply with them. Amendments to the Clean Air Act were passed in 1965, 1966, 1967, and 1969. These amendments authorized the Secretary of Health, Education, and Welfare (HEW) to set standards for auto emissions, expand local air pollution control programs, establish air quality control regions (AQCR), set air quality standards and compliance deadlines for stationary source emissions, and authorize research on low-emissions fuels and automobiles.

The CAA promoted **federalism** with requirements and aid to the states to implement its provisions. Because air pollutants crossed state boundaries, the federal government played an important role in the CAA's implementation and standardization. Furthermore, the CAA promoted public health with health-based air pollutant standards. It also fostered public welfare, since there were secondary standards to protect agriculture, forests, monuments, visibility, and water bodies from the deleterious effects of air pollution. The U.S. Supreme Court upheld the role of the federal government in regulating air pollution because of its regional and national context under the interstate commerce clause.

By 1970, issues under the CAA had been addressed again by Congress. In 1970, President Richard Nixon established the **Environmental Protection Agency (EPA)** by an executive order. Although important legislative precedents had been set, the existing law and amendments were deemed inadequate. Technically another amendment, the Clean Air Act of 1970 was a major revision and set much more demanding standards. It established new primary and secondary standards for ambient air quality, set new limits on emissions from stationary and mobile sources to be enforced by both state and federal governments, and increased funds for air pollution research. The 1970 amendments required a 90% reduction in emissions from new automobiles by 1975, established a program to require the best available control technology at major new sources of air pollution, and established a program to regulate air toxics. It was soon discovered that the deadlines set were overly ambitious (especially those for auto emissions). To reach these standards in such a short period of time, the auto industry would face serious economic limitations and seemingly insurmountable technological challenges. These issues resulted in the 1977 CAA amendments, which adjusted the auto emission standards, extended the deadlines for the attainment of air quality standards and added the **Prevention of Significant Deterioration program**.

Sen. Edmund Muskie (ME-D) stated that the legislation prioritized public health above technological and economic considerations: "The first responsibility of Congress is not the making of technological or economic judgments—or even to be limited by what appears to be technologically or economically feasible. Our responsibility is to establish what the public interest requires to protect the health of persons. This may mean that people and industries will be asked to do what seems to be impossible at the present time. But if health is to be protected, these challenges must be met."

At that time, this was a bipartisan point of view; Republicans also favored the bill in spite of its demands on industry. For instance, Sen. Winston Prouty (VT-R) described the 1970 amendments, stating, "For the first time, air quality standards will take precedence over objections of economic impracticality and technical impossibilities." Congress did not amend the Clean Air Act during the 1980s, in part because President Ronald Reagan's administration placed economic goals ahead of environmental goals.

In 1990, after a lengthy period of inactivity, the federal government believed that they should again revise the CAA due to growing environmental concerns. The Clean Air Act of 1990 addressed five main areas:

1. It decreased exposure to six so-called **criteria pollutants:** carbon monoxide (CO), nitrogen dioxide (NO_2), sulfur dioxide (SO_2), ozone (O_3), particulate matter of 10 microns or less (PM_{10}) and lead (Pb).

2. It limited sources and risks of exposure to 188 enumerated hazardous air pollutants.
3. It prevented significant deterioration of air quality in wilderness areas and national parks.
4. It controlled acid rain.
5. It curbed the use of chemicals that deplete the stratospheric O_3 layer.

The 1990 CAA amendments also included provisions to classify **nonattainment areas** or localities where air pollution levels persistently exceed **National Ambient Air Quality Standards** (Section 1.3) or that contribute to ambient air quality in a nearby area that fails to meet standards. The CAA tailored deadlines, tightened auto and other mobile source emissions standards, required reformulated and alternative fuels in the most polluted areas, established a new program of technology-based standards, required a state-run permit program for the operation of major sources of air pollutants, and updated enforcement provisions, including authority for EPA to assess administrative penalties.

Figure 1.1 illustrates accomplishments of the CAA over the past forty years, and Figure 1.2 illustrates progress in controlling CO. However, the challenges of reducing O_3 pollution continue, Figure 1.3 demonstrates. The Clean Air Act is authorizing legislation and may include authorized appropriations for clean air

FIGURE 1.1   Comparison of growth areas and emissions, 1970–2008

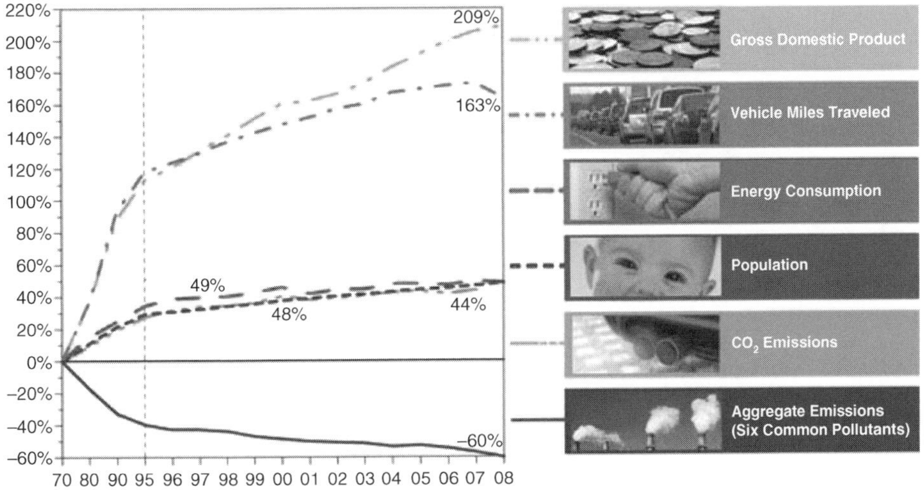

Source: The Environmental Protection Agency.

FIGURE 1.2   CO air quality, 1980–2007

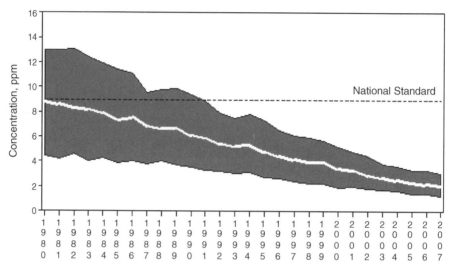

Note: There was a 75% decrease in national average.
Source: The Environmental Protection Agency.

FIGURE 1.3   Ozone air quality, 1980–2007

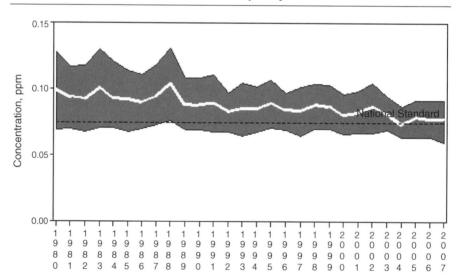

Note: There was only a 21% decrease in the national average. The CAA has been very successful in reducing some criteria such as CO whereas others such as ozone are more intractable.
Source: The Environmental Protection Agency.

programs for a period of time after which they need to be reauthorized. House rules require enactment of an authorization before an appropriation bill can be considered, but this requirement can be waived and frequently has been. The act's legal authorities to issue and enforce regulations are considered to be permanent and do not need reauthorization.

National Ambient Air Quality Standards

Title 1 of the CAA 1970 amendments established National Ambient Air Quality Standards (NAAQS) for pollutants considered harmful to public health and the environment. These pollutants included CO, NO_2, SO_2, total suspended particulates (that became (PM_{10}) in 1987 and $PM_{2.5}$ in 1997), hydrocarbons (removed in 1983), oxidants (became O_3 in 1979), and Pb (since 1976). The NAAQS were designed to protect public health and welfare with an adequate margin of safety. The CAA requires the EPA to review the scientific data upon which the standards are based and revise the standards, if necessary, every five years. The EPA has been increasingly challenged in meeting this five-year review. The Office of Research Development prepares a criteria document summarizing the research

FIGURE 1.4   Air quality changes from 2007 ozone rollbacks

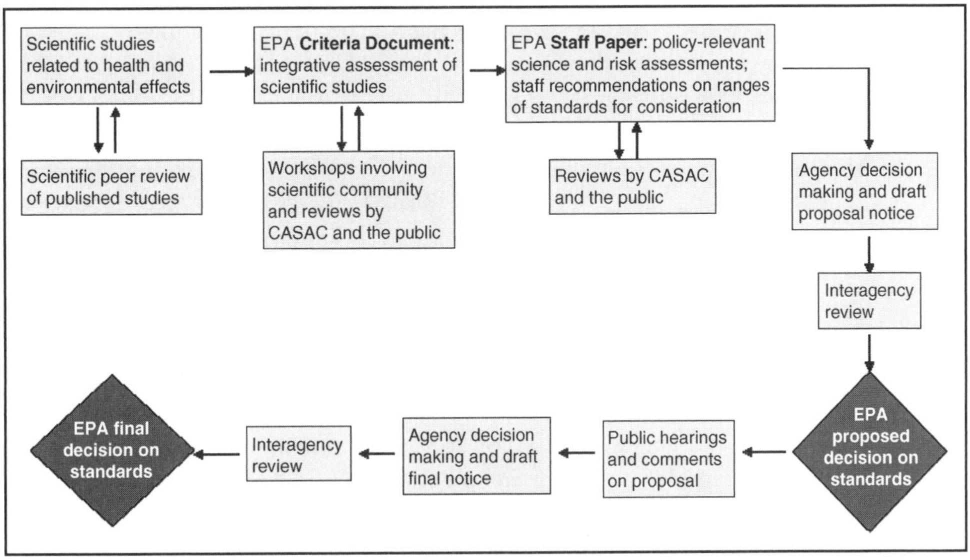

Source: The Environmental Protection Agency.

and implications for regulation using various standards. The Office of Air Quality Planning and Standards uses the EPA staff to prepare a staff paper listing all of the health-related research papers that are relevant to the standard-setting process. These often number more than 2,000 and result in a voluminous staff paper. The staff paper is an evaluative document that assesses the implications for standard setting of information in the criteria document and presents staff recommendations for NAAQS decision making.

The 1970 CAA amendments authorized the National Institute for Environmental Sciences to conduct air pollution research including toxicology, air pollutant measurement and characterization, animal studies, clinical and translational studies, and epidemiological studies. Also, the EPA has funded air pollution research through their Science to Achieve Results (STAR) grant program and centers like their Particulate Matter Center grants. The EPA also shares funding with industries with a stake in air pollution control at the Health Effects Institute (HEI) based in Boston. HEI has a research committee that reviews all applications and a review committee that reviews the results and final reports prior to publication as HEI documents. These funding agencies provide resources for air pollution scientists to conduct research that provides the science behind the regulatory framework. These appropriations provide material support to scientists, establish a cadre of experts, and train future researchers through graduate programs and postdoctoral fellowships.

The federal regulatory agencies have considerable leeway in developing and enforcing standards. During the past eight years, standard setting has slowed, and much of the NAAQS' work has been done under court order, whereby environmental organizations have sued the EPA for missing deadlines or failing to regulate. The presidential budget may curtail agency activities by reducing or eliminating budget items, or Congress can increase or decrease appropriation. More interesting is the regulatory strategy to justify not regulating. The EPA under the administration of George W. Bush decided that CO_2 was not covered under the CAA, and after losing litigation on this interpretation at the Supreme Court, decided to publish a lengthy Advanced Notice of Proposed Rule-Making trying to justify not regulating. It stated explicitly that the CAA was not the proper law to do this. It used the CAA NAAQS, whereby any emitter of more than 250 tons of primary pollutant would have to be regulated. With this interpretation, most buildings would need to comply, resulting in every conservative organization decrying the expansion of big government. The agency, however, could take a targeted approach and focus on coal-fired power plants, for example, where there would be a huge benefit with less cost. The regulatory process allows many entry points for citizens or organizations to write letters on proposed regulations, present data to CASAC meetings, or even petition the administrator directly. These efforts are best made through organizations that have standing such as the American Lung Association or American Thoracic Society.

Clean Air Scientific Advisory Committee

The **Clean Air Scientific Advisory Committee (CASAC)** reviews both the criteria document and the staff paper and adds its own critique. The CASAC takes public testimony of these documents and digests their findings and that of the primary literature before recommending a range of standards for the EPA administrator to consider. The EPA administrator has the authority to ignore or accept their recommendations. The CASAC must have a physician, an individual with expertise on air pollution measurement, and a representative from the state air pollution bureaus. Executive Order 12866 requires the EPA to prepare regulatory impact analyses. Cost and technological feasibility cannot be considered in setting NAAQS, but costs and benefits can be considered in developing control strategies. The EPA must submit the regulatory impact analyses to the Office of Management and Budget for review.

State Implementation Plans

While the CAA authorizes the EPA to set NAAQS, the states are responsible for establishing procedures to attain and maintain the standards. The states adopt plans known as **State Implementation Plans (SIPs)** and submit them to the EPA to ensure that they meet statutory requirements. SIPs are based on emission inventories and computer models to determine whether air quality violations will occur. States must develop monitoring plans for air pollution levels; these may be funded by the EPA. If the SIP shows that standards may be exceeded, the state may be required to impose additional controls on existing sources. Proposed new and modified sources must obtain state construction permits in which the applicant has to show that anticipated emissions will not exceed allowable limits. Three years after EPA implements final NAAQS rule designations, states are required to submit SIPs to EPA that detail how areas will be brought into attainment. EPA reviews the SIPs to determine their adequacy to meet statutory requirements and achieve attainment of the standards.

If states do not meet the requirements of NAAQS, the federal government seeks to attain compliance in a number of ways. First, in nonattainment areas, emissions from new or modified sources must also be offset by reductions in emissions from existing sources. Second, EPA can impose a 2-to-1 emissions offset within eighteen months for the construction of new polluting sources in states where the SIP is inadequate and can impose a ban on most federal highway grants six months later. An additional ban on air quality grants is discretionary, and ultimately, a Federal Implementation Plan may be imposed if the state fails to submit or implement an adequate SIP.

SIPs and Transportation

Demonstrating conformity of transportation plans and SIPs is required in nonattainment areas at least every three years. Nonattainment plans must provide for implementation of all reasonable available control measures. Control technology guidelines exist, for example, the SIP may designate HOV (high occupancy vehicle) lanes on highways to encourage carpooling, or SIPs may increase the number of vehicle inspections to monitor air pollution. Title II on mobile sources contains procedures for setting emissions standards for cars, trucks, off-road vehicles, lawn mowers, chain saws, construction vehicles, locomotives, and marine motors, in order to control CO, VOCs (volatile organic compounds), NOx (NO and NO_2), and O_3. The 1990 CAA amendments reduced the automobile standard for hydrocarbons by 40% and NOx by 50%. A 2001 EPA rule for heavy duty vehicles required a 90% reduction in PM_{10} by 2007 and NOx by 2010. For ozone, nonattainment requirements were assessed to ninety-seven areas, with only Los Angeles categorized as "Extreme," with goals to be set for attainment of a one-hour level of 0.12 ppm by 2010. These goals have been updated by the 0.08 standard for ozone over eight hours, the updated standard of 0.075, and the pending review of this level by the administrator of the EPA. In addition, several iterations of requirements were set for gasoline formulation: first methyl tert butyl ether (MTBE) was favored, but after this additive was noted to contaminate ground water, this high oxygen standard was replaced with ethanol, a renewable fuel. Lead was removed from gasoline in 1990 and sulfur content was further restricted by more than 90% by 2004.

Section 209(b) of the CAA granted California the authority to develop its own vehicle standards as long as they are at least as stringent as federal standards. Section 177 allows other states to adopt California's stricter standards; New York, Maine, Massachusetts, and Vermont have done so.

Permit Requirements

The 1990 amendments to the CAA added Title V, which required states to administer a comprehensive permit program for the operation of sources emitting air pollutants. Sources subject to the permit requirements generally included those that emit 100 tons per year of any regulated pollutant; however, in non-attainment areas, the permit requirements may also include sources of VOCs as low as 10 tons per year. States collect annual fees to cover the costs of the permits and their air pollution control programs. The permit defines how much of which air pollutants a source is allowed to emit. As part of the permit process, a source must prepare a compliance plan and certify compliance. State and local governments enforce the CAA. They issue most permits, monitor compliance, and conduct the majority of inspections. The CAA also provides for citizen suits both against persons and corporations alleged to have violated emissions standards or permit requirements. There may also be claims against EPA in cases where the administrator has failed to perform an action that is not discretionary under the CAA. The EPA has authority to assess administrative penalties, charge violators with felonies in some instances rather than misdemeanors, and pay $10,000 awards to persons supplying information leading to convictions under the CAA.

Hazardous Air Pollutants

Section 112 in the 1990 amendments established a program for protecting the public health and environment from exposure to toxic air pollutants. Under this section, EPA was required to establish **Maximum Achievable Control Technology (MACT)** standards for 188 pollutants and to specify categories of sources subject to regulations. The second major provision directed EPA to set health-based standards to address situations in which a significant residual risk of adverse health effects remained after installation of MACT. Third, EPA was to establish standards for stationary "area sources" that were responsible for 90% of the emissions of hazardous air pollutants (HAPs). Last, EPA was to establish a Chemical Safety and Hazard Investigation Board to investigate accidents involving releases of hazardous substances. Owners and operators had to prepare risk management plans including hazard assessments, measures to prevent releases, and response programs.

During 1993 in the United States, 3.7 metric tons of air toxics were emitted, with 41% derived from mobile sources, 35% from area sources, and 24% from local stationary sources. Taking into account the health and risk information and the extent of human exposure and toxicity, EPA has considered twenty-one mobile source air toxics (MSATs). These include acetaldehyde, benzene, formaldehyde, 1,3-Butadiene, acrolein, polycyclic aromatic hydrocarbons, diesel, arsenic, chromium, dioxin/furan, ethyl benzene, n-hexane, lead, manganese, mercury, MTBE, naphthalene, nickel, styrene, toluene, and xylene. Funding for the HAPS program has been inadequate with the EPA having few resources to accomplish a HAPS regulatory program resulting in the inspector general of the EPA releasing a critical report in 2010. The Inspector General Act of 1978 provides an executive oversight of federal agencies' performance, especially to legal mandates required by congressional authorizing legislation.

New Source Performance Standards

Section 111 of the CAA requires EPA to establish nationally uniform technology-based standards, for categories of new industrial facilities that would prevent dirty industries from locating in states or communities with lax standards. The standards also set up the new source review (NSR) to apply to modifications of existing facilities but left ambiguities as to what was a modification as opposed to routine maintenance of a facility. "Routine maintenance" to cover investments up to 20% of the value of the facility was exempted from NSR. NSR was to apply particularly to nonattainment areas.

Prevention of Significant Deterioration

The Prevention of Significant Deterioration program reflects the principle that areas where air quality is better than that required by NAAQS should be protected from significant new air pollution even if NAAQS would not be violated. Class I areas are wilderness areas and national parks; allowable increments of new pollution in these areas would be very small. Class II areas are all attainment areas (areas considered to have air quality as good as or better than the NAAQS), and Class III are slated for development but not to exceed the NAAQS. Visibility is primarily affected by ozone, NOx, and PM, which is described as regional haze, especially in Grand Canyon and Great Smoky Mountains national parks. The 1990 amendments to the CAA established a Grand Canyon Visibility Transport Commission composed of governors from each state in the affected region, an EPA designee, and a representative of each of the national parks or wilderness areas in the region. The amendments specifically mention a requirement that states impose best available retrofit technology on existing sources of emissions impairing visibility. The EPA promulgated in 1999 the Regional Haze Rule, which established a sixty-five-year program to return 156 national parks and wilderness areas to their natural visibility conditions (baseline 2000–2004 to natural visibility conditions by 2065).

Clean Air Interstate Quality Rule

In 2004, EPA proposed the **Clean Air Interstate Quality Rule (CAIR)** to reduce interstate transport of fine PM and ozone by focusing on twenty-eight states and the District of Columbia that contributed to downwind states in nonattainment of these NAAQS. The EPA proposed a model cap and trade program for SO_2 and NOx, compounds that contribute to PM and ozone. These efforts were aimed at power plants in phased reductions for 2010 and 2015. EPA monitoring showed that numerous counties were in violation of $PM_{2.5}$ and ozone annual standards across the eastern United States due to regional contributions from sources distant to these areas. EPA proposed a regional emissions cap on SO_2 of 3.9 million tons together with a NOx emissions cap of 1.6 million tons by 2010, and 2.7 million tons for SO_2 and 1.3 million tons for NOx by 2015 (70% and 60% reductions from 2003 respectively). In 2008, this rule was struck down by the U.S. Court of Appeals for the D.C. Circuit because it considered the rule fatally flawed due to regional caps rather than a state-by-state approach. With appeals from environmentalists, the EPA, some utilities, and state air regulators, the court reinstated the rule at the end of 2008 with the understanding that this would be revised to meet the court's objections. In 2010 the EPA promulgated the transport rule that would target power plant pollution in thirty-one eastern states and the District of Columbia. EPA estimated that the rule would cost $2.8 billion to implement and would result in $120–$290 billion in benefits—largely from improvements in respiratory health. When fully implemented in 2014, the rule would improve public health by avoiding 14,000 to 36,000 premature deaths; 21,000 cases of acute bronchitis; 23,000 nonfatal heart attacks; 26,000 hospital and emergency room visits; 1.9 million days of missed work or school; 240,000 cases of aggravated asthma; and worsening of 440,000 upper and lower respiratory symptoms. The transport rule would reduce SO_2 emissions by 71% over 2005 levels by 2014, and NOx emissions by 52%. The Cross-State Air Pollution Rule (CSAPR) was finalized July 7, 2011.

The National Environmental Policy Act

In addition to the Clean Air Act, the **National Environmental Policy Act (NEPA)** was the other key law emanating from the environmental movement of the 1960s and 1970s. Rachel Carson had published *Silent Spring*, discussing how DDT and other pesticides had entered the environment, for example, causing thinning of the egg shells of the bald eagle and preventing hatching of the chicks. Bald eagles became rare in the United States, and other song birds were threatened. Many years later, EPA's main meeting hall has been named the Rachel Carson Great Room. Senator Gaylord Nelson began the Earth Day celebrations in April 22, 1970, highlighting the environmental threats and crises on the horizon.

The National Environmental Policy Act was signed into law in 1969 with the following purposes:

- To declare a national policy that will encourage productive and enjoyable harmony between man and his environment
- To promote efforts that will prevent or eliminate damage to the environment and biosphere and stimulate the health and welfare of humans
- To enrich the understanding of the ecological systems and natural resources important to the nation, and
- To establish a Council on Environmental Quality

NEPA created the environmental impact statement (EIS), in which the responsible official has to report on the environmental impact of the proposed action, any adverse environmental effects that cannot be avoided, alternatives to the proposed action, and the relationship between local short-term uses of humans' environment and long-term productivity, and any irreversible commitments of resources. This was a major change in placing environmental harm up to the level of cost-benefit ratios for proceeding with governmental projects. It created a federal Council on Environmental Quality (CEQ) ostensibly to coordinate environmental actions among federal agencies. The CEQ was to prepare regulations for the EIS, prepare an annual report, and coordinate federal environmental activities. The annual report was an incredible compendium of environmental data and actions, but it was terminated after the Republican takeover of Congress in 1997 by Newt Gingrich when he orchestrated passage of the Federal Reports Sunset law. No further annual reports of federal environmental agencies' work were issued after 1997.

If the federal action was not major, an environmental assessment (EA) could be issued rather than a full EIS. In 2006 there were 542 EISs: the U.S. Forest Service had the most at 144; this was probably because of logging and road activities. Others were the U.S. Army Corps of Engineers with 56, the Federal Energy Regulatory Committee with 32, the Bureau of Land Management with 42, the National Park Service with 34, and the Federal Highway Administration with 66.

A natural extension of the EIS is the use of health impact assessments (HIA) to examine the effects that a policy, program, or project may have on the health of a population.[4] HIAs offer great potential for promoting health by encouraging decisions that protect and enhance health and health equity. Major transportation projects may consider the health effects of air pollution or injury prevention, but the influence of road design on physical activity and obesity are often not considered. A bicycle lane may thus be considered. Educational HIAs could promote walking to school and avoiding areas of intense air pollution or noise. The Bureau of Land Management considered the health of Native populations in redesigning their EIS for the Northeast National Petroleum Reserve in Alaska, withdrawing some land from leasing for oil and gas development and instituting new pollution monitoring controls. HIAs are also used by local and state governments encouraging proactive decisions and planning to improve the public's health.

Summary

The Clean Air Act is the monumental environmental law that focuses Americans' attention on the environment. It provides for science-based regulation for clean air, especially ozone and particulate matter. These regulations are carried out by states, and they implement policy to control pollution from stationary sources such as power plants and transportation sources. The Environmental Protection Agency has implemented special programs for diesel engines, new source pollution attainment, prevention of air deterioration in pristine areas, and integration with multiple pollutants. In celebration of its fortieth anniversary, EPA Administrator Lisa Jackson stated that in 2010 alone, the Clean Air Act NAAQS for fine particulate and ozone had prevented more than 160,000 cases of premature mortality, 130,000 heart attacks, 13 million lost work days, and 1.7 million asthma attacks. The National Environmental Policy Act turns attention to land and water where activities of the federal government must consider adverse environmental impacts before embarking on such activities.

Key Terms

Clean Air Act (CAA)

Clean Air Interstate Quality Rule (CAIR)

Clean Air Scientific Advisory Committee (CASAC)

Criteria pollutants

Donora Fog

Environmental Protection Agency (EPA)

Federalism

London Fog

Maximum Achievable Control Technology (MACT)

National Ambient Air Quality Standards (NAAQS)

National Environmental Policy Act (NEPA)

Nonattainment areas

Prevention of Significant Deterioration program

State Implementation Plans (SIPS)

Discussion Questions

1. What are the major provisions of the Clean Air Act?
2. What are National Ambient Air Quality Standards and how are they created?
3. What are the requirements of state implementation plans?
4. Which pollutants are considered especially hazardous?
5. What are New Source Performance Standards?
6. How is the government attempting to stop the deterioration of protected areas?

The author thanks Daniel Greenbaum for permission to use parts of the Clean Air Act chapter published in *Environmental and Occupational Medicine*, 4th ed., by Lippincott, Williams and Wilkins.

CHAPTER 2

PARTICULATE MATTER

LEARNING OBJECTIVES

- To understand what particulate matter is
- To become familiar with the health effects of particulate matter
- To understand public policies regarding particulate matter

Particulate matter (PM), a mixture of solid particles and liquid droplets found in the air, can be natural or anthropogenic. Natural sources of particles include crustal or surface particles dispersed by the wind, pollen from plants, and sea spray. Anthropogenic sources include products of combustion, such as mobile sources, industrial power plants, factories, refineries, forest fires and/or agricultural sources, and secondary sources that are condensation from aerosols.

Characteristics and Deposition

The size of the particles is important because particle size affects exposure. Particles that are >10 microns are generally non-respirable. Particles <10 to 2.5 microns are coarse and are inhaled into the large airways, <2.5 microns, referred to as "fine particulate," can reach the lung's alveolar spaces, and <0.1 microns, referred to as "ultrafine particles," can reach the distal lung and have an affinity for absorption.

The respiratory system's defenses against inhalable particles can be grouped into three lines of defense successively encountered by particles that enter the airways. The first line of defense for the lower respiratory tract is impaction, sedimentation, and diffusional deposition of particles suspended in the inspired air as it passes through the nose, nasopharynx, pharynx, and larynx and the conducting airways, that is, the tracheobronchial tree. The deposition of particles along the air passages reduces their penetration into the more vulnerable gas-exchanging structures, that is, the respiratory bronchioles, alveolar ducts, and alveoli in the periphery of the lung.

The second line of defense is provided by the fluids (surfactant, mucous) that line the airways and gas exchange structures and by the clearance mechanisms that physically remove particles from their surfaces. The respiratory tract fluids constitute a physical barrier to the contact of particles on airway surfaces with the bronchial and alveolar epithelia; these fluids may also represent a chemical buffer when they contain substances that give them detoxifying and bactericidal capabilities. In addition, the secretions that coat the ciliated epithelia of the conducting air passages of the upper and lower airways form a viscoelastic fluid. The cilia beat within the less viscous sol layer, propelling particles remaining on the more viscous gel layer along a mucociliary "escalator" to the larynx, where they are swallowed and eliminated via the gastrointestinal tract or expectorated. The third line of defense, resident alveolar macrophages, scavenge particles from the surfaces of the alveoli, digest them and/or remove them via the mucociliary escalator.

There are several mechanisms by which particles are deposited in the respiratory tract: impaction, gravitational sedimentation, Brownian diffusion, and interception. Deposition by **impaction** occurs at airway bifurcations when a particle, owing to its momentum and the aerodynamic forces exerted on it by the stream of air in which it is carried, fails to make the turn into either of the daughter branches and affects the bifurcation. **Gravitational sedimentation** is the settling of particles onto airway surfaces under the force of gravity. For particles <2.5 microns in diameter, the gravitational effects that cause sedimentation and impaction are less influential, and they are more affected by the random thermal kinetic buffeting (**Brownian diffusion**) of the gas molecules in the air around them. Sedimentation increases with airway length and is independent of branching angle; deposition from impaction increases with the branching angle and is independent of airway length. **Interception** occurs when long fibers travel like a spear into the lower respiratory tract (see Figure 2.1 illustrating deposition by size of particle).

The size distribution of ambient particles has several modes: coarse, accumulation (includes fine). and ultrafine, as shown in Figure 2.2.

Coarse mode particles include resuspended road dust, windblown dust, and sea spray. Particles in the **accumulation mode** are primarily emitted

FIGURE 2.1   Site of particle deposition

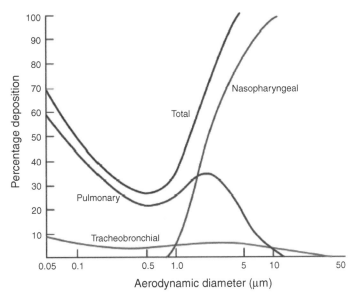

Source: Adapted from Annals of American Conference of Governmental and Industrial Hygienists. Reprinted with permission from The Bloomberg School of Public Health at Johns Hopkins University.

FIGURE 2.2   Idealized size distribution showing fine and coarse particles and the nucleation, Aitken, and accumulation modes that comprise fine particles

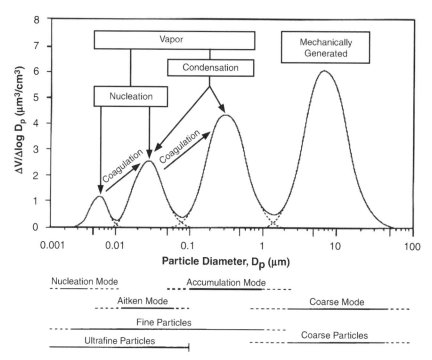

Source: Reprinted with permission from the Environmental Protection Agency.

from combustion processes, formed from coagulation of smaller particles from the nucleation and Aitken modes (aerosol droplets <100 nm), or formed secondarily in atmospheric reactions. The **nucleation mode** consists largely of combustion-related vapors that condense into particles that make up the **Aitken mode**. The coarse mode contains particles from approximately 2–100 μm in diameter and typically contributes the most mass. Particles in the accumulation mode range from approximately 0.1 to 1.0 μm in diameter and collectively have the most surface area. PM mass is contained almost entirely in the coarse and accumulation modes. Particles in the ultrafine region are smaller than 0.1 μm in diameter (with nucleation mode particles ranging up to 0.01 μm in diameter and Aitken mode particles from 0.01 to 0.10 μm in diameter) and contain the largest number of particles; the ultrafine mode generally contributes only a negligible amount to PM mass.

There can also be marked concentration differences between urban and non-urban locations. In the United States, annual average $PM_{2.5}$ concentrations in largely urban areas have recently ranged from 4 to 28 $\mu g/m^3$ (median 13 $\mu g/m^3$). Urban PM concentrations in the United States tend to be higher in eastern regions of the country than in western regions, except for California. Urban concentrations decreased 10% and rural areas by 20% nationally from 1999 to 2003; only the northeast region showed no decrease in annual $PM_{2.5}$ concentration over that short period of time.

Health Effects

History

Air pollution episodes that occurred in the middle of the twentieth century were responsible for deaths that ranged from a few excess deaths to several thousand, depending to a large extent on the size of the population exposed. In the most well-known of these episodes, the London Fog of 1952, an estimated 3,500 excess deaths occurred over a period of a few days, with possibly several thousand more in the ensuing weeks. While the pollution mix in London during this fog was complex, it is likely that particulate air pollution was largely responsible for the excess deaths. These episodes demonstrate that exposure to urban air pollution can, in extreme cases, cause death.

Epidemiological Studies

Several studies have confirmed associations between increased PM concentrations and increased cardiopulmonary mortality. They found that for each 10 $\mu g/m^3$ increase in PM_{10}, mortality increased by a fraction of a percent (2, 3, 4, 5, 6, 7, 8, 9). In spite of the small effect of PM increases, the public health impact could be large if seen across broad populations. Thus, increasing ambient PM concentrations represent a fairly significant risk in terms of mortality.

Similar studies have established other health dangers that are associated with increased PM, including increased for lung cancer and heart disease. The American Cancer Society Air Pollution Study was initiated by C. Arden Pope and colleagues based upon a cohort of 1.2 million individuals enrolled in the fall of 1982.[1] A subgroup of 552,138 adults lived in 151 United States metropolitan areas that could be matched to air pollution data collected under the auspices of the Environmental Protection Agency (EPA). The relationships of sulfate and particulate matter air pollution to all-cause, lung cancer, and cardiopulmonary mortality were examined in this subgroup using multivariate analysis controlling for smoking, education, and other risk factors up to 1989. Deaths due to air pollution were 15%–17% more prevalent in the most polluted communities as compared to the least polluted ones. In a follow-up of this cohort until 1998, when 22.5% of the cohort died, $PM_{2.5}$ data were collected and estimated with mortality risk ratios estimated by a Cox proportional hazard regression model. Significant mortality associations were found for each 10 $\mu g/m^3$ increase in $PM_{2.5}$ for ischemic heart disease, dysrhythmias, heart failure, and cardiac arrest, and in nonsmokers, pneumonia and influenza.[2] Each 10 $\mu g/m^3$ elevation in fine particulate air pollution was associated with approximately a 4%, 6%, and 8% increased risk of all-cause, cardiopulmonary, and lung cancer mortality, respectively[3] (see Figure 2.3). Since PM has fallen over the past two decades, Pope and colleagues compiled data on life expectancy, socioeconomic status, and

FIGURE 2.3   Lung cancer, cardiopulmonary mortality, and long-term exposure to fine particulate air pollution

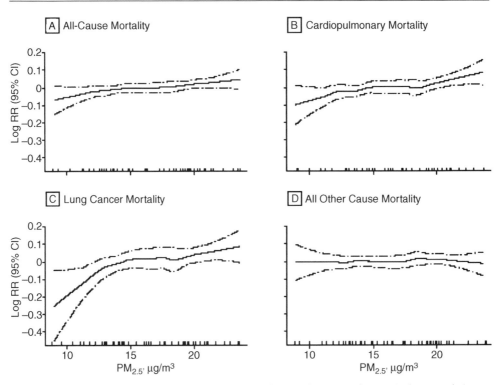

Note: Vertical lines along x-axes indicate relative risk and abscissa plots; mean fine particulate population; mean fine particles measuring less than 2.5 μm in diameter; RR, relative risk; and CI, confidence interval.
Source: Reprinted with permission from The Journal of the American Medical Association.

demographic characteristics for fifty-one U.S. metropolitan areas with matching data on fine particulate air pollution for the late 1970s and early 1980s and the late 1990s and early 2000s.[4] They found that a decrease of 10 $\mu g/m^3$ in $PM_{2.5}$ was associated with an estimated increase in mean ($\pm SE$) life expectancy of 0.61$\pm$0.20 year ($p = 0.004$). Reductions in air pollution accounted for as much as 15% of the overall increase in life expectancy in the study areas.

At the same time the American Cancer Society cohort was being assembled, investigators at the Harvard School of Public Health established a longitudinal study on the health effects of air pollution in six cities. The Harvard Six Cities Study was a sixteen-year prospective cohort study of 8,111 adults living in the northeastern and midwestern United States beginning in the 1970s. The study reported that $PM_{2.5}$ was positively associated with overall mortality, cardio-pulmonary causes, and lung cancer.[5] (See Figures 2.4 and 2.5.) There was a 26%

FIGURE 2.4   Annual average concentrations of $PM_{2.5}$ in the Harvard Six Cities Study

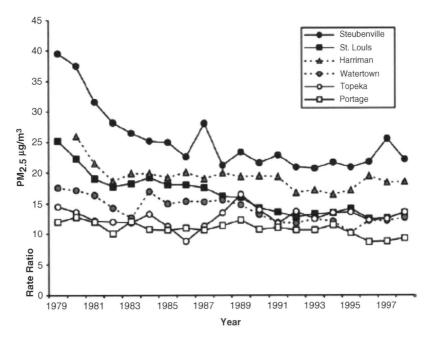

Note: Six Cities monitoring data for available years 1980–1988 and $PM_{2.5}$ estimated from Aerometric Information Retrieval System and extinction data for years where Six Cities data were not available.
Source: Reprinted with permission from the American Journal of Respiratory and Critical Care Medicine.

FIGURE 2.5   Estimated adjusted rate ratios for total mortality and PM$_{2.5}$ levels in the Six Cities Study by period

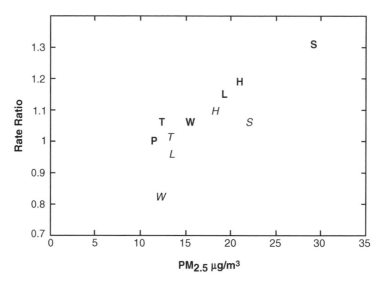

Note: P denotes Portage, WI (reference for both periods); T Topeka, KS; W Watertown, MA; L St. Louis, MO; H Harriman, TN; S Steubenville, OH. A term for Period 1 (1 if Period 2, 0 if Period 1) was included in the model. **Bold letters** represent Period 1 (1974–1989) and *italicized letters* represent Period 2 (1990–1998). In Period 1, PM$_{2.5}$ (g/m3) is defined as the mean concentration during 1980–1985, the years where there are monitoring data for all cities (18). In Period 2, PM$_{2.5}$ is defined as the mean concentrations of the estimated PM$_{2.5}$ in 1990–1998.
Source: Reprinted with permission from the American Journal of Respiratory and Critical Care Medicine.

difference in overall mortality between the most polluted city (Steubenville, Ohio) and the least polluted city (Portage, Wisconsin). An eight-year extended follow-up confirmed the increased mortality rate ratios of 1.27 for lung cancer and 1.28 for cardiovascular deaths, with declines in PM$_{2.5}$ in the more polluted towns associated with declines in mortality.[6] These data suggested that the mortality effect was not cumulative and that air pollution controls were associated with a public health benefit. This was more pronounced in cardiopulmonary mortality than lung cancer.

These studies were followed by publication of the National Morbidity and Mortality Air Pollution Study (NMMAPS) by Jonathan Samet, M.D., and colleagues where they assessed the effects of five major outdoor air pollutants on daily mortality rates (a time-series study) in twenty U.S. metropolitan areas from 1987 to 1994.[7] The pollutants were PM$_{10}$, ozone, sulfur dioxide, carbon monoxide, and nitrogen dioxide. They found a small 0.5% increase of all-cause mortality per 10 µg/m^3 increase in PM$_{10}$. This small increase was later revised downward to 0.2% after revisions were made in the statistical modeling. The data were analyzed with a generalized additive model (GAM) using the GAM function in S-plus (with default convergence criteria previously used and with more stringent criteria) and with a generalized linear model (GLM) with natural cubic splines. With the original method, the estimated effect of PM_{10} on total mortality from nonexternal causes was a 0.41% increase per 10 $\mu g/m^3$ increase in PM_{10}; with the more stringent criteria, the estimate was 0.27%; and with GLM, the effect was 0.21%. The risk was highest in the Northeast and for cardiovascular and respiratory causes of death. Seasonal ozone (June, July, August) had an increase of 0.41% per 10 ppb in overall mortality. There were no significant associations with CO, SO_2, or NO_2. PM declined 20% during these years as indicated by 799 monitoring sites. Key socioeconomic factors did not affect the association between PM_{10} levels and the risk of death in linear regression models.

These NMMAPS data were then correlated to Medicare hospitalizations for 1999 through 2002 for 204 U.S. urban counties with 11.5 million Medicare enrollees (ages >65 years) living an average of 5.9 miles from a $PM_{2.5}$ monitor.[8] They reported a short-term increase per 10 $\mu g/m^3$ $PM_{2.5}$ for hospitalizations for stroke, ischemic heart disease, heart rhythm, heart failure, exacerbations of chronic obstructive pulmonary disease (COPD), and respiratory tract infections with no increase in injuries (a negative control group that has no discernible relation to air pollution). Cardiovascular risks tended to be higher in counties located in the eastern region of the United States, especially the Northeast, South, and Midwest. There is a greater sulfate concentration of PM in the East and more nitrate in PM in California, which probably reflects power plant sources in the East and traffic in California. The mechanisms for these adverse outcomes is thought to be that $PM_{2.5}$ initiates inflammatory responses in the lower respiratory tract, causing release of cytokines that have local and systemic consequences. Particulate matter promotes inflammation and exacerbates underlying lung disease and reduces the efficacy of lung defense mechanisms.

Moolgavkar used data for Los Angeles County, California, for 1987–1995 and found that $PM_{2.5}$ was significantly associated with risk for hospital admissions for cardiovascular disease in persons ages 65 years or older.[9] In Europe, the Air Pollution and Health: A European Approach (APHEA 1 and 2) found epidemiological evidence that short-term exposure to PM and ozone impacted daily hospital admissions and emergency room (ER) visits for asthma (greater effect in children than adults) and COPD in eight cities.[10] The Swiss Cohort Study on Air Pollution and Lung Diseases in Adults (SAPALDIA) correlated PM_{10} measurements to lung function in 4,742 participants over an eleven-year period.[11] They found a linear correlation with FEV_1 from 5 to 45 $\mu g/m^3$, providing support for World Health Organization recommendations for annual PM_{10} standards of 20 $\mu g/m^3$, and a decline in PM_{10} over the eleven years 5.3 μg was associated with significant reductions in annual levels of decline in lung function (FEV_1).

The California Air Resources Board has funded air pollution studies to provide data on the unique circumstances of California smog and develop a rationale to justify expenditures and strategies to reduce emissions. The Children's

FIGURE 2.6 Community-specific proportion of 18-year-olds with FEV₁ below 80% of the predicted value vs. average levels of pollutants, 1994–2000

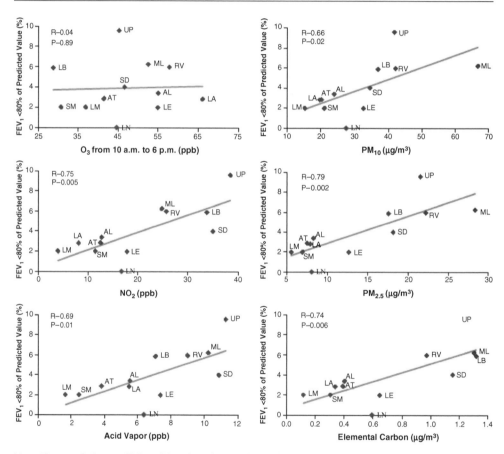

Note: The correlation coefficient (R) and P value are shown for each comparison. AL denotes Alpine, AT Atascadero, LE Lake Elsinore, LA Lake Arrowhead, LN Lancaster, LM Lompoc, LB Long Beach, ML Mira Loma, RV Riverside, SD San Dimas, SM Santa Maria, and UP Upland. O₃ denotes ozone, NO₂ nitrogen dioxide, and PM₁₀ and PM₂.₅ particulate matter with an aerodynamic diameter of less than 10 μm and less than 2.5 μm, respectively.

Source: Reprinted with permission from The New England Journal of Medicine.

Health Study begun at the Department of Preventive Medicine at the University of Southern California enrolled schoolchildren in the fourth grade in twelve communities in the Los Angeles basin. There were two cohorts enrolled in 1993 and 1996 (total $n = 3840$), and an annual questionnaire and pulmonary function test were obtained. Air pollutants measured included hourly ozone, NO_2, PM_{10}, two-week integrated samples for $PM_{2.5}$, and acid vapor. Gauderman and colleagues reported on 1,759 children who had eight years of pulmonary function data where they could compare residence in high- versus low-polluted communities. Deficits in the growth of forced expired volume in the first second (FEV_1) were associated with NO_2, acid vapor, $PM_{2.5}$, and elemental carbon. The percent predicted FEV_1 at age 18 <80% of normal values was 4.9 times as great in those children from the highest $PM_{2.5}$ communities versus the lowest (7.9% versus 1.6% respectively). (See Figure 2.6.)[12]

These data were then reanalyzed for 1,445 children who had eight years of data with proximity to a freeway and lung growth; sensitivity analyses showed a significant adverse effect for residence closer than 500 meters to a freeway and growth of FEV_1.[13] (See Figure 2.7.) By 18 years of age, there was a substantially

FIGURE 2.7   Percentage predicted lung function at age 18 vs. residential distance from a freeway

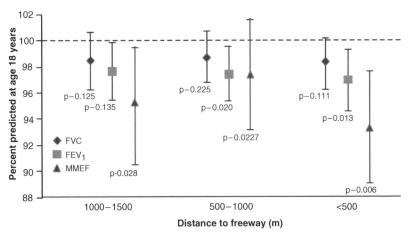

Note: The horizontal line at 100% corresponds to the referent group, children living >1,500 meters from a freeway.

Source: Reprinted with permission from Gauderman WJ, Vora H, McConnell R, Berhane K, Gilliland F, Thomas D, Lurmann F, Avol E, Kunzli N, Jerrett M, and Peters J. Effect of exposure to traffic on lung development from 10 to 18 years of age: a cohort study. Lancet 2007; 369:571–577.

lower attained FEV_1 for those who lived closest to a freeway than those who lived at least 1,500 meters from a freeway. Residence within 75 meters of a major road increased asthma risk with an odds ratio of 1.29 (95% confidence interval 1.01–1.86), prevalent asthma, and wheeze; background rates were observed 150–200 meters from a major road.[14] In analyses of those who had left the Los Angeles area, those who moved to a less polluted area had less loss of pulmonary function.[15]

Since traffic is a major source of pollutants, numerous studies have attempted to identify adverse health effects among persons exposed to traffic. In the Netherlands, environmental scientists investigated a random sample of 5,000 persons enrolled in a national diet and cancer study (ages 55–69 years), beginning in 1986, with their home addresses and plotted distance to a major road using Cox's proportional hazard models with follow-up until 1994. The relative risk for cardiopulmonary mortality was 1.95 (95% confidence interval [CI] 1.09–3.52) with living near a major road.[16] All-cause mortality was 1.41 for living near a major road after adjusting for age, sex, education, occupation, and active and passive smoking. One would think that asthmatics would be more susceptible to traffic-related exposure, especially black smoke from diesel engines. McCreanor et al. designed such a study by recruiting sixty asthmatics into a randomized crossover study walking for two hours on polluted Oxford Street restricted to diesel-powered buses and taxicabs versus two hours in pleasant Hyde Park.[17] Their FEV_1 was reduced by 6.1% and forced vital capacity (FVC) was reduced 5.4% (both $p < 0.05$) after walking on Oxford Street, and moderate asthmatics had greater reductions. Sputum was collected after the walk and measurement of the inflammatory mediator, myeloperoxidase, was 24.5 ng/ml after walking on Oxford Street compared to 4.2 ng/ml after walking in Hyde Park. These associations were significant for ultrafine particles, elemental carbon, and NO_2 but only trended to significance for $PM_{2.5}$ (see Figure 2.8). Another important study of children exposed to traffic with measurements of pulmonary function and induced sputum found microscopic carbonaceous particles within alveolar macrophages that correlated with increased PM_{10} exposure and reduced FEV_1. For example, each increase in 1.0 μm^2 in carbon in the alveolar macrophage was associated with a 17% decrease in FEV_1 predicted[18] (see Figure 2.9).

Air pollution intervention studies have documented declines in air pollutant levels and improved health outcomes. In 1987 in Utah Valley, Utah, there was a thirteen-month labor strike at the local steel mill. PM_{10} dropped approximately 15 $\mu g/m^3$, and total deaths declined 3.2%.[19] Acute bronchitis and asthma exacerbations for preschool-aged children declined by half after the strike compared to before. Dublin, Ireland, had declining air quality during the 1980s after a switch from oil to the much cheaper and more readily available bituminous coal for domestic space and water heating.[20] Periods of high air pollution were

FIGURE 2.8   Mean percentage changes in FEV₁ and FVC during and after exposure on Oxford Street and in Hyde Park

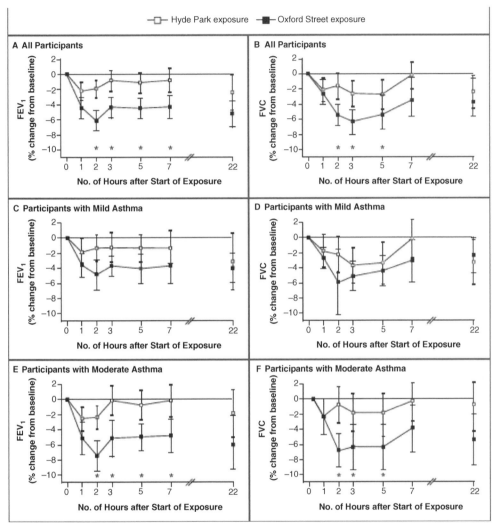

Note: Percentage changes from initial values in the forced expiratory volume in 1 second (FEV₁) and forced vital capacity (FVC) are shown for all the study participants (Panels A and B, respectively), those with mild asthma (Panels C and D, respectively), and those with moderate asthma (Panels E and F, respectively). Asterisks denote $p < 0.05$ for the difference in values between Oxford Street and Hyde Park exposures. I bars represent 95% CI.

Source: Reprinted with permission from The New England Journal of Medicine.

FIGURE 2.9 Associations between carbon in airway macrophages and lung function in healthy children

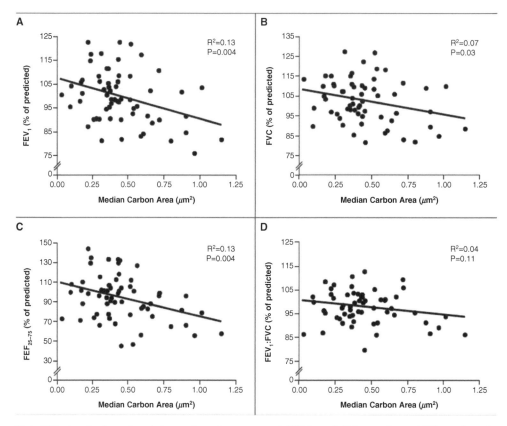

Note: FEV_1 denotes forced expiratory volume in one second, FVC forced vital capacity, and FEF_{25-75} forced expiratory flow between 25% and 75% of the FVC.
Source: Reprinted with permission from The New England Journal of Medicine.

associated with increased in-hospital respiratory deaths. On September 1, 1990, the Irish government banned coal within Dublin. Mean black smoke fell by two-thirds and SO_2 by a third. In comparing the six years after the intervention to the six years before, there was a 5.7% decline in the death rate; cardiovascular deaths fell by 10.3% and respiratory deaths fell by 15.5%. (See Figure 2.10.)

Since the ongoing hypothesis is that PM causes inflammation in the lower respiratory tract, Ghio and Devlin tested this directly by instilling PM into the lung through a fiberoptic bronchoscope.[21] Twenty-four nonsmoking volunteers had a left bronchoalveolar lavage (BAL) followed by 10 ml of saline extract of PM_{10}

FIGURE 2.10   Effect of air-pollution control on death rates in Dublin, Ireland: An intervention study

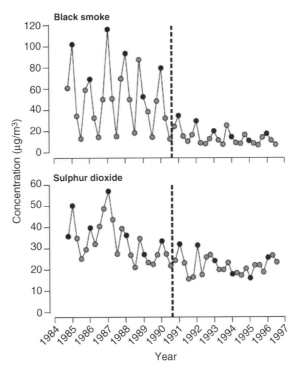

Note: Seasonal mean black smoke (upper) and sulphur dioxide (lower) concentrations, September 1984–96. Vertical line shows date sale of coal was banned in Dublin County Borough. Black circles represent winter data.
Source: Reprinted with permission from The Lancet.

collected on a filter near the Utah Valley steel mill, with one-third receiving extract from 1986 before the strike, one-third 1987 filters during the strike, and one-third 1988 filters after the strike. Twenty-four hours later they were lavaged at the challenge site and a right middle lobe control saline site. There were significantly more total cells and neutrophils in 1986 and 1988 before and after the strike compared to 1987 during the strike and to the normal saline controls. The inflammatory cytokines TNF-α, IL-8, and IL-1β were also increased similarly to the inflammatory cells. Analysis of the PM extracts showed significantly more metal content in 1986 and 1988, including iron, copper, zinc, lead, and nickel. This study was reproduced in Germany with increased reactive oxidant species measured in recovered bronchoalveolar lavage related to instilled PM high in metal content.[22]

In vitro studies of macrophages or normal human bronchial epithelial cells when exposed to PM release inflammatory cytokines and demonstrate induction of the transcription factor NF-κB. $PM_{2.5}$ stimulates normal human bronchial epithelial cells to release macrophage inflammatory protein-3α that is the ligand for CCR6, which is expressed on immature dendritic cells.[23] Theoretically, recruitment of immature dendritic cells to the airway where PM deposits can result in their maturation via GM-CSF, which is also released. Diesel exhaust particulate induces such normal human bronchial epithelial cell–dendritic cell interaction to release a third factor, thymic stromal lymphopoietic factor, that attracts and activates Th2 lymphocytes that release the characteristic cytokines IL-4, IL-5, and IL-13 that causes asthma exacerbation.[24]

Cardiovascular Disease and Particulate Matter

How does $PM_{2.5}$ cause cardiovascular disease? Anthony Seaton, M.D., proposed in 1995 that fine particles provoked alveolitis with release of cytokines capable of exacerbating lung disease and increasing blood coagulability.[25] Phagocytosis of $PM_{2.5}$ by alveolar macrophages releases cytokines in rabbits that stimulate the bone marrow to release neutrophils and monocytes.[26,27] Particulate matter may cause a form of systemic inflammatory response syndrome (SIRS) that causes endothelial activation and up-regulation of surface adhesion molecules that are critically important for leukocyte recruitment into atherosclerotic plaques.[28] (See Figure 2.11.)

Rats breathing $PM_{2.5}$ for five hours have increased reactive oxidant species and antioxidant enzymes in their lung tissues.[29] Using transgenic mice lacking ApoE(-/-), atherosclerosis and vascular inflammation developed on high-fat chow with exposure to $PM_{2.5}$ for six hours per day, five days per week, for six months as shown by increased thoracic and abdominal plaque: $PM_{2.5}$ 41.5% versus air 26.2% ($p < 0.001$) or normal chow $PM_{2.5}$ 19.2% versus 13.2%.[30] Mice fed high-fat chow and exposed to $PM_{2.5}$ had marked increases in macrophage infiltration, induced nitric oxide synthase expression, increased reactive oxidant species, and had more lipid content in the aortic arch. Ultrafine particles may have an even greater effect in these mice in causing atherosclerotic plaques.[31]

Human clinical and epidemiological studies of air pollution and heart disease have been more challenging. Increases in PM_{10} and $PM_{2.5}$ particles were significantly associated with increases in C-reactive protein, a measure of systemic inflammation that was collected repeatedly in a German panel study of fifty-seven male patients with coronary heart disease.[32] Peters and colleagues studied whether exposure to air pollution while stuck in heavy traffic would increase the

FIGURE 2.11 Systemic response to ambient particulate matter: Relevance to chronic obstructive pulmonary disease

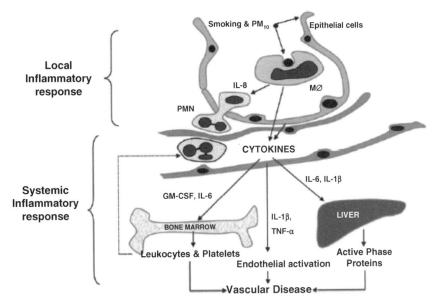

Note: Proposed mechanisms of lung inflammation induced vascular disease. Inhaled cigarette smoke or ambient particles are processed by alveolar macrophages and lung epithelial cells. These cells produce proinflammatory mediators such as cytokines that promote a local inflammatory response in the lung that are thought to contribute to the exacerbation of chronic obstructive pulmonary disease and asthma and promote lung infection. These inflammatory mediators also translocate into the circulation and induce a systemic inflammatory response. This response includes stimulation of the marrow to release leukocytes and platelets, activation of the acute phase response with the production of procoagulation factors, and activation of endothelium. Together these effects could precipitate or aggravate underlying vascular disease with the development of acute cardiovascular events such as acute coronary thrombosis, arrhythmias, and heart failure.
Source: Reprinted with permission from the Proceedings of the American Thoracic Society.

risk of myocardial infarction (heart attack).[33] They collected case histories of 691 subjects with heart attacks in Germany who survived 24 hours and obtained diaries of their activities over the previous four days prior to the heart attack. They found an increased odds ratio (OR) of exposure to traffic in an automobile, on public transport, or riding a bicycle at least one hour prior to the heart attack (OR 2.92 95% CI 2.22–3.83; P <0.001). They did extensive correlations with PM_{10} and gaseous air pollutants, but extensive analyses of these associations did not reach significance. Long-term exposure to traffic within 100 meters of living near a road was assessed in a case-control study of the Worcester, Massachusetts,

Heart Attack Study.[34] They had 5,049 confirmed cases between 1995 and 2003; population controls were drawn from Massachusetts resident lists. Using logistic regression they found a 5% increase in the odds of acute myocardial infarction near a major roadway (95% CI 3–6%). In a cohort of 3,239 nonsmoking adults followed in California for twenty-two years, correlates were made for residence and work and air pollution variables.[35] Only females had statistical associations between coronary heart disease and $PM_{2.5}$, increasing relative risk (RR) to 1.42 (95% CI 1.06–1.90). Ozone increased the relative risk to 2.00 in a two-pollutant model (95% CI 1.51–2.64). The NIH's Women's Health Initiative enrolled 65,893 postmenopausal women without previous cardiovascular disease from 36 U.S. metropolitan areas from 1994 to 1998 and followed them up for a median of six years.[36]

There were 1,816 women who had one or more fatal or nonfatal cardiovascular events, including death, from coronary or cerebrovascular disease, coronary revascularization, myocardial infarction, and stroke. Each 10 $\mu g/m^3$ of $PM_{2.5}$ exposure was associated with a 24% increase in the risk of cardiovascular event (Hazard Ratio 1.24; 95% CI 1.09–1.41) and a 76% increase in the risk of death from cardiovascular disease (Hazard Ratio 1.76; CI 1.25–2.47). There was a larger within-city difference related to exposure differences than between cities.

A controlled, double-blind, randomized, crossover study of twenty men with prior heart attacks, but currently stable, had exposure to dilute diesel exhaust (300 $\mu g/m^3$) of filtered air for one hour with moderate exercise.[37] Exercise-induced ST-segment depression (an electrocardiographic sign of oxygen deprivation of heart muscle) was present in all patients, but there was a greater increase in the ischemic burden during exposure to diesel exhaust. Exposure to diesel exhaust did not aggravate preexisting vasomotor dysfunction, but it did reduce the acute release of endothelial plasminogen activator (a mediator of fibrinolysis that dissolves blood clots). As shown in Figure 2.12, diesel particulate exacerbated electrocardiographic indicators compared to filtered air. In a further measure of atherosclerosis related to air pollution, carotid artery intima-media thickness was determined by ultrasound in 798 participants from vitamin E and B atherosclerosis intervention trials.[38] Their residential areas were geocoded to annual $PM_{2.5}$ concentrations. For a cross-sectional exposure contrast of 10 $\mu g/m^3$ $PM_{2.5}$, carotid intima-media thickness increased by 5.9% (95% CI 1–11%). The strongest association of $PM_{2.5}$ with carotid intima/media thickness was in women >60 years of age, which was 15.7%. There may be genetic susceptibility to air pollution exposures, for example, those lacking the gene glutathione S-transferase M1, which encodes an enzyme scavenger of oxygen-free radicals, have an increased sensitivity to inhaled particulate matter as shown by greater changes in heart rate variability.[39]

FIGURE 2.12   Myocardial ischemia during intervals of exercise-induced stress and exposure to diesel exhaust or filtered air

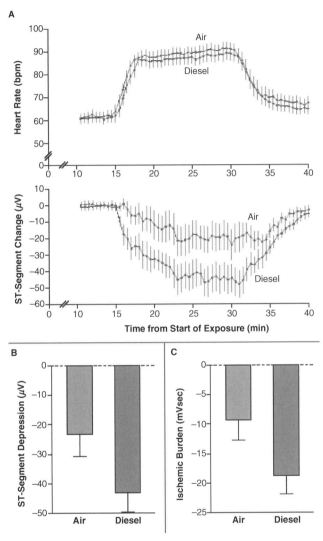

Note: Ischemic and thrombotic effects of dilute diesel exhaust inhalation in men with coronary heart disease. Panel A shows the average change in the heart rate and in the ST segment in lead II. Panel B shows the maximum ST-segment depression during inhalation of diesel exhaust as compared with filtered air ($p = 0.003$), and Panel C shows the total ischemic burden during inhalation of diesel exhaust as compared with filtered air ($p < 0.001$); the values in Panels B and C are averages of the values in leads II, V2, and V5. In all three panels, lower line indicates exposure to diesel exhaust, and upper exposure to filtered air. T bars denote standard errors, and mVsec millivolt seconds.

Source: Reprinted with permission from The New England Journal of Medicine.

Patients with automatic implantable cardioverter defibrillators (AICDs) have been used to study short-term effects of PM and other ambient pollutants on arrhythmias in a population subgroup that might be expected to be especially susceptible. AICDs store information on previous arrhythmias that can then be utilized to evaluate the relationship between arrhythmia onset and PM concentration. Initial evidence that short-term increases in PM (and NO_2) concentrations were associated with arrhythmias was reported in a study from Boston.[40]

Recent studies have also explored associations with outcomes of pregnancy. Only some of these have focused on the short-term associations with PM. As in time-series studies of total and more specific causes of mortality, associations between short-term increases in PM concentrations and infant mortality, especially respiratory mortality and death from sudden infant death syndrome, have been reported.[41] Recently, PM_{10} averaged over the previous six weeks, or at a few individual days (lags) before delivery, has been associated with preterm birth in a time-series study.[42] A New Jersey Department of Health statewide study linked birth certificate and maternal/newborn hospital discharge summaries for all singleton births from 1999 to 2003 with a gestational age of 37–42 completed weeks and a birth weight >500 grams with air pollution data from a monitoring station within 10 km of residence for $PM_{2.5}$, NO_2, CO, and SO_2.[43] There were significant increased risks for small for gestational age (fetal growth ratio >0.75 and <0.85, 88,678 births) and first and third trimester $PM_{2.5}$ exposure, and first, second, and third trimester for very small for gestational age (fetal growth ratio <0.75, 114,411 births) and NO_2 concentrations. This suggests an adverse effect of traffic on birth outcome after controlling for known risk factors.

At least two time-series studies indicate that PM of crustal origin may not cause mortality. In both Spokane, Washington,[44] and Salt Lake City, Utah,[45] high-PM concentrations attributed to windy conditions that result in suspension of crustal PM in air were not associated with mortality, whereas PM on other days was associated with mortality.

Rather than focus on effects of specific components of PM, focusing on effects of particles emitted from specific sources could potentially help to identify particularly toxic forms of PM.[46] Factor analysis approaches have been used in a few health studies in an attempt to parcel daily PM concentrations into their relative source contributions. Data from the U.S. Six Cities Study that included measurements of elemental chemical species of fine PM were used to estimate daily mortality effects associated with separate sources of ambient PM.[47] Of all sources, PM from motor vehicle exhaust was more consistently associated with daily mortality than was PM from coal combustion. Crustal PM was not associated with mortality. PM size, independent of chemical composition, could conceivably play a role in determining toxicity. In epidemiological studies, partly due to the use of PM data from monitoring networks used for regulatory purposes, PM has typically been classed by size into total suspended particles (TSP) and its inhalable fraction (PM_{10}), which has in turn been divided into coarse ($PM_{10-2.5}$), and fine ($PM_{2.5}$) fractions.

Respiratory Effects of Concentrated Ambient Particles

Concentrated ambient particles (CAPs) exposures in healthy and asthmatic individuals have demonstrated an absence of respiratory symptoms, or changes in spirometry, with particle concentrations of up to 311 $\mu g/m^3$.[48,49] In these studies, healthy participants had a mild increase in bronchoalveolar lavage neutrophils at 18 hours after CAPs exposure relative to filtered air. In one study, no significant effect was found on spirometry or induced sputum cell counts in elderly individuals with and without COPD exposed to CAPs and NO_2. However, decrements in maximal mid-expiratory flow and arterial saturation associated with CAPs exposure were seen, suggesting an effect on small airways. Surprisingly, a greater effect was found in the healthy individuals. Induced sputum in asthmatics, young healthy participants, and elderly participants with and without COPD contained decreased numbers of columnar epithelial cells after CAPs exposure relative to filtered air suggesting a potential effect on bronchial epithelial cells.

In controlled exposure studies in healthy and asthmatic volunteers, diesel exhaust increases airway hyper-responsiveness to methacholine and airway resistance in patients with mild asthma[50,51] increases sputum neutrophil counts, and bronchial tissue mast cell, neutrophil, and lymphocyte counts. In addition, diesel particulate exposure (DE) increases expression of IL-6, IL-8, and the adhesion molecules ICAM-1 and VCAM-1. Simultaneous exposure to allergen and DE has been hypothesized to be a potential cause of greater allergic sensitization and prevalence of allergic disorders.[52] With high-level exposures and nasal instillations in humans, investigators have demonstrated the ability of DE (or traffic exposure) to augment later allergic effects (antibody class switching, Th2 skewing of cytokines, and neo-antigen effects).[53] More recent studies suggest that the diesel particle is responsible for the allergic sensitization.[54]

Particulate Matter and Public Policy

There are six criteria pollutants established by the EPA: ozone, particulate matter, carbon monoxide, nitrogen oxides, sulfur dioxide, and lead. Of these, PM is unique in not being a specific chemical compound or element. Each NAAQS consists of an indicator, an averaging time, a form and a level. PM_{10} supplanted TSP as the indicator in 1987. $PM_{2.5}$ was added as an indicator in 1997. PM averaging times include both a 24-hour average and an annual average. Forms of the standards relate to the specific statistics that are calculated in determining area attainment with the NAAQS. Separate NAAQS are set to protect public health (the primary standard) and to protect welfare (the secondary standard); welfare effects include effects on visibility and flora. Since 1987, the primary and secondary PM NAAQS have been identical. Review of the NAAQS is mandated to take place every five years.

The latest EPA PM review was completed in 1997, at which time the 24-hour and annual levels for PM_{10} were maintained at concentrations of 150 $\mu g/m^3$ and 50 $\mu g/m^3$ respectively. At that time, the first 24-hour and annual levels for $PM_{2.5}$ were set at concentrations of 65 $\mu g/m^3$ and 15 $\mu g/m^3$ respectively. Because of the wealth of scientific health data that has accumulated since that time indicating that effects can occur well below those concentrations, it became imperative that the next review would recommend reductions in these levels. In 2005, the State of California Air Resources Board approved revised ambient air quality standards that were substantially more stringent that those of the EPA, with 24-hour and annual PM_{10} concentrations of 50 and 20 $\mu g/m^3$, respectively, and an annual $PM_{2.5}$ concentration of 12 $\mu g/m^3$. Recommended limit values of the European Union to be met in 2005 for 24-hour and annual PM_{10} were 50 and 40 $\mu g/m^3$, respectively, with recommended further reduction in the annual level to 20 $\mu g/m^3$ by 2010.

EPA was sued over the 1997 PM standards by the American Trucking Association; the D.C. Circuit Court of Appeals, in a split decision, held that the new public health air quality standards for PM were unconstitutional and an improper delegation of legislative authority to the EPA. EPA appealed the court's decision all the way to the U.S. Supreme Court. In a landmark decision in February 2001, the Supreme Court upheld EPA's authority to set national air quality standards that protect millions of people from the harmful effects of air pollution. The Supreme Court also affirmed that the Clean Air Act does not allow the EPA to consider cost when setting national ambient air quality standards but requires the EPA to set those air quality standards at levels necessary to protect the public health with an adequate margin of safety and to protect public welfare from adverse effects. This was an important case for interpretation of the constitutional basis for the EPA to enforce clean air standards to protect the public's health.

The EPA staff paper recommended two choices for the administrator to consider: (1) an annual $PM_{2.5}$ standard at the current level of 15 $\mu g/m^3$, together with a revised 24-hour $PM_{2.5}$ standard in the range of 35–25 $\mu g/m^3$;

alternatively, (2) an annual standard of 14–12 $\mu g/m^3$ together with a revised 24-hour $PM_{2.5}$ standard to provide supplemental protection against episodic localized or seasonal peaks, in the range of 40 to 35 $\mu g/m^3$. The Clean Air Scientific Advisory Committee (CASAC, comprised of one member of the National Academies, one physician, and one member of State Pollution Control agencies) evaluated the EPA criteria document for $PM_{2.5}$ including health effects, exposure trends, and policy considerations and recommended that the administrator strengthen the 24-hour standard from 65 to 35 $\mu g/m^3$ and the annual standard from 15 $\mu g/m^3$ to the range of 13–14 $\mu g/m^3$. The CASAC recommendations were not unanimous, however. The Environmental Health Policy Committee of the American Thoracic Society (ATS) and the American Lung Association (ALA) coordinated their recommendations to lower the 24-hour standard to 25 $\mu g/m^3$ and the annual standard to 12 $\mu g/m^3$.[55] To achieve these levels, the ATS wrote a letter to the administrator and obtained co-sponsorship from other professional societies, including the American College of Cardiology, the American Academy of Pediatrics, the American Association of Cardiovascular and Pulmonary Rehabilitation, and the National Association for the Medical Direction of Respiratory Care. The American Medical Association House of Delegates introduced a measure and passed the recommendation for the ATS recommendation levels. Separately, other health organizations supported lowering the standard including the American College of Chest Physicians, the American College of Preventive Medicine, and the American Public Health Association. Next, in a telephone call at the CASAC public hearing, the ATS provided verbal support for lowering the standard. EPA held public hearings in several sites around the country, and the ATS coordinated academic pulmonologists testifying at the hearings so that each one would have a public record of support. Lastly, the EPA administrator allowed the ATS and ALA to present their data and interpretations in a personal interview. They met personally with Administrator Steven Johnson and his advisors in the Rachel Carson Great Room and argued emphatically that there was a scientific consensus justifying a lowering of the standard.[55] The EPA did not follow the CASAC recommendations by leaving the annual standard intact, although the EPA did lower the 24-hour standard to 35 $\mu g/m^3$. PM_{10} was still regulated. The American Farm Bureau immediately sued the EPA from the industry side, stating that $PM_{2.5}$ was being regulated twice by overlapping PM_{10} and $PM_{2.5}$ standards and that farms should only have a coarse standard of $PM_{10-2.5}$ that, furthermore, was nontoxic. On the other side, thirteen states, the District of Columbia, the ALA, Environmental Defense, and the National Parks Conservation Council all joined with briefs arguing the opposite that the EPA unlawfully used uncertainty to justify ignoring the scientific consensus recommending a more protective standard.

Going forward, the EPA plans an Advanced Notice of Public Rulemaking (ANPR) and Integrated Science Assessment to incorporate the criteria document and staff paper.

Summary

Particulate matter less than 2.5 microns in size is able to penetrate deep into the lungs and has proved to be toxic to human cells. Epidemiologic studies have demonstrated increased cardiopulmonary mortality and hospitalizations. Regulations have proven contentious, since there are many sources, including transport and stationary, especially coal-fired power plants.

Key Terms

Accumulation mode

Aitken mode

Brownian diffusion

Course mode

Gravitational
   sedimentation

Impaction

Interception

Nucleation mode

Particulate matter
   (PM)

Discussion Questions

1. What is particulate matter?
2. What are some of the health effects of increased ambient concentrations of particulate matter?
3. How do the courts play a role in regulating particulate matter?
4. What is the EPA's current role in particulate matter regulation?

The author thanks Sverre Vedal, M.D., and Jeffrey H. Sullivan, M.D., for permission to use parts of the Particulate Matter chapter published in *Environmental and Occupational Medicine*, 4th ed., by Lippincott, Williams and Wilkins.

CHAPTER 3

OZONE

LEARNING OBJECTIVES

- To understand what ozone is and where it comes from
- To become familiar with the health effects of ozone
- To understand how ozone is regulated by the government

Ozone (O_3) forms from reactions on nitrogen oxides (NOx) and volatile organic hydrocarbons (VOCs) with ultraviolet energy from sunlight catalyzing the reaction. Each VOC can produce different amounts of ozone. For example, one kilogram of ethane produces half the amount of ozone as one kg of formaldehyde. Levels of ozone tend to be highest on warm, sunny, windless days. Ozone concentration peaks in the morning and/or afternoon and declines in the evening following rush hour peaks. Among the sources of VOCs are motor vehicles (about 40% of emissions); industrial processes, particularly the chemical and petroleum industries; any use of paints, coatings, and solvents (another 40% for these sources combined). Service stations, pesticide application, dry cleaning, fuel combustion, and open burning are other significant sources of VOCs. Ozone is a powerful oxidant and respiratory tract irritant in adults and children, causing shortness of breath (dyspnea), chest pain when inhaling deeply, wheezing, and cough. Since 1980, ozone levels have dropped 21% as the Environmental Protection Agency (EPA) and state and local governments have worked together to improve air quality. A large and reasonably consistent body of knowledge has accumulated on the effects of O_3 on respiratory symptoms, respiratory function and airway inflammation in humans, especially on transient responses to acute exposure.[1]

Other lung function responses to acute and subacute exposure that have been studied, largely in animals, include mucociliary and early alveolar zone particle clearance, functional responses in macrophages and epithelial cells, and changes in lung cell secretions. Structural changes in the smaller conductive airways and the more proximal gas exchange region have been associated with "subchronic" and chronic animal exposure protocols. Chronic effects may result from cumulative damage or from the side effects of adaptive responses to repeated daily or intermittent exposure.

Health Effects

Pulmonary Function

Inhalation of O_3 causes concentration-dependent mean decrements in exhaled volume and flow rate during forced expiratory maneuvers. In 1972, David Bates, M.D., showed that subjects exposed to ambient O_3 levels while exercising also exhibited pulmonary function changes.[2] In a study of 846 urban children (ages 4–9 years) with asthma, Mortimer et al.[3] showed that the greatest effect on peak expiratory flow rate (PEFR) occurred with a two-day lag, with an even greater effect for a five-day distributed lag. They collected data from eight U.S.

cities with an O_3 mean of 48 ppb and maximum of 58 ppb. Respiratory symptoms were associated with O_3 or NO_2 levels.

It is also well established that repeated daily one- or two-hour exposures, at a level that produces a functional response with a single exposure, results in an enhanced response on the second day, diminishing responses on days 3 and 4, and virtually no response by day 5.[4,5] This functional adaptation to exposure disappears about a week after exposure ceases. Inflammation, as indexed by polymorphonuclear cells (PMNs), fibronectin, and IL-4 in lavage fluid, was also attenuated by multiday exposures.[6] For repeated 6.6 hour per day exposures to 120 ppb O_3, the peak functional response occurs on the first day, with progressively lesser responses after the second, third, and fourth days of exposure. However, responsiveness to methacholine challenge peaked on the second day and remained elevated throughout all five days of exposure,[7] and there were protracted changes in small airway function. For patients with asthma, O_3 can cause a further increase in responsiveness. The persistent changes in airway responsiveness and small airways function are an important health effect.

Kinney and colleagues studied 154 Tennessee schoolchildren by measuring lung function on as many as six occasions during a two-month period in the late winter and early spring.[8] Child-specific regressions of lung function versus maximum 1-hour O_3 concentration during the previous day indicated significant associations. Because children in school may be expected to have relatively low activity levels, the relatively high response coefficients may be due to potentiation by other pollutants or to a low level of seasonal adaptation. Kingston-Harriman, Tennessee, is notable for its relatively high levels of aerosol acidity. In a study of children with moderate to severe asthma at a summer camp in the Connecticut River Valley,[9] decrements in peak expiratory flow rates were associated with ambient O_3 concentrations. The level of physical activity of the asthmatic children was low, and hence their O_3 intake was low and they had less reserve functional capacity. The level of health concern for these functional decrements is high.

Field studies of functional responses of adults engaged in recreational activities outdoors in the presence of varying levels of O_3 have also been performed. Spektor et al.[10] made pre- and post-exercise respiratory function measurements on thirty young adults who were engaged in daily outdoor exercise for about one-half-hour per day in an area with regional summer haze but no local point sources. The magnitudes of the functional decrements per unit of ambient O_3 concentration was similar to those observed in volunteers exposed while exercising vigorously for one or two hours in controlled chamber exposure studies. Functional decrements in proportion to ambient O_3 concentrations have also been reported for competitive cyclists in the Netherlands[11] and hikers on Mount Washington, New Hampshire.[12] The hikers on Mount Washington with a history of asthma or wheeze had fourfold greater responses to O_3, $PM_{2.5}$, and aerosol acidity than the others. The average pollutant levels were quite low, with O_3 averaging 4.0 ppb, $PM_{2.5}$ at 10 $\mu g/m^3$, and acidity at 0.3 $\mu g/m^3$ (H_2SO_4 equivalent). Brauer reported that pulmonary function in fifty-eight outdoor farm workers in British Columbia during the summer had reductions associated with O_3 mean of 54 ppb and a maximum of 84 ppb.[13] Ozone was related to reduced evening peak expiratory flow rates when measured twice a day over two weeks in the summer with a five-day cumulative lag exposure showing the greatest effect in 473 nonsmoking women (ages 19–43 years) in Virginia.[14] The morning peak expiratory flow rate decrements were related to exposure to $PM_{2.5}$ and acid. Mail carriers had PEFR measured twice per day also for six weeks; the night PEFR reduction was related to 8-hour O_3 levels with a lag of 0–2 days controlling for PM, temperature, humidity, sex, age, and disease status.[15]

Inflammation

Folinsbee and colleagues undertook a 6.6-hour chamber exposure study of adult volunteers to 120 ppb O_3. Moderate exercise was performed for 50 minutes every hour, for 3 hours in the morning and again in the afternoon.[16] The investigators found that the pulmonary function decrements became progressively greater after each hour of exposure, reaching average values of about 400 ml for forced vital capacity (FVC) and about 540 ml for forced expiratory volume in one second (FEV_1) by the end of the day (Figure 3.1). The effects were

FIGURE 3.1   Mean ±SE of FVC (dashed lines) and FEV$_1$ (solid lines) after each of six 1-hour exercise periods

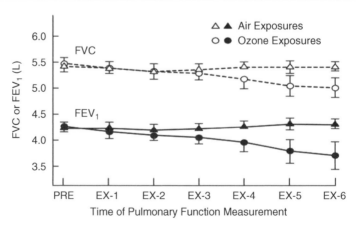

Source: Reprinted with permission from Environmental and Occupational Medicine. Ed: William N. Rom.

FIGURE 3.2   Relationship between ozone-induced neutrophilia in the distal airways during the late-acute response and concentration breathing rate and exposure time (CVT)

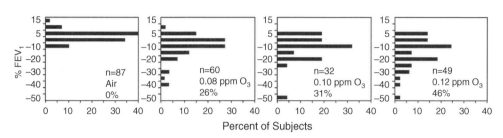

Note: The distribution of response for eighty subjects exposed to clean air and at least one of 0.08, 0.10, or 0.12 ppm ozone (O_3) is shown here. The O_3 exposures lasted 6.6 hours, during which time the subjects exercised for 50 minutes of each hour with a 35-minute rest period at the end of the third hour. Decreases in forced expiratory volume in 1 second (FEV_1) are expressed as percentage change from baseline. For example, the bar labeled "−10" indicates the percentage of subjects with a decrease in FEV_1 of >5% but ≤10%, and the bar labeled "5" indicates improvement in FEV_1 of >0% but ≤5%. Each panel of the figure indicates the percentage of subjects at each O_3 concentration with a decrease of FEV_1 in excess of 10%.
Source: Reprinted with permission from the American Journal of Respiratory and Critical Care Medicine 2004; 169:1092.

transient in that there were no residual function decrements on the following day. The decrements in FEV_1 after 6.6 hours' exposure to 120 ppb averaged 13%. Follow-up studies involved 6.6-hour exposures at concentrations of 80, 100, and 120 ppb. The results at 120 ppb confirmed the previous findings, whereas those at 80 and 100 ppb showed smaller changes, which however also became progressively greater with duration of exposure.[17]

McDonnell et al. modeled the data from sixty-eight healthy nonsmoking adults studied using this protocol at the EPA Chapel Hill, North Carolina, laboratory and reported that for exposure at 120 ppb for 6.6 hours, 46% (95% CI 30–65%) would have an FEV_1 decrement ≥10% (18). Figure 3.2 illustrates the decrements in pulmonary function with increasing O_3 exposures.

Airway Reactivity and Inflammation

Ozone is an irritant gas and increases airway reactivity that can be measured by responsiveness to inhaled methacholine. Not all subjects have airway hyper-reactivity, and asthmatic and atopic individuals may be more susceptible. Ozone may interact with particles and other gaseous pollutants to increase bronchial hyper-reactivity. The follow-up tests by Horstman and coworkers[18] in healthy subjects, involving 6.6-hour exposures to 80, 100, and 120 ppb, indicated 56, 89, and 121% increases in methacholine responsiveness, respectively. Seven asthmatic subjects were exposed to 1 hour of ozone at 0.12 ppm followed by allergen; the low dose of O_3 increased bronchial responsiveness to allergen, reducing by almost two-thirds the amount of allergen required to produce a 15% decline in FEV_1.[19] Jorres et al.[20] exposed twenty-four subjects with mild stable allergic asthma, twelve subjects with allergic rhinitis without asthma, and ten healthy subjects to 250 ppb O_3 or filtered air (FA) for 3 hours with intermittent exercise. In the subjects with asthma, FEV_1 decreased by 13%, and the dose of methacholine or allergen more than doubled after O_3 compared with filtered air. In the subjects with rhinitis, mean FEV_1 decreased by 7.8% and 1.3% when O_3 or filtered air, respectively, were followed by allergen inhalation. Seltzer and colleagues exposed 10 healthy subjects to air or ozone at 0.4 or 0.6 ppm and followed up with bronchoalveolar lavage (BAL) 3 hours later.[21] Exposure to ozone caused more bronchial hyper-reactivity, increased methacholine responsiveness, increased neutrophils and prostaglandins in the BAL, and responses were greater with the higher dose of ozone.

The EPA established a Health Effects Research Laboratory at their Research Triangle Park, North Carolina, facility where ozone-induced inflammation in the lower airways could be studied directly using tools such as bronchoalveolar lavage.[22] They demonstrated an exposure–response relationship at three levels of exposure also demonstrating inter-individual variation.

They first began with 0.4 ppm O_3 exposure to eleven healthy adults for 2 hours with exercise followed by BAL the next day. Neutrophils increased eightfold, and biochemical changes in the BAL fluid included increases in neutrophil elastase, fibronectin, and prostaglandins. They also included a nasal lavage (NL) and noted an increase in neutrophils immediately after the NL and also the next day at the time of the BAL.[23] Next was a lowering of the O_3 dose to 0.10 or 0.08 ppm O_3, with exercise for a longer time period of 6.6 hours followed by BAL the next day.[24] Both exposure levels caused inflammation in the lower respiratory tract with increased neutrophils, prostaglandins, fibronectin, interleukin-6, and decreased alveolar phagocytosis. These studies were validated by Aris and colleagues at the University of California-San Francisco, where fourteen volunteers were exposed to 0.20 ppm O_3 for 4 hours with exercise and BAL performed of the proximal airway to assess the irritant nature of O_3 gas.[25] They found increases of neutrophils and the same biochemical parameters including interleukin-8 that is chemotactic for neutrophils. They also did mucosal biopsies for histology documenting the infiltration of neutrophils after O_3 exposure compared to filtered air. The time course of O_3-related effects after exposure to 0.3 ppm for 1 hour on three separate days showed FEV_1 declined immediately; the proximal airway neutrophilia peaked at 6 hours and continued until the next day.[26] To bring these findings into a real-life scenario, Kinney and colleagues reported on fifteen U.S. Coast Guard joggers on Governor's Island in New York Harbor, comparing an ambient summer ozone exposure to that in the winter using BAL.[27] BAL fluids in the summer had higher levels of lactic dehydrogenase and IL-8 and prostaglandin E2. Asthmatics may be especially sensitive to the irritant properties of inhaling O_3 for 6 hours and engaging in exercise.[28] Five asthmatics and five normals exposed to 0.20 ppm O_3 in chamber studies had no change in FEV_1 but developed significant increases in next day BALs of neutrophils from 1% to 12%, IL-6, and IL-8. In these chamber studies, there was considerable inter-individual variability, and methacholine tests for bronchial hyper-reactivity were unable to predict those who might respond to O_3. In a study of fourteen asthmatics exposed to O_3 at 0.20 ppm for 1 hour with exercise, there was no additional effect from allergen exposure including pulmonary function, BAL neutrophils, or cytokines, that is, a negative study, but a subgroup of nine individuals were more sensitive to allergen exposure and had more neutrophilia.[29] A meta-analysis from twenty-one publications illustrated in Figure 3.3 shows a linear relationship between neutrophils at 6-hour or 18-hour post-O_3 exposure BALs.[30]

FIGURE 3.3   BAL neutrophils and ozone exposure

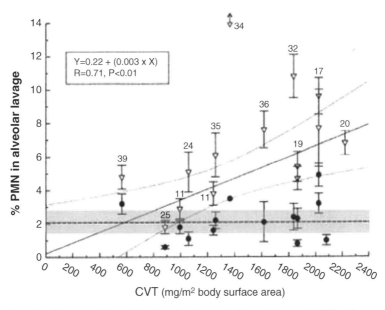

$$Y = 0.22 + (0.003 \times X)$$
$$R = 0.71, P < 0.01$$

% PMN in alveolar lavage

CVT (mg/m² body surface area)

Source: Reprinted by permission of the American Journal of Respiratory and Critical Care Medicine.

Two weeks of pretreatment of inhaled budesonide (a corticosteroid) with 800 μg twice a day provided no protection against inhaled O_3 in terms of pulmonary function, methacholine reactivity, or neutrophil recruitment.[31] Samet et al.[32] studied the pulmonary effects of O_3 on healthy adults with and without dietary supplementation of antioxidants and found that the antioxidants reduced the O_3-induced functional decrements but not its effect on increasing neutrophils and IL-6 in BAL fluid.

Short-term, one-hour exposures of alveolar macrophages to 0.4 ppm O_3 in vitro increased release of inflammatory cytokines IL-1β, IL-6, IL-8, and TNF-α approximately fourfold over control without any loss in cell viability.[33] Rats exposed to a single dose of O_3 had increased proliferation of bronchial and alveolar epithelial cells as measured by proliferating cell nuclear antigen (PCNA). Corticosteroids reduced this from 19.2% to 10.9% (p <0.5) and reduced the neutrophil influx.[34] Using transgenic knockout mice exposed to O_3 in chamber studies, matrix metalloproteinases (MMPs) were noted to have a role in O_3 mediated lung injury with MMP-9 having a protective role but MMP-7 did not.[35]

Also, tumor necrosis factor-α receptor, the transcription factor NF-κB, and the signaling pathways to the nucleus were all essential for the inflammatory effects of O_3 as elucidated by O_3 exposure to transgenic mice lacking these genes.[36]

Epidemiological Studies of Populations Exposed to Ozone in Ambient Air

Observational studies of the influence of O_3 on human health are often difficult to interpret because the population is also exposed to other pollutants in the ambient air that could affect the responses observed, or to other environmental challenges that may produce comparable effects, such as environmental tobacco smoke, other pollutants in indoor air, and allergens found in indoor and outdoor air.

Grades 1 and 2 schoolchildren in Austria were studied across the summer for three successive years, and an O_3 effect was detected on reducing FEV_1 or lung growth.[37] In the Children's Health Study from Southern California, a new diagnosis of asthma was sought among 3,535 children with no history of asthma in twelve communities followed longitudinally.[38] Six communities had increased O_3 concentration, and 265 children reported a new diagnosis of asthma over five years of follow-up. In six communities with high O_3 concentration, the **relative risk (RR)**—the risk of an event (or of developing a disease) relative to exposure—of developing asthma in children playing three or more sports was 3.3 (95% CI 1.9–5.8) compared to children playing no sports. Sports had no effect in areas of low O_3 concentrations (RR 0.8, 0.4–1.6). Time spent outside was associated with a higher incidence of asthma in areas of high O_3 (RR 1.4, 1.0–2.1) but not in areas of low O_3. Exposure to pollutants other than O_3 did not alter the effect of team sports. Children inside the school have exposure to only 15% of O_3 concentrations outdoors due to central air conditioning, but when they play outside they are exposed to daily peak O_3 exposures. School absences for respiratory tract illness increased 63% in association with a 0.02 ppm increase in O_3.[39] Further investigation of gene–environment interaction was pursued in this closely monitored cohort of children and their exposure to air pollutants.[40] Airway oxidative stress is a cardinal feature and antioxidant enzymes exist to neutralize effects of reactive oxidant species (ROS). Antioxidant enzymes include heme oxygenase, superoxide dismutases, and catalase; these enzymes have functional polymorphisms that may predispose to asthma development. Children eligible for this study from the Southern California Children's Study included 576 Hispanic and 1,125 non-Hispanic, with 1,690 who developed new-onset asthma. Heme oxygenase short alleles were associated with a reduced risk of asthma in non-Hispanic whites, and Hispanic children with Catalase-262 T allele had an increased risk for asthma (Hazard Ratio 1.78, $p = 0.01$). Other susceptibility studies have shown that persons >65 years old have a 2.7-fold increase in deaths per 10 ppb O_3; blacks have 2.8-fold increase in deaths compared to non-blacks; women >60 years had a 1.9 increase compared to men; a 1.7-fold increase per 10 ppb increase in O_3 occurs for atrial fibrillation; and an increased risk of reduced FEV_1 with O_3 exposure occurs with obesity.

Ambient ozone has been a particular hazard for children who play outdoors, especially in the summer season when school is over, ozone is peaking, and automobile traffic increases. In Virginia, 691 infants were enrolled in a time-series study over the 1995 summer; for every interquartile-range increase in same-day 24-hour O_3, wheeze increased 37%.[41] Among infants of asthmatic mothers, same-day 24-hour O_3 increased the likelihood of wheeze to 59% and of difficulty breathing to 83%. Mortimer and colleagues followed a cohort of 846 inner-city asthmatic children observing that those with low birth weight had increased respiratory symptoms, and greater decline in morning percentage peak expiratory flow rate compared to normal birth weight in relation to O_3.[42] Pediatric emergency room (ER) visits during the summers of 1993–1995 in Atlanta were correlated by zip code to O_3 and PM_{10} with more than 6,000 asthma visits.[43] There was a linear correlation of O_3 exposure trends comparing >100 ppb versus <50 ppb OR (odds ratio) = 1.23, $p = 0.003$, similar to findings for PM_{10}. In 1996, Atlanta hosted the Summer Olympics and the city rerouted traffic during the games. Friedman et al. performed an ecologic study comparing the seventeen days of the games to the four-week periods before and after for children's acute care.[44] Asthma acute care events declined more than 40% using several databases including the Georgia Medicaid claims file, and peak daily O_3 concentrations decreased 28% with traffic declining 23% during the games. An epidemiologic study of 271 asthmatic children <12 years attending a summer camp in southern New England correlated respiratory symptoms (wheeze increase by 35% and chest tightness by 47%) with a 50 ppb increase in 1 hr O_3.[45] O_3 >0.063 ppm for an 8-hour peak on the same day was associated with a 30% increase in chest tightness (OR 1.64 95% CI 1.23–2.17). One-day lags were also associated with persistent cough and shortness of breath (OR 1.33, 95% CI 1.09–1.62). These data were significant only for the half of the cohort who used maintenance medication. Increased bronchodilator use was associated with the highest level of same-day O_3. Neither respiratory symptoms nor bronchodilator use were associated with $PM_{2.5}$. Thus asthma severity can divide the group into two levels of vulnerability to air pollution O_3. A two-year longitudinal study of eighty-six inner city school children in Detroit found striking 8-hour peak O_3 association with upper respiratory infection, and the subgroup of asthmatic children on corticosteroids had significant associations with both O_3 and PM and reduced FEV_1.[46] Most (thirty-one) of Atlanta's hospitals' emergency departments participated in the Study of Particles and Health in Atlanta (SOPHIA) 1993–2000, in which 11% of 4.5 million ER visits were due to respiratory causes.[47] PM_{10}, O_3, NO_2, and CO were individually associated with 1%–3% increases of upper respiratory infection visits per standard deviation increase of pollutant; a 20 ppb increase of NO_2 was associated with a 3.5% increase of chronic obstructive pulmonary disease (COPD) visits. The risk ratios for asthma visits were strongest for lags of five to eight days, and with O_3 were strongest at lags of one and two days. The associations for asthma were stronger in summer months for O_3 and $PM_{2.5}$. Asthma hospitalizations in children from birth to age 19 years were correlated to residence air pollutant levels from California Air Resources Board from 1983 to 2000; they found a time-independent, constant effect of ambient levels of O_3 and quarterly hospital discharge for asthma.[48]

Decreased lung function and increased respiratory symptoms, including exacerbation of asthma, occur with increasing ambient O_3, especially in children. In an analysis of respiratory hospital admissions in fourteen Canadian cities, Burnett et al.[49] showed that the effect was greatest at a one- or two-day lag but greatest of all for a distributed lag over four days. They studied hospital admissions from 1980 to 1994 in Toronto for acute respiratory admissions in children <2 years of age using daily time-series to adjust for influences of day of the week, season, and weather. There was a 35% increase (CI 19–52%) in daily admissions for respiratory diagnoses associated with a 5-day moving average daily 1-hour maximum O_3 concentration of 0.045 ppm during May to August. Neonatal respiratory morbidity in eleven Canadian cities was found to be related to gaseous pollutants reaching an independent effect of 9.61% of all pollutants combined.[50] Modifying factors, such as ambient temperature, aeroallergens, and other co-pollutants (for example, particles) also can contribute to this relationship. Ozone air pollution can account for a portion of summertime hospital admissions and emergency room visits for respiratory causes. It has been estimated from these studies that O_3 may account for roughly one to three excess summertime respiratory hospital admissions per 100 ppb O_3, per million persons. A recent study by Yang et al.[51] reported significant associations between O_3 respiratory hospital admissions for children less than three years of age and for the elderly in Vancouver, Canada, where the 24-hour average O_3 concentration was only 13 ppb.

In a Denver epidemiological study covering July to August between 1993 and 1997, daily measures of temperature, PM_{10}, and gaseous pollutants were compared to concurrent data on hospital admissions for ages >65 years.[52] The results suggested that O_3 was associated with an increase in the risk of hospitalization for acute myocardial infarction, coronary atherosclerosis, and pulmonary heart disease. A cross-over study of thirty-six U.S. cities tabulated respiratory hospital admissions and ozone and PM_{10} data for 1986–1999.[53] During the warm season, the two-day cumulative effect of a 5 ppb increase in O_3 was a 0.27% (95% CI 0.08–0.47%) increase in COPD admissions and a 0.41% (95% CI 0.26–0.57%) increase in pneumonia admissions. There were increases of 1.47% in COPD and 0.84% for pneumonia for a 10 $\mu g/m^3$ increase in PM_{10} for the same time period.

Mortality

Thurston and Ito[54] evaluated data from earlier time-series mortality studies that had not corrected for ambient temperature. The combined analysis yielded a RR = 1.036 per 100 ppb increase in daily 1-hr maximum O_3 (95% CI 1.023–1.050). However, the subset of studies that specified the nonlinear nature of the temperature–mortality association yielded a combined estimate of RR = 1.056 per 100 ppb (95% CI 1.032–1.081). This indicates that past time-series studies using linear temperature–mortality specifications have underpredicted the premature mortality effects of O_3 air pollution. For studies of O_3, weather control is a particular problem because high O_3 days are generally quite hot. Schwartz used a case-crossover approach where he matched a day by temperature with date of death with O_3 as the independent variable.[55] In a study of more than one million deaths in fourteen U.S. cities, he found that while matching on temperature, there was an association of 0.23% (CI 0.01–0.44%) with a 10 ppb increase in maximum hourly O_3 concentrations. The finding was restricted to summer months, was not affected by PM, and was similar in magnitude to seasonal matching and controlling for temperature with regression splines. Findings of increased mortality from O_3 epidemiological studies are important because mortality dominates the cost–benefit analyses when crafting a health standard. The National Mortality and Morbidity Air Pollution Study (NMMAPS) used EPA's Atmospheric Information Retrieval System (AIRS) data on ambient O_3 from ninety-five U.S. communities to correlate to daily mortality data.[56] A positive association was found in all but two communities, and a statistically significant association was shown for seven communities and for the ninety-five as a whole.[57] The ninety-five-community effect was strongest on the same day, and highly significant for one- and two-day lags, as well as being even stronger when the distributed lag over six days was considered (see Figure 3.4). National and community-specific effect estimates of the short-term effects of O_3 on mortality were robust to inclusion of PM_{10} or $PM_{2.5}$ in time-series models.

The EPA contracted with three independent groups of scientists to perform meta-analyses of different groups' approaches to studying exposures to O_3 and mortality. Bayesian hierarchical models were used in all three analyses, and PM interaction with O_3 was generally found to be unimportant. Ito and colleagues used data from fourteen U.S. cities, thirteen Canadian cities, and twenty-one European cities excluding NMMAPS and found a combined estimate of 0.39% (95% CI 0.26–0.51%) per 10 ppb increase in 1-hour daily maximum O_3.[58] Because during this time, air conditioning was not prevalent in Europe, the prevalence of air conditioning in North America reduced the exposure–mortality association. Bell et al. used NMMAPS and pooled data from thirty-nine time-series studies with 144 effect estimates with lags, age groups, cause-specific mortality, and concentration metrics.[59] In the meta-analysis, a 10 ppb increase in daily O_3 at single day or two-day average of lags 0, 1, or 2 days was associated with an 0.87% increase in total mortality (95% CI 0.55–1.18%) with higher rates for cardiovascular and respiratory mortality. The NMMAPS estimate was consistently higher due to more aggressive adjusting for effects of weather. Levy et al. evaluated seventy-one time-series studies relating to O_3 including seven U.S. cities and many worldwide cities, finding that total mortality increased by 0.41% per 10 ppb O_3.[60] Brisbane, Australia, and Mexico City do not have seasonal effects, and have the highest O_3 mortality associations. A recent report of European data summarized data from twenty-three regions with mortality data over a three-year period.[61] There was an association between O_3 and mortality only in the summer, with a mean increase in 0.33% in total mortality, 0.45% in cardiovascular deaths, and 1.13% in respiratory deaths per 5 ppb O_3 (twice as high for 10 ppb). In a study of forty-eight U.S. cities between 1989 and 2000, mortality during June–August was correlated to various lags and corrected for

FIGURE 3.4 Bayesian city-specific and national average estimates for the percentage change (95% CI) in daily mortality per 10 ppb increase in 24-hour average O$_3$ for ninety-five U.S. communities (NMMAPS)

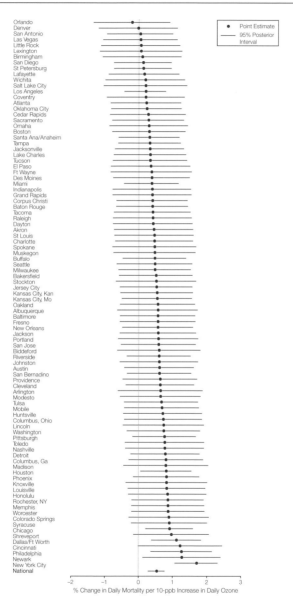

Source: Reprinted with permission from The Journal of the American Medical Association 2004; 292:2372–2378.

temperature and other pollutants to determine if O_3 exposure only moves forward otherwise susceptible elderly with chronic cardiopulmonary disease mortality.[62] The authors found a 0.3% (95% CI 0.2–0.4) increase in total mortality for a 10 ppb increase in 8-hour O_3 at lag 0 during the summer months. The association of ozone with daily deaths was not due to short-term mortality displacement. Risk assessments using the single day of O_3 exposure are likely to underestimate rather than overestimate, the public health impact.

Long-term ozone exposure 1977–2000 and mortality was evaluated from eighteen years' follow-up with the American Cancer Society II cohort correlated to air pollution data from ninety-six metropolitan statistical areas in the United States.[63] In two-pollutant models, $PM_{2.5}$ was associated with the risk of death from cardiovascular causes, whereas ozone was associated with the risk of death from respiratory causes. The estimated relative risk of death from respiratory causes that was associated with an increment in ozone concentration of 10 ppb was 1.040 (95% CI 1.010–1.067) or roughly 2.9% increase in respiratory cause of death from O_3. [here]

Nitrogen Oxides

Nitrogen dioxide (NO_2) is a precursor to the formation of O_3, and controls for the O_3 standard must take into account this key NAAQS-regulated pollutant. Nitrogen dioxide usually is referred to as NOx because there are other gases involved, including nitric oxide NO, nitrous oxide N_2O, nitrogen peroxide (NO_2 and N_2O_4), and nitrogen trioxide N_2O_3. Sources include inner cities with automobile and truck traffic, electrical utilities, refineries, and gas-fired indoor ranges. Annual average outdoor concentrations decreased 41% from 1980 to 2006 and average maximum hourly concentrations in the United States were about 30 ppb with peaks to 200 ppb, especially near high-traffic roads. An annual average standard of 53 ppb was set in 1971.

These are irritant gases similar to ozone. Chamber studies of normal volunteers exposed to NO_2 levels at 7,500 ppb for 1–2 hours reported increased non-specific airway hyper-responsiveness.[64] Levels as low as 300 ppb could reduce pulmonary function in asthmatics after exposure to 30–60 minutes with exercise. COPD patients during exercise have increased airways resistance at 1,600 ppb. Indoor exposure to NO_2 from gas stoves has been associated with increased respiratory illnesses in children <2 years of age in selected households in the Harvard Six Cities Study. There was no change in pulmonary function, but wheeze and shortness of breath were increased compared to households using electric stoves. In Tucson, Arizona, asthmatic children had significant declines in peak flow associated with gas stoves. A meta-analysis of respiratory illness in children related to NO_2 exposure found a 20% increase in the risk of respiratory illness per 15-ppb increment in indoor NO_2 exposure.[6] Epidemiology studies linked NO_2 within the current standard to reduced lung function, increased asthma symptoms, and increased emergency hospital visits.[65,66,67,68] Clinical studies demonstrated increased airway responsiveness to allergen challenge in patients with asthma.[68] In January 2009 the EPA promulgated a new 1-hour NO_2 standard at the level of 100 ppb. The form for the 1-hour standard would be the three-year average of the 98th percentile of the annual distribution of daily maximum 1-hour average concentrations.

The Ozone Standard in NAAQS

The ozone standard affects a larger percentage of the population than any other air quality standard. About half the U.S. population, or 156 million people, live in ozone **nonattainment areas** (locality where air pollution levels persistently exceed **National Ambient Air Quality Standards [NAAQS]**). A U.S. NAAQS of 120 ppb for O_3 using a 1-hour averaging time not to be exceeded more than once per year was established in 1979. It was based principally on the expectation that ambient exposure was characterized by relatively sharp afternoon peaks. However, it has been shown that ambient O_3 concentrations in New Jersey often have broad daytime peaks—maximum 8-hour averages close to 90% of peak 1-hour levels. Thus ozone standards of 1 hour are not relevant since exposure occurs over 6–8 hours. In 1997, the EPA administrator promulgated a revised O_3 NAAQS with an 8-hour average concentration limit of 0.08 ppm, not to be exceeded more than three times a year.

Before EPA could promulgate the 1997 rule for O_3, it was sued by the American Trucking Association, which argued that EPA should have considered economic factors in setting the revised standard. In 2002, the U.S. Supreme Court unanimously ruled against that argument, with Justice Antonin Scalia writing the opinion, "Were it not for the hundreds of pages of briefing respondents have submitted on the issue, one would have thought it fairly clear that this text does not permit the EPA to consider costs in setting the standards." However, a cost-benefit analysis is required by Executive Order 12866 for agencies to prepare prior to promulgating a regulation. Agencies must prepare cost-benefit analyses for regulations that are likely to have "an annual effect on the economy of $100 million or more or adversely affect in a material way the economy, productivity, competition, jobs, the environment, public health or safety, or State, local, or tribal governments or communities." The White House Office of Management and Budget (OMB) is responsible for enforcing these provisions, and within OMB, the Office of Information and Regulatory Affairs (OIRA) reviews agency regulations and cost-benefit analyses. Agencies release the final product of their assessment as a **regulatory impact analysis (RIA)**. The outcome of the RIA is a net benefit calculation—the difference between estimated costs and estimated benefits. All agency assessments, including the RIA itself, involve assumptions and uncertainties of varying degrees of significance. In the O_3 NAAQS, it was very difficult to cost account repeated exposures on health outcomes and to account for technological innovation moving forward. The benefits calculation for the O_3 RIA for a statistical life saved in the year 2020 yielded a $6.6 million benefit to society. From the NMMAPS study estimates, if a standard of 0.070 were in effect in 2020, then reduced exposure would save between 670 and 4,300 lives in that year, with a net benefits range of minus $17 billion to $16 billion. OIRA in OMB consistently called into question the scientifically based causal relationship between ground-level ozone exposure and premature mortality. These are political considerations subject to the occupant in the White House and the direction and priorities of his or her political party. Although presidential appointments to OMB and OIRA are subject to confirmation by the Senate, a recess appointment circumvents this approval process. Thus the OIRA forced EPA to include figures assuming no causal relationship between O_3 and a health outcome; OIRA could extend the lower limit of the benefits range for each regulatory alternative. Thus for critics of regulation, the White House and industry representatives, the RIA could provide ammunition against a more stringent standard. For example, upon release of the O_3 RIA, the National Association of Manufacturers (NAM) stated, "If we're going to move forward with something so very expensive, we think we need more certainty." Cost-benefit analysis should be an especially minor tool in the considerations of public health rulemakings. OIRA has the power to edit proposed rulemaking and change scientific emphasis with the perverse outcome of elevating costs, thus providing a vehicle for industry to undermine support for improved health outcomes envisioned by Congress in establishing the Clean Air Act (CAA) and oversight of EPA.

The National Academy of Sciences (NAS)[69] reviewed the scientific data and risk estimates, concluding that the mortality evidence of O_3 exposure was strong. The NAS is considered a politically neutral forum of expertise in interpreting science. The report concluded that the O_3-associated deaths were not due to confounding effects of temperature or other secondary pollutants.

From 2000 to 2002, 36%–57% of ozone monitors each year failed to meet the standard. The EPA staff paper on January 30, 1997, stated that scientific evidence provided strong support for lowering the existing limit of 0.08 ppm. Under this standard, a level of 0.084 was still within compliance. They recommended that the EPA administrator set the standard within the range of 0.80 to 0.060 ppm. "The overall body of evidence on ozone health effects clearly calls into question the adequacy of the current standard." The World Health Organization (WHO) and Canada use 0.060, and the U.K. goal is 0.050 ppm. The EPA also assessed the ozone secondary standard that was identical to the 1997 primary standard. Ozone affects both tree growth and crop yields, and the damage from exposure is cumulative over the growing season. EPA staff recommended a new seasonal (three-month) average for the standard that would cumulate hourly ozone exposures for the daily 12-hour daylight window.

The Clean Air Scientific Advisory Committee (CASAC) ozone sub-committee unanimously called for EPA to set the primary 8-hour limit at a level between 0.070 and 0.060 ppm in 2006 after reviewing 2,000 pages of data, and a secondary standard to have an upper limit of 15 ppm-hours. On June 20, 2007, the EPA proposed tightening the standard to 0.070–0.075 but left open the possibility of retaining the current standard of 0.085 or lowering it to 0.060. Before issuing the final rule, the EPA allowed for written comments, public hearings, and meetings with the EPA administrator. The ATS Environmental Health Policy Committee recommended a level of 0.060 ppm for the 8-hour standard with a letter to the EPA administrator stating that the evidence for lowering the standard was "compelling" and that there was unanimous consensus among respiratory scientists that left no doubt or uncertainty. Industry groups (American Chemistry Council) formed broad coalitions (NAAQS Business Coalition) to oppose the tighter standard, saying the science was too uncertain and the current standard had not been given a chance to go into effect. They stated that background ground-level ozone was 0.040 ppm, which was higher than EPA assumptions. Oil and agriculture stakeholders and the NAM met with representatives of the EPA and the White House OMB to discuss the final ozone proposals. "Raising the primary and secondary standard will put a lot of rural communities out of attainment for the first time ever," stated the American Corn Growers. The National Association of Manufacturers rallied opposition to the new standards and publicized a letter by 11 governors protesting the proposed EPA rule. The California Air Resources Board set a state standard of 0.070 ppm but this had no force unless certified by the EPA; California has 8 of 10 counties with the highest concentration of ozone in the U.S. with San Bernardino County being number one. Clean Air Watch, an advocacy group, stated that it was seeing a real industry blitz aimed at stopping EPA from setting tougher ozone standards.

EPA Administrator Steven Johnson agreed to meet with the chief executive officer and one other person from several environmental groups. Representatives from eleven groups attended the meeting, including the American Lung

Association (ALA), the American Thoracic Society, American Academy of Pediatrics, the American Public Health Association, Environmental Defense, and the Natural Resources Defense Council. The environmental and health groups rejected industry arguments that the health impacts of ozone were reversible by citing the possible mortality effects of ozone. "Premature death is not a reversible health effect," the ALA commented. EPA Administrator Johnson requested information on background levels of ozone, one asthma study, and a chamber study. Schildcrout et al. in the asthma study evaluated criteria pollutants on daily symptoms and rescue inhalers among 990 children in eight North American cities during 1993–1995. They found that lags in CO and NO_2 were positively associated with both measures of asthma exacerbation.[70] Opponents of a stronger ozone standard apparently used this in meetings with the EPA, since it found no significant effect of ozone on worsening asthma in the children in eight cities during the year-long study of five of the NAAQS criteria pollutants. The authors stated this "finding" as "not unexpected" and cited twelve other studies that showed that ozone had been repeatedly found to harm children with asthma. The authors offered a reasonable explanation for the anomaly: that on average, only twelve children were observed on any given day, making the effects of O_3 harder to capture, that is, the study may have been underpowered to detect any effect of ozone.

The other study reviewed by the EPA administrator was the Adams chamber study, which was a study of thirty healthy young adults at the University of California–Davis, where they were exposed for 6.6 hours to O_3 with moderate exercise.[71,72] Consistent with prior studies, Adams reported statistically significant effects of O_3 on FEV_1 and respiratory symptoms responses at 0.08 ppm. Below 0.08 ppm, Adams[72] reported significant O_3 effect only on a total symptom score for the triangular 0.060 ppm O_3 protocol following 6.6 hours of exposure (see Figure 3.5). The author was principally interested in evaluating the pattern of responses at each hourly time interval and conducted a two-way analysis of variance with repeated measures that was not significant compared to filtered air. A conservative test, the Scheffé post hoc test, was used by the author to minimize type I errors (rejecting the null hypothesis of no difference) when performing multiple comparisons; however, this method may increase type II error (false negative) for the simple evaluation of pre- to post-exposure effects of O_3 versus filtered air on FEV_1. In contrast, EPA staff's evaluation of pre- to post-exposure effects found that there was a lack of an overlap in the range of responses (that is, means and standard error) at 0.060 ppm O_3 versus filtered air at 6.6 hour, and that this was suggestive of a statistically significant effect on FEV_1. Consistent with common practice for comparing pre- and post-exposure responses to test for whether or not O_3-related effect was significant, the paired

FIGURE 3.5   Effects of ozone on FEV$_1$ in healthy young adults

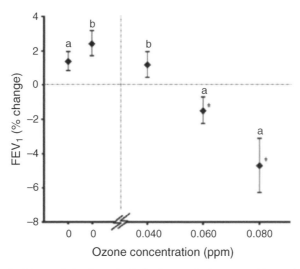

Source: Reprinted with permission from the United States Environmental Protection Agency.

t-test was statistically significant (p <0.01) different from filtered air.[73] The paired t-test has been the conventional statistical test used by investigators of chamber studies comparing short or long exposure to filtered air for a group of individuals (See Figure 3.6). The CASAC O$_3$ panel scrutinized this difference and supported the use of the paired t-test approach as the preferred method for analyzing the pre- minus post-exposure lung function responses.

Adams[71,72] modeled pulmonary function response data from both 2-hour and 6.6-hour exposure studies and the recovery times following the end of exposures and reported that FEV$_1$ and symptom recovery rates were related to total O$_3$ dose (product of concentration, ventilation rate, and duration of exposures).

The Adams study was reproduced by Schelegle and colleagues in 2009 with thirty-one healthy adults who completed five 6.6-hour chamber exposures with mean O$_3$ concentrations of 60, 70, 80, and 87 ppb. Statistically significant decrements in FEV$_1$ and increases in total subjective symptoms scores were measured after exposure to mean concentrations of 70, 80, and 87 ppb O$_3$.[74]

During March 2008 EPA set the new primary O$_3$ 8-hour standard at 0.075 ppm and the new secondary standard at a form and level identical to the primary standard. The Bush White House, at the last minute, held up the announcement because EPA had proposed to lower the secondary standard further. EPA estimated the health benefits between $2 billion and $19 billion, including preventing cases of bronchitis, aggravated asthma, hospital and

FIGURE 3.6   Hour-by-hour changes in FEV$_1$

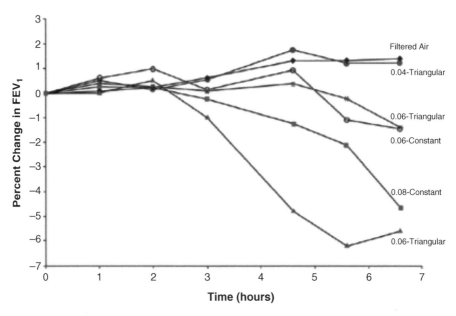

Source: Reprinted with permission from Adams WC. Comparison of chamber 6.6-h exposures to 0.04–0.08 PPM Ozone via square-wave and triangular profiles on pulmonary responses. Inhalation Toxicology 2006; 18:127–136.

emergency room visits, nonfatal heart attacks, and premature death. EPA's RIA showed that benefits were greater than the costs of implementing the standards that ranged from $7.6 billion to $8.5 billion. EPA stated that states and local communities have three years to comply and twenty years to meet the new standard. Going forward, EPA stated that the new standard would prevent more than 260 premature deaths, 890 heart attacks, and 200,000 missed school days every year starting in 2020. EPA looked at the health-related benefits for attaining the 8-hour standard that had been in effect during 2000, 2001, and 2002. The average of the health impacts across the three years included reductions of 800 premature deaths, 4,500 hospital and emergency department admissions, 900,000 school absences, and >1 million minor restricted activity days for costs estimated at $5.7 billion.[75] The assumed hourly background of O$_3$ of approximately 40 ppm reduced impacts approximately 30%–60%, which is why industry pushed for the assumption of 40 ppm as the true background level. The new ozone standard was challenged in federal district court on May 27, 2008, as not strict enough by five environmental groups, fourteen states, and two cities, with industry groups under the Ozone NAAQS Litigation Group suing to have the standard relaxed. In September 2009, the Obama EPA told the court that they would reconsider the Bush-imposed ozone NAAQS in part because it rejected CASAC's recommendation (range 60–70 ppb) for an even tighter limit than 75 ppb.

Summary

Ozone is an irritant gas formed from the oxidation of volatile organic compounds and NOx by the action of sunlight, thus peaking during the day. Adverse health effects noted are increases in mortality, changes in lung inflammation, pulmonary function, and adverse effects on children with asthma. Regulating ozone requires an 8-hour standard that protects susceptible individuals. Nearly half of U.S. counties are unable to meet the standard, which will require notable efforts on traffic and stationary sources such as refineries.

Key Terms

National Ambient Air Quality Standards (NAAQS)

Nonattainment areas

Ozone

Regulatory impact analysis (RIA)

Relative risk (RR)

Discussion Questions

1. What are some of the sources of ozone?
2. Why is ozone harmful to human health?
3. Who typically favors and disfavors ozone regulation?
4. What branches of government play a role in ozone regulation?
5. How is ozone currently regulated by the government?

The author thanks Morton Lippmann, Ph.D., for permission to use parts of the Ozone chapter published in *Environmental and Occupational Medicine*, 4th ed., by Lippincott, Williams and Wilkins.

CHAPTER 4

SULFUR DIOXIDE AND ACID RAIN

LEARNING OBJECTIVES

- To understand the health impact of sulfur dioxide exposure
- To understand how acid rain is formed and the history of its study
- To become familiar with the environmental hazards of acid rain
- To comprehend efforts to reduce production of sulfur dioxide and other acid rain causing pollutants

Sulfur dioxide (SO_2) is a colorless, highly soluble, and reactive gas. About 65% of SO_2 released in the air comes from electric power plants, with 35% from metal processing, industrial sources, and fuel combustion sources. SO_2 can dissolve in water or water vapor to form various acidic sulfates. Point sources from smoke stacks from industrial and electric power plants disperse SO_2 in a 20 km radius, resulting in levels of 0.2–0.3 ppm as 1-hour averages in North America. Outdoor ambient concentration of SO_2 has decreased 54% from 1983 to 2002, largely as a result of reductions in power plant and industrial emissions. The reduction in emissions has been from 31,161,000 tons in 1970 to 18,867,000 tons in 1999, largely due to flue gas desulfurization from adding calcium oxide (lime) that reacts with SO_2 to form calcium sulfite (see Figure 4.1). More stringent regulation limits on the amount of sulfur in fuels will reduce ambient SO_2 further following the 2007 diesel truck regulations. Indoor space heaters that burn kerosene are a source of indoor air pollution from SO_2. Since ambient SO_2 levels have been declining compared to ozone, particulate matter (PM), and hazardous air pollutants, there has been less emphasis on controlling SO_2 for health effects.

FIGURE 4.1 SO_2 air quality, 1980–2007

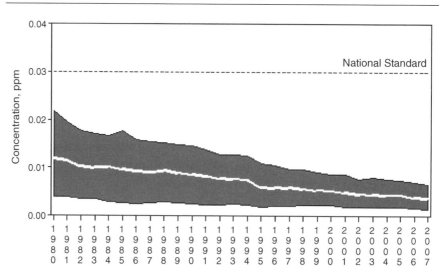

Note: Based on annual arithmetic average. National trend based on 147 sites.
Source: U.S. Environmental Protection Agency. Reprinted with permission from the National Atmospheric Deposition Program (NRSP-3). 2009. NADP Program Office. http://nadp.sws.uiuc.edu.

SO_2 is an important chemical precursor in the formation of sulfate-containing PM, and acidic aerosols (acid rain), both of which have substantial impacts on health and ecology.[1] Mixtures of combustion-related gases in the atmosphere, such as SO_2 from power plants and industrial facilities, and nitrogen oxides from power plants, automobiles, and other combustion sources, cause "nucleation" or formation of fine and ultrafine particles in ambient air. Secondary formation of PM, with the recognized precursors primarily SO_2 and nitrogen oxides, represent a substantial fraction of the total PM exposure in the northeastern United States. SO_2 can mix with industrial ultrafine particles to form larger fine particles. SO_2 can be absorbed or scrubbed in the nasal turbinates, with only 2% reaching the glottis. This increases in exercise with mouth breathing, where SO_2 can be absorbed in the aqueous lining of the respiratory epithelium and can reach the lower respiratory tract, where its irritant properties can cause bronchoconstriction and airway inflammation.

Acid rain is a broad term referring to a mixture of wet and dry deposition (deposited material) from the atmosphere containing higher than normal amounts of nitric and sulfuric acids. The precursors, or chemical forerunners, of acid rain formation result from both natural sources, such as volcanoes and decaying vegetation, and human-made sources, primarily emissions of sulfur dioxide (SO_2) and nitrogen oxides (NOx) resulting from fossil fuel combustion. In the United States, roughly two-thirds of all SO_2 and one-quarter of all NOx come from electric power generation that relies on burning fossil fuels like coal. Acid rain occurs when these gases react in the atmosphere with water, oxygen, and other chemicals to form various acidic compounds. The result is a mild solution of sulfuric acid and nitric acid. When sulfur dioxide and nitrogen oxides are released from power plants and other sources, prevailing winds blow these compounds across state and national borders, sometimes over hundreds of miles. Acid rain can have harmful effects on plants, aquatic animals, and infrastructure.

SO$_2$ Health Effects

In several studies, SO_2 exposure has been linked with increased mortality due to all causes and to lung cancer specifically. For example, the study of the American Cancer Society cohort that reported the link between mortality and criteria air pollutants, the relative risk (RR) of all-cause mortality from sulfate exposure was 1.25 (95% CI [confidence interval] 1.13–1.37) and was higher at the county level with an RR of 1.5.[2] The National Mortality and Morbidity Air Pollution Study (NMMAPS) also analyzed SO_2 and found no significant associations with total mortality.[3] An international study of pulp and paper workers with 40,704 SO_2-exposed workers found a reduced overall standardized mortality ratio of 0.89 (95% CI 0.87–0.96) but a marginally increased rate of 1.08 for lung cancer (95% CI 0.98–1.18).[4] After adjustment for occupational co-exposures, the lung cancer risk was increased compared with unexposed workers (rate ratio = 1.49; 95% CI 1.14–1.96). There was a suggestion of a positive relationship between weighted cumulative SO_2 exposure and lung cancer mortality. These confirm that SO_2 exposure increases mortality.

SO_2 is a respiratory irritant with exposures at 10 ppm, causing cough, dyspnea, irritation of the eyes and throat, and reflex bronchial constriction. In July 1990, Hong Kong introduced a requirement that all power plants and road vehicles had to use fuel oil with a sulfur content no greater than 0.5% by weight.[5] In the ensuing twelve months, there was a reduction in seasonal deaths followed by a peak in the cool season death rate between thirteen and twenty-four months, returning to the expected pattern during years 3–5. There were declines in the average annual trend in deaths from all causes (2.1%, $p = 0.001$), respiratory 3.9%, and cardiovascular 2.0%. The average gain in life expectancy per year of exposure to the lower pollutant concentration was twenty days for females and forty-one days for males. In the two years after the intervention, there was a reduction in chronic bronchitic symptoms and bronchial hyper-responsiveness in children. SO_2 declined 45% over five years and respirable particulates declined for two years.

In twelve Canadian cities, daily SO_2 concentrations were significantly associated with daily mortality, with an average concentration of only 5 µg/m³.[6] In a district of Chongqing, China, daily mortality was analyzed from January through December 1995 for associations with daily ambient sulfur dioxide and fine particles.[7] Particulate matter less than 2.5 µm in diameter ($PM_{2.5}$) was monitored for seven months, while SO_2 was monitored for the entire year. The investigators found positive associations between daily ambient SO_2 concentrations and mortality from respiratory and cardiovascular disease. For example, the effect of a 100 µg/m³ (0.04 ppm) increase in daily SO_2 concentrations was a relative risk of 1.20 (95% CI 1.11–1.30) for cardiovascular mortality, with up to a three-day lag. The SO_2 association remained robust when controlled for $PM_{2.5}$. No associations were observed between daily ambient $PM_{2.5}$ concentration and any cause of mortality. A weakness of this study was the absence of measurements of carbon monoxide, ozone, or nitrogen dioxide. Chongqing is surrounded by mountains, is one of China's largest cities at 30 million people, and uses high-sulfur coal for energy, with sulfur ranging from 4% to 12%.

In a report on the European Air Pollution Health Effects Approach (APHEA-II) study, Sunyer et al. assessed the short-term effects of SO_2 levels on hospital admissions for cardiovascular diseases in seven European areas.[8] Daily numbers of cardiovascular admissions increased 0.7% (95% CI 0.1–1.3 per each 10 $\mu g/m^3$ increase of SO_2), particularly ischemic heart disease, rose significantly with increased SO_2 levels of the same day and the day before among subjects younger than 65 years. This remained significant after adjusting for PM_{10} changes. Study subjects >65 years had significant cardiovascular daily admissions only for PM_{10} (1.3%, CI 0.7–1.8 per each increase in 10 $\mu g/m^3$ of PM_{10}). This study supports a role for SO_2 pollution triggering ischemic cardiac events. A study in Toronto of 7,319 admissions for asthma in children ages 6 to 12 years covering 1981–1993 found that sulfur dioxide concentrations were related to asthma hospitalizations in girls and CO exposure and asthma hospitalizations in boys.[9] Nitrogen dioxide was positively associated with asthma admissions in both sexes. The lag time was two to three days for CO and NO_2 for boys and six to seven days with girls for SO_2 and NO_2. These effects remained after adjustment for PM. Ware et al. analyzed data from the Harvard Six Cities Study.[10] Pollutant measurements available at that time were total suspended particulates [TSP], total suspended particulates that are less than 100 m, SO_2, and total sulfates. In preadolescent children, cough was significantly associated with all three pollutants. Lower respiratory illness and bronchitis were associated with TSP.

Lee et al. evaluated the relationships between low birth weight and air pollution in South Korea.[11] Low birth weight tended to increase with CO exposure between months 2 and 5 of pregnancy, PM_{10} with months 2 and 4, and exposure to SO_2 and NO_2 in pregnancy during months 3 to 5. A retrospective cohort study in Taiwan examined 92,288 full-term births in relation to SO_2 exposure during the first trimester. Higher exposure levels, exceeding 0.011 ppm, were associated with a 26% increase in risk for low birth weight in term pregnancies, compared with exposures to SO_2 less than 0.007 ppm.[12] No significant elevated risk was observed for other air pollutants.

Studies using human exposure chambers with normal subjects exposed to SO_2 show effects at 1–2 ppm, including reduced forced expiratory volume in 1 second (FEV_1), and respiratory symptoms, and asthmatics show bronchoconstriction from 0.5 to 0.1 ppm. Sulfuric acid aerosol exposure to nonsmoking healthy volunteers with exercise was not associated with an inflammatory response assessed by bronchoalveolar lavage, and there was no evidence for alteration in antimicrobial defense.[13] Carlisle and Sharp reviewed the role of athletic exercise in increasing the risks of exposure to outdoor ambient air pollution, specifically carbon monoxide, nitrogen oxides, ozone, PM, volatile organic compounds, and sulfur dioxide,[14] and they found that asthmatics were approximately tenfold more sensitive to SO_2 than nonasthmatics, placing the threshold for effects below the 24-hour National Ambient Air Quality Standard of 0.14 ppm. Individuals with asthma breathing 0.5 ppm of SO_2, with exercise, may experience as much as a 100% increase in airways resistance with as little as 5 minutes of exposure. It is possible that SO_2 may be one of the triggers for exercise-induced airway constriction in people with asthma. The overall incidence of exercise-induced bronchospasm across all sports and sexes in a recent survey of Olympic winter sports athletes was reported as 23%.[14] Forty-seven subjects with asthma, ages 18 to 39 years, were screened for SO_2 sensitivity with a 10-minute exposure to 0.5 ppm SO_2 with moderate exercise.[15] Twenty-five of forty-seven subjects, or 53%, had a drop in $FEV_1 \geq 8\%$. Severity of asthma was not a predictor for SO_2 responsiveness in this group. Studies of both humans and animals have demonstrated that exposures to sulfur dioxide and acidic aerosols alter mucociliary clearance. The removal of inhaled particles from the airways depends on the intact function of ciliated epithelium and its overlying mucous layer. Resting exposure to sulfur dioxide levels as low as 1.0 ppm reduced nasal mucous flow rates.

Bronchoalveolar lavage has been used to evaluate responses to exposure to sulfur dioxide in humans.[16] Twenty-two healthy nonsmokers were exposed to 8 ppm SO_2 for 20 minutes, with light exercise during the last 15 minutes of exposure. There were mild upper-airway symptoms during exposure, with minimal reductions in lung function. Bronchoscopy 24 hours after exposure showed reddened airways, and bronchoalveolar lavage fluid showed increases in macrophages, lymphocytes, and mast cells. These findings suggest that SO_2 at high concentrations causes inflammation in the distal airways in healthy subjects.

SO_2 exposure in combination with other pollutants may enhance the effects of allergen exposure in people with asthma. Rusznak and colleagues exposed thirteen mild atopic asthmatic subjects[17] for 6 hours to air or a combination of 0.4 ppm NO_2 plus 0.2 ppm SO_2. Subjects underwent three separate exposures to the combination of gases, with allergen challenge after exposure, immediately, 24, or 48 hours after exposure. The investigators found that exposure to NO_2 plus SO_2 decreased the dose of allergen required to produce a 20% fall in FEV_1, at all of the post-exposure time points. These findings suggested that environmental peaks of SO_2 exposure, when combined with NO_2, may enhance allergen responsiveness in asthmatics. The effect persisted over a period of 24–48 hours and was maximal 24 hours after exposure to these air pollutants.

Health Policy: National Ambient Air Quality Standards

There are two primary U.S. NAAQS (National Ambient Air Quality Standards) for SO_2. The short-term (24-hour) standard is set at 0.14 ppm (0.365 mg/m^3) and is not to be exceeded more than once per year per air pollution control district. The long-term standard specifies an annual arithmetic mean not to exceed 0.03 ppm (0.080 mg/m^3). These standards do not address very short-term exposures to SO_2. It is well established that even brief exposures to SO_2 during exercise, such as 15 or 20 minutes, can cause significant lung function impairment in people with asthma. Because of this, the United Kingdom has established a 15-minute standard for outdoor SO_2 exposure of 0.1 ppm (100 ppb). On June 2, 2010, the Environmental Protection Agency (EPA) strengthened the primary NAAQS for sulfur dioxide (SO_2), establishing a new 1-hour standard at a level of 75 parts per billion (ppb). The EPA revoked the two existing primary standards of 140 ppb evaluated over 24 hours and 30 ppb evaluated over an entire year, because they do not add additional public health protection given a 1-hour standard at 75 ppb. EPA estimated that the revised standard would yield health benefits between $13 billion and $33 billion, including reduced hospital admissions, emergency room visits, work days lost due to illness, and cases of aggravated asthma and chronic bronchitis. The benefits include preventing 2,300 to 5,900 premature deaths and 54,000 asthma attacks a year. The estimated cost in 2020 to fully implement the new standard would be approximately $1.5 billion. EPA also set minimum requirements that inform states on where they are required to place SO_2 monitors; approximately 163 SO_2 monitoring sites nationwide would be required. The American Petroleum Institute recommended a 1-hour standard of 400 ppb, arguing that EPA's epidemiological evidence was inconsistent and insufficient and, further, that adverse effects were reversible and transient similar to a variety of common stimuli.

Acid Rain

Acid rain—the result of emissions of sulfur and nitrogen oxides—is one of the few ecological issues that has captured the interest of scientists, politicians, lawmakers, industry, and the general public alike. The concept of acid rain appeared in the literature more than 100 years ago. An English chemist in an 1872 publication entitled "Air and Rain: The Beginnings of Chemical Climatology" made reference to the acidic nature of rain water collected and analyzed from England.[18] However, it wasn't until the late 1960s and early 1970s that this environmental problem was brought to the attention of scientists and the public, particularly in North America and Western Europe. The next two decades saw an exponential rise in interest about—and research on—acid rain. During this era of acid rain research, our understanding of the atmospheric chemistry, patterns of deposition, and ecological and environmental effects of acidic deposition grew dramatically.

Acid rain crosses geographic and political boundaries (for example, state, national, and international); thus its environmental, economic, political, and legal ramifications are extraordinarily complex and often vexing. *Acid rain* is the popular term for rain, snow, sleet, and hail that is abnormally acidic due to human activities, primarily the burning of fossil fuels. Acid rain is caused by the emissions of gaseous sulfur oxides (SO_2) and nitrogen oxides that originate from the combustion of coal, oil, and other organic matter and from smelting processes.[19] These primary pollutants (that is, those emitted directly from smokestacks or tail pipes of combustion engines) are further oxidized and then hydrolyzed in the atmosphere to form secondary pollutants, such as the strong mineral acids, sulfuric (H_2SO_4) and nitric (HNO_3).[20]

Natural sources of sulfur oxides include volcanic activity and sea spray. In many parts of the world, the burning of fossil fuels is the primary source of SO_2 in the atmosphere. In fact, in the eastern United States it is estimated that more than 90% of sulfur emitted to the atmosphere is the result of human activity. In 1970, three-fourths of anthropogenically produced sulfur dioxides were from fuel combustion, including electric utilities concentrated primarily in the midwestern United States, especially the Ohio and Tennessee river valleys. Approximately one-fourth were from industrial processes, such as chemical and petroleum industries, but by 2002, the major source of SO_2 was fuel combustion (85%), while industrial processes declined to 9%. Recently, oxygen isotope fingerprinting localized anthropogenically formed SO_4 pollutant in fine particulate from ship smoke observing 4%–25% of the annual fine particulate may originate from sulfate particles from ships burning 2.4% sulfur-containing bunker oil.[21] An estimated 60,000 cardiopulmonary and lung cancer deaths occur from this source of pollution, primarily in ports in Europe and Asia.[22] California and the European Union are mandating 0.1% sulfur marine distillate for ships in their coastal waters by 2012 and 2010, respectively.

Nitrogen oxides (generally referred to as NOx) are the other important precursors to acid rain. Nitrogen oxide emissions are the result of either (1) thermal reactions when combustion temperatures are raised high enough to oxidize atmospheric N_2 (thermal NOx) or (2) the oxidation of nitrogenous compounds in fuel (fuel NOx), though fossil fuels (for example, coal or oil) normally contain much lower concentrations of nitrogen than of sulfur. Thus an important source of the nitrogen for NOx emissions is often atmospheric nitrogen (N_2). The resultant NOx can be deposited to surfaces as NO_2 or further oxidized, often through reacting with hydroxyl radicals, and hydrolyzed to nitrate (NO_3^-) and nitric acid (HNO_3).

The acid-base status of a solution is the result of its complete chemistry, not simply its hydrogen ion, sulfate, nitrate, and chloride content. The pH of precipitation, then, is a result of its total ionic composition, which is in turn a result of the sulfur and nitrogen content as well as other substances that are emitted to the atmosphere, react, and subsequently are delivered to the Earth's surface in precipitation. In fact, some of these compounds are important in neutralizing the acidity in rain. For example, reduced nitrogenous compounds such as ammonia and ammonium (NH_3 and NH_4^+), which are the result of both combustion and agricultural activities, often combine with NO_3^- as NH_4NO_3 or sulfate as $(NH_4)_2SO_4$ and are transported long distances. Atmospheric calcium, sodium, potassium, and magnesium, often referred to as *base cations*, are a result of sea spray, the suspension of dirt and dust particles, anthropogenic emissions, and a variety of other sources. They can neutralize the acidity of precipitation.

Sulfur and nitrogen oxides may be transported long distances in the atmosphere either as primary pollutants or as secondary pollutants. An early solution to local air pollution problems in urban and industrialized areas was to increase the height of chimneys and smokestacks in order to reduce local, ground-level concentrations of particulate air pollutants ("The solution to pollution is dilution"). One of the results of this control measure was that air pollutants, particularly gases, were introduced into the atmosphere at a greater height and thereby were transported greater distances downwind. The average height of chimneys and smokestacks increased dramatically within the United States after about 1950: more than 400 smokestacks taller than 60 m were built in the 1970s, and many were extended to greater than 300 m in height. Local pollution issues were therefore transformed into regional air pollution problems. This fact led to one of the most contentious and politically vexing aspects of the acid deposition issue. That is, pollutants generated in one area could be deposited in a far distant area with little recourse for the recipients. Moreover, it was difficult to trace quantitatively the individual sources of the pollutants.

Research since the 1970s at locations such as the Hubbard Brook Experimental Forest (HBEF) in New Hampshire, which has the longest continuous record of precipitation chemistry in North America, has shown that although rain and snow may account for much of the total deposition to a variety of ecosystems, in some regions dry deposition and/or cloud, fog, or rime ice deposition can contribute approximately one-third to two-thirds of the total depositional load.[23,24,25] For example, dry deposition averages about 25% of total sulfur deposition at the HBEF. For several sites in other parts of North America, dry deposition can contribute, on average, 50% of the total deposition of sulfur and nitrogen. For many high-elevation or coastal areas in the northeastern United States, cloud or fog water accounts for 50%–80% of the total sulfur and nitrogen deposited. The relative contribution of each of these processes (wet, dry, and cloud) depends on many factors, such as frequency and amount of rain and snow, presence of cloud cover, the condition and architecture of impaction surfaces, elevation, and wind speeds.[26]

Throughout much of the world, acid deposition is a result of sulfuric and nitric acids—strong mineral acids—that tend to release hydrogen ion (H^+), which is a measure of acidity. Acidity is usually expressed as pH: the greater the concentration of the H^+, the lower the pH and the more acidic. Early in the acid rain debate, in the absence of much actual data, the "background" pH of precipitation was considered to be approximately 5.[6]

In the early 1980s, a group of scientists measured the chemistry of rainwater collected from some of the most remote locations on Earth to test this assumption.[27,28,29] They surmised that, in the absence of appropriate historical data, rain water from these locations was likely to be as representative of "preindustrial" rain as possible. Indeed, their data showed that the chemical concentrations from these sites were the lowest in the world and suggested that the background pH of rain is more likely 5.1 to 5.3 rather than 5.6, or about 10 times less acidic, and less concentrated in sulfate and nitrate than average annual rain collected from the northeastern United States. The additional acidity (between pH 5.6 and 5.1–5.3) was thought to be the result of natural emissions of S and N from, for example, volcanoes, lightning, wild fires, and stratospheric transport, in combination with other cations and anions in solution. They found that precipitation in remote sites was far more likely to be dominated by naturally occurring organic acids, such as formic and acetic acids, than that collected from eastern North America. Thus preindustrial rain has been shown to be quite different from postindustrial rain, and it is clear that human activities have led to acid deposition.

In the United States, the trend for acid rain has been increasing since the 1950s, with most of the increase in the northeastern United States and acidity spreading into the Midwest. In 2011, the average pH of rain throughout North America, Europe, and other parts of the world is between 4 and 5 (100 μEq/L and 10 μEq H+/L, respectively),[30] though historically, precipitation events have been reported with pHs much lower than this (for example, pH 2.85 at HBEF). The changing trends in emissions of NOx and SO_2 have influenced the relative proportions of sulfuric and nitric acid in rain water: to wit, the ratio of sulfur to nitrogen in rain has shifted from 2:1 in 1980 to 1:1 in 2000.[31]

Monitoring programs exist that are designed to measure and quantify atmospheric deposition in its various forms. Most of these programs were begun in the late 1970s in North America and until the past decade included only rain monitoring. One of the goals of these wet deposition-monitoring networks has been to gather sufficient data to quantify the deposition of pollutants and nutrients over large geographic regions. As a result, data now exist that show the geographic distribution of deposition of various ions in precipitation. It is clear from these data that for the United States wet deposition of various pollutants and nutrients varies across the country. For example, there are much higher rates of sulfate and nitrate deposition in most of the eastern versus western United States. This pattern is, in part, a result of proximity to sources, predominant wind direction, and amount of precipitation deposited.

Cloud water is another form of wet deposition. Although continuous records for cloud water deposition are quite rare, we do know that cloud water samples collected from remote locations in North America show similar geographic patterns to rain water and are often several times more acidic (lower in pH) and more concentrated in other ions than rain water collected at the same time from those same locations. In addition, average cloud water from the northeastern United States is about 40 times more acidic than rainwater from remote areas of the world. Extremely acid (<pH 3.0), regional cloud events have been measured, and cloud water pHs often occur in the 3 range.[19] At times these acidic cloud water events have occurred in combination with high concentrations of other air pollutants such as ozone.

There now exist approximately 250 EPA wet deposition-monitoring locations under the National Atmospheric Deposition Program and approximately 80 air chemistry monitoring locations where dry deposition is estimated. Many of the wet and dry monitoring sites have been co-located in an effort to provide information on total (wet plus dry) deposition over a wide geographic region. Although the data are somewhat spatially limited, they have been used to model total deposition over the northeastern United States, showing generally higher total deposition in the northeastern United States compared to the western United States and a difference in the form (dry versus wet) and species (for example, SO_2 versus wet sulfate) deposition by region.

Environmental Effects of Acid Rain and Deposition

The first and most obvious effects of acid deposition were observed in freshwater ecosystems.[32] Tens of thousands of lakes and streams in North America and Europe are more acidic than they were a few decades ago as a result of acid deposition.[33,34] These freshwaters are in sensitive areas with hard bedrock, thin acid soils, and little acid-neutralizing capacity, and their **acidification** has resulted in losses of fish and other aquatic organisms.[35] The evidence showing that strong mineral acidity has caused ecological changes has come from many sources, including (1) historical changes in chemistry and biology of freshwaters, (2) experimental manipulations, and (3) measurements made in aquatic ecosystems receiving acid deposition.[19] For example, analyses of historical changes in alkalinity of lakes in the Adirondack Mountain region of New York state showed highly significant acidification of a large number of those lakes during recent decades. Approximately 80% of 274 lakes studied became acidified during the past 50 to 60 years.[34] These changes were attributed to acid deposition and were not explainable by other factors such as changes in land use. In the Adirondacks, the Department of Environmental Conservation has found that fish populations are endangered in more than half of all the lakes and ponds in the region and more than 200 lakes have become totally fishless.

Indeed, surface water acidification as a result of acid rain has had demonstrable effects on organisms at several trophic levels, including fish, zooplankton, and benthic organisms.[36] The chemical constituents that consistently appear to have an effect on freshwater organisms, and that are a result of acid deposition, are monomeric aluminum (Al^{3+}), calcium, and hydrogen (as indicated by pH). Fish as well as invertebrates are affected by acidification, primarily through physiologic disturbances. In waters where mobile, monomeric aluminum species are present, direct effects on gills (for example, lesions and disturbance of respiratory function) and ion regulation disturbances have been observed.[37] The danger to fish populations is particularly acute during the spring, when acid stored in melting snow causes rapid decreases in pH values, a condition known as "spring shock." Moreover, liming of acidic lakes has not been able to restore lakes' fish and biota due to the complexity of the chemistry accompanying the acidification process. In response, fish taken from acidic waters in New York, Canada, and Sweden have higher levels of mercury in them due to acid mobilizing mercuric ions and conversion to methyl mercury and bioamplification in the food chain.

Acidification also presents dangers to long-lived species, such as trees, and highly heterogeneous systems, such as soils. Within the context of other simultaneous stresses, such as disease, ozone, and drought, the effect of acidification can be difficult to quantify in general but particularly difficult when effects exhibit significant time lags. Demonstrating cause and effect of acid deposition has been more difficult in the case of terrestrial ecosystems than for acidic deposition's effects on aquatic ecosystems. Nonetheless, recent data suggest a link between atmospheric deposition and leaching of calcium from red spruce needles and sugar maple decline in parts of the northeastern United States.[38] Nitrogen saturation, a condition in which the nitrogen inputs to an ecosystem exceed the capacity of the system to "use" the nitrogen, are being documented and include soil acidification and impacts on plant and ecosystem productivity.[39]

Soils require hundreds to thousands of years to develop. Exchange sites on negatively charged clay particles in soils often are dominated by such ions as aluminum, calcium, magnesium, potassium, and sodium. Excess hydrogen ions from acidic deposition has been shown to displace these cations, which are subsequently removed from the soil through leaching.[40] This displacement represents a change in the nutrient and acid-base status of the soils, since calcium, for example, is an essential plant nutrient that is usually taken up by plant roots from the soil. Rain at pH 4.6 can affect soils in ways that rain at pH 5.6 cannot. For example, common alumina minerals are essentially insoluble at pH 5.6 but are quite soluble at 4.6—in fact, 1,000 times more soluble. Increased leaching of aluminum from soil occurs at these lower pHs, and dissolved aluminum is toxic to organisms. In addition, a build-up of aluminum in the soil can affect a plant's biogeochemical function as well as result in toxicity. We now know that some soils in regions of high acid deposition are significantly affected by acid deposition.[19] **Forest decline** can be defined as a measurable reduction in the health of a forest ecosystem, which is characterized by unexpected changes in growth, reproduction, and death of trees, and has been noted in many parts of the industrialized world. In the areas affected by acid rain, forest trees are dying, generally unhealthy, or growing slowly. This condition has become widespread in Europe and parts of North America.[41] Many, if not most, terrestrial ecosystems are likely to be stressed simultaneously by acid rain, acid cloud or fog water, ozone, toxic metals, the global climate, hydrocarbons, disease, exotic pests, as well as land use changes. Interactive effects of various pollutants as well as the interaction between pollutants and other stresses have been proposed as causes of forest decline. Another complicating factor is that many years may be required before symptoms of stress become obvious as damage to trees or forests. Although these interactions are admittedly complex and it is difficult, if not impossible, to assign absolute cause and effect, it is clear that air pollution can stress forest ecosystems.

Acid Rain and Environmental Policy

The 1990 CAA (Clean Air Act) amendments specifically addressed acid rain and proposed to reduce sulfur dioxide emissions by 50% by the year 2000, based on 1980 levels; actual reductions were closer to 40%. The reductions employed the

"cap and trade" program designed to achieve environmental objectives while providing affected industries wide latitude in choice. This program was the first to set a national pollution cap and to allow power plants to meet their obligations either by reducing their emissions or purchasing emission "allowances" from other sources that reduce emissions beyond their obligations. Each source affected was required by the program to install continuous emissions-monitoring systems to accurately measure emissions. Hourly data was required to be submitted to EPA each quarter. An enhanced auditing system launched in 2002 provided additional assurance of continued high-quality emissions data. Environmental monitoring networks, the National Atmospheric Deposition Program (NADP), and the Clean Air Status and Trends network measure wet and dry deposition and water quality across the country. Sulfur dioxide emissions were projected to decrease to about 10 million tons below the 1980 values by the year 2000, with contributions from electric utilities declining and non-point utility sources and miscellaneous categories increasing. The SO_2 emissions from utilities were 10.6 million tons per year in 2001 compared with 17.3 million tons in 1980. The goal had been 8.9 million tons of SO_2 by 2000 and was above the goal per year due to the ability of sources to bank credits. The reductions were 75% less expensive than projected in 1990. The expected market price for SO_2 allowances was in the range of $579 to $1,935 per ton of SO_2; the actual market price as of January 2003 was $150 per ton. A 2003 Office of Management and Budget study found that the Acid Rain Program accounted for the largest quantified human health benefits—more than $70 billion annually—of any major federal regulatory program implemented in the previous ten years, with benefits exceeding costs by more than 40:1 (see Figure 4.2).

The cap and trade program had two phases with specific power plants under a Phase I cap by 1995–2000 and all point sources under a Phase II cap after 2000. By the time Phase II began, power plants had banked more than 10 million tons of SO_2 emission allowances, primarily by capturing flue gases. They planned to draw down the savings in order to cushion the impact of the more stringent cap in Phase II. Phase II had a total EPA emission allowance of 9.5 million tons per year. The EPA maintains an allowance tracking system that tracks the ownership of all existing SO_2 allowances. Meeting the requirements of the CAA amendments can be made easily by switching to low-sulfur coal from Wyoming, Montana, North Dakota, and the Mountain West compared to eastern coal. To further reduce pollution, plants can install flue gas scrubbers that reduce cost as they achieve greater efficiency.

Pollutants often travel long distances and are chemically transformed in the process between emission and deposition. A logical question and one that has been asked is, What is the relationship between reduction in emission

FIGURE 4.2 The acid rain experience: Unprecedented environmental protection at unmatched cost-efficiency

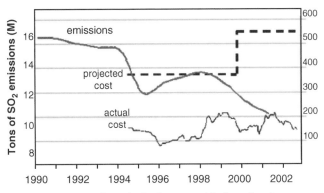

Source: Reprinted with permission from the Environmental Defense Fund.

of primary pollutants that lead to acid deposition and the chemical concentrations and deposition of those components in rain? Data from the long-term precipitation chemistry record at Hubbard Brook Experimental Forest suggest that reductions in SO_2 emission in the United States are reflected in both sulfate concentration and deposition in rainwater, indicating that reduction in emissions is closely related to the amount of sulfur deposited to ecosystems.[19] Similarly, after leaded gasoline was banned in the eastern United States, there was a steep and significant decrease in lead concentration in precipitation at the Hubbard Brook Experimental Forest. These are persuasive examples of how a reduction in source results in decreasing deposition, despite the complicated chemical and transport processes involved between emission and deposition.

Although the CAA amendments addressed emissions, it was not clear that this regulation would be enough to protect ecosystems. Emissions may need to be reduced even more if the goal is to reduce acid rain and its effects. The 1990 CAA amendments focused primarily on reducing sulfur emissions and less on nitrogen emissions. As noted previously, in 2011 at HBEF, the nitric acid inputs in atmospheric deposition are almost as large as the sulfuric acid additions. In the early 1960s, when studies began at HBEF, acidic sulfate contributed approximately 70% and acidic nitrate approximately 15%–20% to the total anion charge of precipitation. With decreased emissions of SO_2, the relative contribution of SO_4^{2-} has declined and NO_3^- increased, so that it is predicted that by 2012, nitric acid will be the dominant acid in precipitation at HBEF.[42] The ecological consequences of this change could be large.

From 2003 on, several competing bills were introduced in the Senate's Committee on Environment and Public Works, but none of these could gain a consensus during the administration of President George W. Bush. The Bush bill was called the Clear Skies Act of 2003. It was a mandatory program that would reduce and cap emissions of SO_2 and NOx and mercury from electric power generation to approximately 70% below 2000 levels. Clear Skies' NOx and SO_2 requirements would affect all fossil fuel-fired electric generators >25 megawatts, and mercury requirements would only affect the subset of units that were coal fired. SO_2 would go from 11.2 million tons in 2000 to 4.5 million tons by 2010 and 3 million tons by 2018, for a 73% reduction. NOx would go from 5.1 million tons in 2000 to 2.1 million tons in 2008 and 1.7 million tons in 2018, for a 67% reduction. NOx would have been more stringent in the eastern half of the country, with thirty-one states allowed 1.58 million tons in 2008 and 1.16 million tons in 2018. Mercury would go from 48 tons to 26 tons in 2010 and 15 tons in 2018, a 69% reduction. Clear Skies would provide human health benefits of $110 billion in 2020, outweighing costs of $6.3 billion. EPA projected 14,000 avoided premature deaths, 30,000 fewer emergency room visits, and 12.5 million fewer days with respiratory symptoms each year under Clear Skies by 2020. The competing Clean Power Act introduced by Sen. Robert Stafford, followed by Sen. Bernard Sanders, both of Vermont, in 2007 had much more stringent reductions: from 2010 to 2012, 2.25 million tons of SO_2, 1.51 million tons of NOx; 2013 and each year thereafter—1.3 million tons of SO_2 and 900,000 tons of NOx, with only 5 tons of mercury to be emitted by 2012. This bill also placed limits on CO_2 emissions as a multipollutant approach. None of these bills emerged from the Environment and Public Works Committee to be debated on the Senate floor.

The EPA under President Barack Obama began planning a more vigorous regulatory effort for the secondary standards of SO_2 and NOx to prevent acid rain under the NAAQS mandate to protect the public welfare. The EPA collaborated with the National Park Service to craft a joint secondary standard to cut NOx and SOx emissions to protect aquatic ecosystems from acidification due to emissions depositing on water. The EPA initial policy assessment stated that SOx and NOx compounds in the atmosphere undergo a complex mix of reactions to form various acidic compounds that lead to ecosystem exposure affecting ecosystem structure and function, especially losses in fish species richness. EPA's integrated science assessment found that the two pollutants and their deposition products jointly impact ecosystems. The policy assessment stated that the existing standards must consider the months- to years-long exposure period during which deposition-related impacts occur. The National Park System supported EPA's proposal to use an Atmospheric Acidification Potential Index

(AAPI) to evaluate a given ecosystem's potential to become acidified. The AAPI would include area-specific characteristics such as deposition, background acid neutralizing capacity (ANC), and other parameters that impact sensitivity.

Summary

SO_2 has adverse health effects related to its irritability for the respiratory tract, affecting both mortality and morbidity with susceptible populations being asthmatics and those with chronic cardiopulmonary diseases. The new lower standard of 75 ppb over 1 hour will reduce these adverse events. SO_2 combines with NOx to cause acid rain, adversely affecting ecosystems in the eastern United States and Western Europe. Although "cap and trade" was immensely successful in reducing acid rain, more needs to be done with a two pollutant model to reverse the decades-long accumulation of acidification.

Key Terms

Acidification

Acid rain

Cap and trade

Forest decline

Sulfur dioxide

Discussion Questions

1. What are some of the health impacts of sulfur dioxide exposure?
2. How is acid rain formed?
3. What are some of the environmental hazards of acid rain?
4. How successful have efforts been at stopping the production of acid rain?

The author thanks Mark W. Frampton, M.D., and Mark Utell, M.D., for permission to use parts of the chapter on sulfur dioxide and Kathleen C. Weathers, Gene E. Likens, and Thomas J. Butler to use parts of the chapter on acid rain published in *Environmental and Occupational Medicine*, 4th ed., by Lippincott, Williams and Wilkins.

CHAPTER 5

ENVIRONMENTAL TOBACCO SMOKE

LEARNING OBJECTIVES

- To understand the historical study of smoking and its link to disease
- To become familiar with the modern scientific findings on the relation between smoking and disease
- To comprehend the health effects of passive smoking and secondhand smoke
- To become familiar with how people can effectively quit smoking
- To understand attempts to regulate smoking and the outlook of smoking in today's world

Cigarette smoking and other tobacco use is a global problem, yet it is one of the most preventable causes of premature deaths in our society. Cigarette smoking accounts for 443,000 deaths annually and $193 billion in health-related economic losses. The three major adult diseases and causes of death are lung cancer (160,000 deaths), ischemic heart disease (82,000), and chronic obstructive pulmonary disease (COPD) (95,000). Cigarette smoking accounts for 30% of all deaths from cancer in the United States and is a major risk factor for cancer of the lungs, larynx, oral cavity, pharynx, and esophagus. Also, cigarette smoking is causally related to cancers of the bladder, pancreas, uterine cervix, kidney, stomach, and acute myeloid leukemia. On average, male smokers lose 13.2 years of life expectancy, and female smokers lose 14.5 years. The prevalence of cigarette smoking among adults in the United States declined from 42.0% in 1965 to 19.9% in 2007 (43.4 million people), with a higher rate among men (23.9%) than among women (18.1%). However, the percentage of Americans who smoke has begun to creep up again, to 20.6 percent in 2008. The prevalence of cigarette smoking varies from a high of 31% in Kentucky to a low of 13% in Utah, since the Mormon Church proscribes tobacco smoking. There are 8.6 million people who suffer from serious tobacco-induced illnesses. Approximately 44% of all cigarettes smoked in the United States are used by individuals who have comorbid psychiatric or substance abuse disorders. Globally, an estimated 4.83 million deaths were caused by cigarette smoking in 2000, and this may rise to 10 million deaths annually by 2020. There are one billion men who smoke and 250 million women who smoke globally; 70% of men in China smoke. The national public health objective of <12% prevalence cigarette smoking by 2010 has not been reached; subgroups <12% include Hispanic and Asian women, men and women with graduate degrees, and men and women >65 years of age.

The History of Smoking and Disease

In 1939, Drs. Alton Ochsner and Michael Debakey presented a case series of lung cancer and attributed the cause to be cigarette smoking. They were preceded by a case series by Dr. James Alexander Miller, the first director of the Bellevue Chest Service, who asserted that the cause of lung cancer was bronchial irritation. He did not make the connection to cigarette smoking. In 1953, Ernest Wynder showed that cigarette smoke condensate caused tumors when applied to the shaved skin of mice. In initiating their pioneering case-control study of lung cancer, Doll and Hill[1] gave equal weight to smoking and to air pollution as possible causes of lung cancer. In 1938, Raymond Pearl reported that tobacco smoking shortened life span.[2] He found that the life span of white male heavy

FIGURE 5.1   Survivorship lines of life tables for white men in three categories of tobacco use, from Raymond Pearl's longevity study

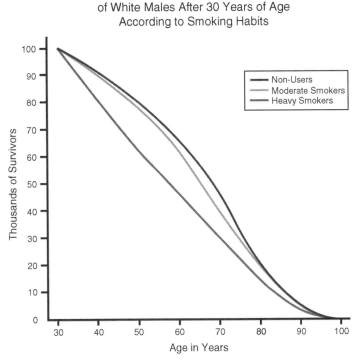

Tobacco and Longevity Survivorship
of White Males After 30 Years of Age
According to Smoking Habits

Source: Reprinted with permission from Pearl R. Tobacco smoke and longevity. Science 1938; 87:216–217.

smokers was reduced by about ten years years, after age 30, compared with non-smokers (see Figure 5.1). Longevity was also lower for moderate smokers. Subsequently, as cohort studies of smokers were carried out, Pearl's observation was repeatedly and readily confirmed. There have been many landmark investigations of smoking and disease: the early case-control studies of lung cancer[3,4] and the cohort studies such as the Framingham study,[5] the British Physician's Study,[6] and the studies initiated by the American Cancer Society.[7] In the United Kingdom, the 1962 report of the Royal College of Physicians[8] concluded that smoking was a cause of lung cancer and bronchitis and a contributing factor to coronary heart disease. In the United States, the 1964 report of the Advisory Committee to the Surgeon General concluded that smoking was a cause of lung cancer in men and of chronic bronchitis.[9] Subsequent reports have led to a progressively lengthier list of diseases caused by smoking.

Tobacco Smoke and Disease

Tobacco smoke in a burning cigarette is generated by the burning of complex organic material, tobacco, additives and paper, at a high temperature, reaching about 1000°C.[9] The resulting smoke, comprising numerous gases and also particles, includes myriad toxic components that can cause injury through inflammation and irritation, asphyxiation, carcinogenesis and other mechanisms. **Active smokers** inhale **mainstream smoke (MS)**, the smoke that is drawn directly through the end of the cigarette. **Passive smokers** (also referred to as **secondhand smokers**) inhale smoke that is often referred to as **environmental tobacco smoke (ETS)**, comprising a mixture of mostly **sidestream smoke (SS)** given off by the smoldering cigarette and some exhaled MS. Concentrations of tobacco smoke components in ETS are far below the levels of MS inhaled by the active smoker, but there are qualitative similarities between ETS and MS. The mainstream smoke emerging from the cigarette is an aerosol containing about 1×10^{10} particles per ml, ranging in diameter from 0.1 to 1.0 μm (mean diameter 0.2 μm). Cigarette smoke is known to contain approximately 4,000 identified compounds. Many of the components are present in higher concentration in SS than in MS, particularly for nitrogen-containing compounds.

Smoking damages nearly every organ in the human body, is linked to at least fifteen different cancers, and accounts for some 30% of all cancer deaths. For many of the diseases caused by smoking, the increases in risk in adult smokers are dramatic. Table 5.1 provides relative risks for dying overall and from major smoking-caused diseases obtained in two studies, the American Cancer Society's Cancer Prevention Studies (CPS) I and II, each of about one million persons.[10] The wide range of relative risk values reflects the strength of smoking as a cause of the different diseases and the relative strengths of other causal factors. For the principal chronic diseases associated with smoking, the effect on disease risk is usually manifest only after a substantial latent period, which represents the time needed for the injury to be sufficient to cause disease and for the underlying process to come to completion, for example, the transformation of a normal cell to a malignant cell. For smoking and lung cancer, for example, incidence rates rise after about twenty years of active smoking.

The relative risk values generally rise with indicators of exposure to tobacco smoke, including numbers of cigarettes smoked and the duration of smoking, and fall after successful cessation. Figure 5.2 illustrates dose–response

Table 5.1 Estimated relative risk for current cigarette smokers ages 35 years or more in CPS I (1959–1965) and CPS II (1982–1988)

Underlying Cause of Death (selected diseases)	CPS I Males	CPSII Males	CPS I Females	CPS II Females
All causes (cancer and other)	1.80	2.34	1.23	1.90
CHD, ages 35 to 64	2.25	2.81	1.81	3.00
CHD, ages ≥65	1.39	1.62	1.24	1.60
Influenza and pneumonia	1.82	0.91		
Bronchitis and emphysema	8.81	5.89		
COPD	9.65	10.47		
Other respiratory diseases[1]	1.99	2.18		
Lung cancer	11.35	22.36	2.69	11.94
Cancer of the esophagus	3.62	7.60	1.94	10.25
Kidney cancer	1.84	2.95	1.43	1.41
Cancer of the larynx	10.00	10.48	3.81	17.78
Cancer of the lip, oral cavity, and pharynx	6.33	27.48	1.96	5.59
Cancer of the pancreas	2.34	2.14	1.39	2.33
Cancer of the bladder and other urinary organs	2.90	2.86	2.87	2.58
Cancer of the cervix uteri	1.10	2.14		

[1]Includes influenza and pneumonia.
Note: CPS, American Cancer Society's Cancer Prevention Studies; CHD, coronary heart disease; COPD, Chronic obstructive pulmonary disease.
Source: Adapted from U.S. Department of Health and Human Services. Reducing the Health Consequences of Smoking. 25 Years of Progress. A Report of the Surgeon General. Washington, DC: U.S. Government Printing Office; 1989.

relationships with the number of cigarettes smoked for coronary heart disease among female participants in the Nurses Health Study.[11] For the cancers caused by smoking, the relative risks tend to decline slowly as the number of years since quitting increases.[12] By contrast, there is an immediate decline in the relative risk for cardiovascular disease, and the levels of former smokers tend to reach those of never-smokers after five to ten years of abstinence. Chronic obstructive pulmonary disease results from sustained excessive loss of lung function in smokers. Fortunately, after cessation, the rate of decline quickly returns to the rate of persons who have never smoked (see Figure 5.3).

Smoking can have negative effects on reproduction. Smoking during pregnancy reduces birth weight by approximately 200 grams on average. The degree of reduction is related to the amount smoked. If a mother who smokes quits this behavior by the third trimester, much of the weight reduction can be avoided. What's more, smoking increases the number of abnormal sperm in men, which

FIGURE 5.2   Dose–response relationships with the number of cigarettes smoked for coronary heart disease among female participants in the Nurses' Health Study

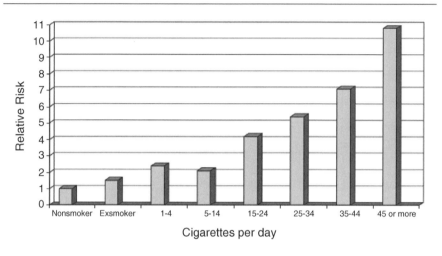

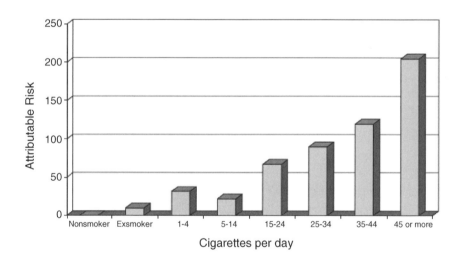

Source: Reprinted with permission from Willett WC, Green A, Stampfer MJ, Speizer FE, Colditz GA, Rosner B, Monson RR, Stason W and Hennekens CH. Relative and absolute excess risks of coronary heart disease among women who smoke cigarettes. N Engl J Med 1987; 317:1303–1309.

FIGURE 5.3   Theoretical curves depicting varying rates of decline of forced expiratory volume in one second (FEV₁)

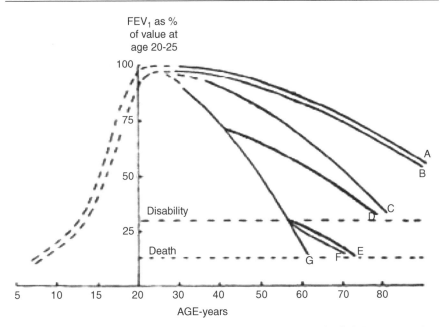

Note: Curves A and B represent never-smokers and smokers, respectively, declining at normal rates. Curve C shows increased declines without the development of COPD. Rates of decline for former smokers are represented by curves D and E for those without and with clinical COPD, respectively. Curves F and G show rates of decline with continued smoking after developing COPD.
Source: DHHS Publication number 90–8416, p. 281, and USDHHS 2004 The Effects of Active Smoking: A Report of the Surgeon General, p. 468. 1990.

can lead to infertility, birth defects, or other complications.[13] Smoking also increases rates of spontaneous abortion, placenta previa, and perinatal mortality, and smoking during pregnancy is now considered to be a cause of sudden infant death syndrome (SIDS). There is more limited evidence suggesting that smoking by the mother may increase childhood cancer incidence for some types of childhood cancer and congenital defects.[13,14]

Smoking can also cause cardiovascular diseases, including coronary heart disease (CHD), abdominal aortic aneurysm, atherosclerotic vascular disease, and cerebral vascular disease (stroke).[15] These conditions have in common the narrowing of the coronary arteries, the blood vessels that carry blood to the heart. Most cases of myocardial infarction (heart attack) result from blockage of the narrowed coronary arteries by thrombus or blood clot. Smoking not only is a cause of the atherosclerosis, which narrows the coronary arteries, but it also increases the tendency of the blood to clot. Studies using Doppler ultrasonography to image the carotid artery have documented a higher rate of thickening in smokers compared with nonsmokers. The mechanisms by which smoking causes stroke are similar to those that lead to myocardial infarction.

Risk for the cardiovascular diseases increases with the number of cigarettes smoked per day and with the duration of smoking. Smoking cessation reduces the risk of the cardiovascular diseases. For coronary heart disease, the risk tends to decline rapidly immediately following cessation. After one year of not smoking, the risk reduces by about half as compared to a current smoker, and after five to ten years is similar to a person who never smoked. In terms of cardiovascular diseases, smoking lower tar and nicotine cigarettes has not been shown to affect risk.

In addition to heart disease, cigarette smoking causes inflammation of the lungs. Smoking causes migration of inflammatory cells into the lungs and release of enzymes that can destroy the lungs' delicate alveoli. Smoking activates the inflammatory process and reduces the efficacy of defenses against inflammation. Unchecked inflammation, sustained over many years, underlies the development of COPD. This disease develops progressively in 10%–15% of smokers.[16,17] Relevant epidemiologic evidence comes from research on the level of lung function in smokers and nonsmokers and on the change of level of lung function over time. Increasing mortality from COPD in smokers has been described in cohort studies as well.[16] The studies show that smokers, in comparison with nonsmokers, have a lower level of lung function on average and that the level of lung function in smokers declines as the number of cigarettes smoked per day increases. Smokers, followed over time, have a faster decline of lung function, on average, than nonsmokers. The rate of decline in smokers reverts to that of nonsmokers following successful quitting. Unfortunately, the damage prior to cessation is mostly irreversible. Mortality rates for COPD are elevated in smokers compared with nonsmokers by approximately tenfold. There is no consistent evidence that risk for this disease is associated with the tar and nicotine yield of the cigarettes smoked.

Substantial epidemiologic evidence exists on respiratory health and health status in relation to smoking. Smoking causes increased occurrence of the cardinal respiratory symptoms—cough (that is, "smoker's cough"), sputum production, wheezing, and dyspnea (shortness of breath). Symptom rates are substantially higher in smokers in comparison with those who have never smoked and tend to increase in frequency with the numbers of cigarettes smoked per day. The Surgeon Generals' reports have repeatedly commented on these associations and ascribed the relationship between smoking and cough and phlegm as causal.

Health Effects of Passive Smoking

The relationship between passive smoking and health has a briefer history. Some of the first epidemiological studies on secondhand smoke or environmental tobacco smoke and health were reported in the 1960s. The initial investigations focused on parental smoking and lower respiratory illnesses in infants; studies of lung function and respiratory symptoms in children soon followed.[18,19] The 1972 report of the Surgeon General was the first to call attention to passive smoking.[20] Hirayama and colleagues reported that among nonsmokers in 91,549 married women, age-adjusted lung cancer mortality rates were lowest for wives of nonsmokers, intermediate for wives of light or ex-smokers, and highest for wives of heavy smokers (>20 cigarettes/day, p <0.01).[21] Another study from two Athens hospitals of lung cancer cases and controls found a risk of lung cancer 2.4 times higher for wives of men who smoked less than a pack per day and 3.4 times higher for wives of heavy smokers, compared with the wives of nonsmokers.[22] By 1986, the evidence supported the conclusion that passive smoking was a cause of lung cancer in nonsmokers. This conclusion was supported in a review by the International Agency for Research on Cancer (IARC), the U.S. Surgeon General, the U.S. National Research Council, and summarized by Fielding.[19,23,24,25] A meta-analysis of all available studies concluded that there was an increased risk of lung cancer associated with environmental tobacco smoke.[26] A now substantial body of evidence has continued to identify new diseases and other adverse effects of passive smoking, including increased risk for coronary heart disease.[27,28,29] Estimates are as high as 53,000 ETS-related deaths per year from heart disease, lung cancer, and respiratory illness, with increased incidence of asthma, chronic bronchitis, respiratory infections, and low-birth weight infants.[30]

ETS exposure has particular adverse effects for infants and children. These include decreased respiratory health, including increased risk for more severe lower-respiratory infections, middle ear disease, chronic respiratory symptoms, and asthma, and a reduction in the rate of lung function growth during childhood. There is more limited evidence suggesting that ETS exposure of the mother reduces birth weight and that child development and behavior are adversely affected by parental smoking.[31] The NHANES III data was used to correlate children's serum cotinine levels with a variety of cognitive and academic abilities, reporting a significant negative linear correlation between cognitive abilities and exposure to ETS.[32] Reduced lung function in children and adolescents has been associated with occasional exposure to ETS.[33] Over a five-year period, maternal smoking effects on their children's pulmonary function was evaluated in 1,156 East Boston children, observing a reduction of 101 ml (7%) compared to children of nonsmoking mothers.[34] However, there is no strong evidence at present that ETS exposure increases childhood cancer risk.

In adults, ETS exposure has been causally associated with lung cancer and ischemic and coronary heart disease.[35,36] In a 1997 meta-analysis, Law et al.[37] estimated the excess risk from ETS exposure as 30% (95% CI [confidence interval] 22, 38%) at age 65 years. Pell and colleagues studied acute coronary syndrome admissions to nine Scottish hospitals for the ten-month period before and after their smoking prohibition.[38] There was a 17% reduction in hospital admissions for acute coronary syndrome compared to 4% in England, which had no such legislation over the same time. The number of hospital admissions for acute coronary syndrome decreased after implementation of this smoke-free legislation; 67% of the decrease involved nonsmokers. Systemic effects of smoking include a low level of inflammation; C reactive protein may be elevated for up to ten years after quitting and is associated with increased risk of atherosclerotic and coronary heart disease.[39]

Negative studies include Enstrom's study of the American Cancer Society cohort covering thirty-nine years in California, finding no effect for secondhand smoke on risk of spousal lung cancer, coronary heart disease, and COPD mortality, although this study had been criticized for misclassification of smoke effects.[40] The SAPALDIA study in Switzerland used questionnaires prospectively in 4,197 never-smoking adults, finding passive smoking to be associated with wheezing apart from colds, chronic bronchitis, dyspnea, and physician-diagnosed asthma.[41] In 200 asthmatics followed for a year, with half having a spouse who smoked, those exposed to ETS had significantly more daily bronchodilator use, intermittent corticosteroid use, more emergency room visits, more acute episodes, and had more absence from work.[42] ETS exposure among police officers in Hong Kong was associated with increased respiratory symptoms, including throat problems, cough, phlegm, and wheezing.[43] A random sample of San Francisco bartenders studied before and after a workplace smoking ban reduced ETS from a median of 28 to 2 hours per week.[44] There was a reduction from thirty-nine (74%) who had respiratory symptoms before to seventeen (32%) after the ban, and pulmonary function also improved. These results were reproduced in Dublin after a ban on smoking in bars with $PM_{2.5}$, dropping 83% accompanied by significant improvement in bartender pulmonary function and respiratory symptoms.[45]

Several panels, including the U.S. National Research Council, the U.S. Surgeon General, and the Environmental Protection Agency, have concluded that secondhand tobacco smoke is a cause of lung cancer.[47,48] The most recent evaluation was carried out by the International Agency for Research on Cancer (IARC). It compiled more than fifty studies of involuntary smoking and lung cancer risk in nonsmokers as well as completing meta-analyses in which the relative risk estimates from the individual studies were pooled. The IARC monograph concluded that there is a significant and consistent association between lung cancer risk in spouses of smokers and secondhand tobacco smoke exposure, with the excess risk being about 20% in women and 30% in men. Workplace exposures to secondhand smoke also increased lung cancer risk in nonsmokers by 12%–19%. Thus, IARC concluded that involuntary smoking (exposure to secondhand smoke or ETS) causes lung cancer in humans.

Lung Cancer Epidemiology

Lung cancer is the most common cause of cancer death in the United States, with more than 200,000 new cases and 160,000 annual deaths. It is estimated that lung cancer causes about 1.2 million deaths annually worldwide. Approximately 90% of lung cancer cases are due to cigarette smoking in populations with prolonged cigarette use. The strongest determinant of lung cancer in smokers is duration of smoking; risk also increases with the number of cigarettes smoked. Smoking causes lung cancer in both men and women. Cessation of smoking at any age avoids the further increase in risk of lung cancer caused by continued smoking (see Figure 5.4). However, the risk of ex-smokers for lung cancer remains elevated for years after cessation, compared to the risk of never smokers. The impact of smoking on lung cancer in the twentieth century in the United States can be seen in Figure 5.5. Cigarette smoking was rare in the early part of the twentieth century, as was lung cancer. Smoking increased due to mass production of cigarettes, increased advertising, and pervasive use of cigarettes by military personnel during World War I. During the twentieth century, smoking rose first among males and then with a twenty- to thirty-year delay among females. Cigarette smoking peaked in the 1950s and 1960s and began to decline after the wave of studies documenting its risks appeared and the publication of the first Surgeon General's report in 1964. Mortality due to lung cancer in men can be seen to follow the curve for smoking prevalence by about thirty years, beginning to decrease in the mid-1990s. Lung cancer became the most common cause of cancer death in U.S. women, surpassing breast cancer in 1988. (Refer to Table 5.1 for the types of cancers caused by cigarette smoking.)

FIGURE 5.4   Cumulative lung cancer risk by smoking status and age at quitting smoking in men in the UK

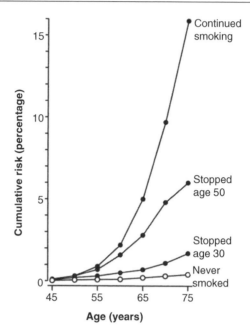

Source: IARC monograph. Lyon, France, International Agency for Research on Cancer, 2004.

Carcinogens in Cigarette Smoke

The range of total carcinogen exposure in smokers is approximately 1.4–2.2 mg/cigarette, which can be compared to the current sales-weighted average nicotine delivery of about 0.8 mg/cigarette. Some of the strongest carcinogens, such as polycyclic aromatic hydrocarbons (PAH), N-nitrosamines, and aromatic amines, occur in the lowest amounts, while some of the weaker carcinogens (such as acetaldehyde and isoprene) occur in the highest amounts. PAH are incomplete combustion products that were first identified as carcinogenic constituents of coal tar.[49] They occur as mixtures in tars, soots, broiled foods, automobile engine exhaust and other materials generated by incomplete combustion.[50] N-nitrosamines are a large class of carcinogens with demonstrated activity in at least thirty animal species. Considerable evidence favors PAH and N-nitrosamines as major etiological factors in lung cancer. PAH are strong,

FIGURE 5.5 Annual adult per capita consumption of cigarettes and major smoking and health events (United States, 1900–1998)

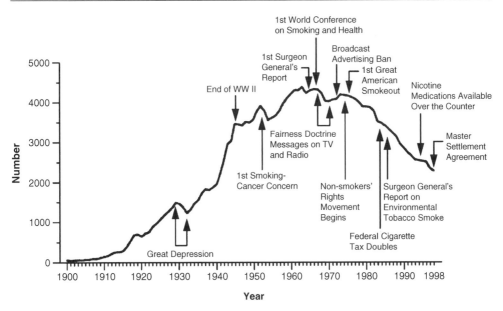

Source: IARC monograph. Lyon, France, International Agency for Research on Cancer, 2004.

locally acting carcinogens, and tobacco smoke fractions enriched in these compounds are carcinogenic. PAH-DNA adducts have been detected in the human lung, and mutations in the TP53 tumor suppressor gene isolated from lung tumors are similar to those produced in vitro by PAH diol epoxide metabolites and in cell culture by Benzo(a)pyrene.[51] Persistent DNA adducts can cause miscoding during replication when DNA polymerase enzymes process them incorrectly.[52] There is considerable specificity in the relationship between specific DNA adducts caused by cigarette smoke carcinogens and the types of mutations which they cause. G to T and G to A mutations are frequently observed.[53] Mutations have been frequently observed in the K-ras oncogene in smokers with lung cancer and in the TP53 tumor suppressor gene in a variety of cigarette smoke-induced cancers. The cancer-causing role of mutations in these genes has been firmly established in animal studies. The K-ras and TP53 mutations observed in lung cancer in smokers appear to reflect DNA damage by metabolically activated PAH, although acrolein can also cause p53 adducts in lung cancer hot spots, and there is far more acrolein in cigarette smoke than PAH. In addition, numerous cytogenetic changes have been observed in lung cancer, and chromosome damage throughout the aerodigestive tract is strongly linked with cigarette smoke exposure. Gene mutations can cause loss of normal cellular growth control functions via a complex process of signal transduction pathways, ultimately resulting in cellular proliferation and cancer.

The most commonly mutated gene found in human cancers is the TP53 tumor suppresser gene.[51] Among the tobacco related cancers, the most extensive database exists for lung cancer, in which mutations in the TP53 gene have been detected in approximately 70% of tumors.[54] In smokers, the mutations are focused in the central part of the gene, which is the DNA binding region that is essential for its function. Smokers have mutations in hot spots of this region that are a characteristic signature, for example, codons 157, 176, 248, 249, 273. Exposure of lung fibroblasts or epithelial cells in vitro to activated PAH results in DNA adducts on the same codons.[51]

Smoking Cessation

Mark Twain stated, "Giving up smoking is easy. I've done it a hundred times." In 2008 it was noted that social networks amplify smoking cessation, with one's spouse, sibling, friend, or coworker, in descending order, influencing a smoker's possibility of smoking cessation, and that smokers over time are increasingly marginalized socially.[55] The Lung Health Study was a randomized clinical trial of smoking cessation and inhaled bronchodilator (ipratropium) therapy in smokers 35 to 60 years of age who were in good health but had evidence of mild to moderate airway obstruction.[56] They enrolled 5,887 smokers at ten clinical centers, with an intervention group of twelve smoking cessation sessions and nicotine gum; the intervention group had smaller declines in FEV_1 than the control group.[57] At five years, 21.7% of special intervention participants had stopped smoking since study entry, compared with 5.4% of usual care participants. At 14.5 years' follow-up, there was a lower mortality in the intervention group, with the hazard ratio for usual care 1.18 (95% CI 1.02–1.37), and differences in death rates were greatest for lung cancer and cardiovascular disease.

Tobacco cessation programs have difficulty exceeding sustained quit rates above 15%, which is the typical success rate of those attempting to stop "cold turkey." Treatment of tobacco dependence with nicotine gum and patches may double this rate.[58] Nicotine is the addictive substance in tobacco, and cigarette manufacturers are very sophisticated at mixing tobacco blends to achieve maximal nicotine delivery via the cigarette. Nicotine has a rather short half-life of about 20 minutes, requiring another cigarette to be smoked to keep blood levels of nicotine at sufficient levels to prevent withdrawal symptoms. Smoking provides an immediate delivery of nicotine to the blood and to the brain, where nicotinic acetylcholine receptors are critical for the development of dependence. The highest levels of these receptors, the $\alpha4\beta2$, are in the reward center of the brain. A treatment strategy is to have a competitor for this receptor that doesn't or only partially activates it; varenicline, a plant alkaloid cytisine, is such a drug.[59] This drug had a higher sustained quit rate in comparative clinical trials with bupropion or nicotine-replacement therapy.

Policy Controls on Tobacco and Cigarette Smoking

There are more than twenty states that have laws prohibiting smoking in public places—notably bars, restaurants, and workplaces.[60] Minnesota began this trend in 1975 by enacting a law stating that public places had to have nonsmoking areas, but it took until 2008 to ban smoking entirely. The major state-level policy on smoking is the attorneys general (AGs) lawsuit against U.S. tobacco companies (Brown and Williamson, Lorillard, Philip Morris, RJ Reynolds) reclaiming tobacco-attributable health care costs.[61] The AGs proposed a $368.5 billion settlement by forty-six states, but this was negotiated downward to approximately $206 billion to be paid over twenty-five years. This master settlement agreement restricted tobacco advertising (included a ban on cigarette advertising on billboards; an end to the use of cartoons to promote tobacco; a ban on T-shirts, hats, and apparel bearing a tobacco product name; limits on athletic and music sponsorships; a prohibition on free samples to underage consumers and a ban on packs of fewer than twenty cigarettes [which are more affordable for kids]; a requirement that producers pay fines if smoking rates among youth did not decline; and an indemnification of U.S. tobacco companies against personal injury lawsuits). Unfortunately, the vast majority of states spend only a sliver of their money on programs aimed at preventing young people from smoking and helping older smokers quit. The Centers for Disease Control and Prevention recommends that states contribute one-fifth of the money they receive for anti-tobacco programs. In 2006, states allocated to prevention and cessation programs, 3% of the $8.1 billion that they stood to receive from the tobacco companies.[62] To pay for the anti-tobacco programs required under the master settlement agreement, tobacco companies raised the price of cigarettes 45 cents a pack, which has probably led to a 4%–5% decrease in demand.[62] New York City expanded its tobacco program in 2002 by passing the New York City Smoke-Free Air Act, which increased taxes on cigarette packs 32%, to nearly $7 a pack.[63] All indoor workplaces, including bars and restaurants, were made smoke free. Here is an example to give an idea of the impact of such bans: a smoking bar in New York had PM$_{2.5}$ levels 50 times higher than the entrance to the Holland Tunnel, and a nonsmoking bar had levels equal to Central Park's Great Lawn. Hard-hitting print and broadcast anti-tobacco advertising campaigns were initiated. Nicotine replacement was made available free of charge, and over two years there was a drop of 200,000 smokers or 3% in the smoking rate. Support for the Smoke-Free Air Act increased from 52% in 1999 to 73% in 2002.

The Food and Drug Administration (FDA) had been prevented from regulating nicotine as a drug for many years, primarily because the tobacco industry obfuscated the fact that nicotine was addictive and manipulated the nicotine delivery to enhance addiction. In 1995, President Bill Clinton announced that FDA analyses supported the finding that the nicotine in cigarettes and smokeless tobacco products is a drug and that these products were drug delivery devices under the terms of the act. FDA Commissioner David Kessler tried unsuccessfully to regulate nicotine, but he was able to obtain many confidential documents by the tobacco industry aimed at thwarting FDA regulatory efforts.[64] These documents showed that the tobacco companies manipulated the amount of nicotine in cigarettes. FDA regulation of tobacco would generate $28–$43 billion in health benefits versus $180 million in costs, plus $149–$185 million per year in operating expenses. In *FDA v. Brown and Williamson Tobacco Corp* in 2000, the U.S. Supreme Court ruled 5–4 that since Congress had developed a separate regulatory structure for tobacco outside of the FDA, it never intended to give the agency regulatory authority over tobacco. The Court majority also held strongly for commercial free speech.

In response, Congress wrote the Family Smoking Prevention and Tobacco Control Act, which gave the FDA broad authority to regulate the manufacture of tobacco products as well as the sale, distribution, and promotion of tobacco products in order to protect public health.[65] Tobacco manufacturers would have to provide lists of ingredients, which could be regulated or banned if found harmful by the FDA. The labels *light, mild,* and low would be subject to regulation, and fruit, spice, or other flavorings that appeal to children would be banned. Menthol would not be banned, but it could be regulated if found to be harmful. Philip Morris supported this act, but it was opposed by the smaller tobacco companies because the act solidified Philip Morris's lead or dominant position while restricting the activities of its competitors. On July 30, 2008, the U.S. House voted 326 to 102 in favor of this bill.

In August 2006, U.S. District Court Judge Gladys Kessler issued her opinion on the U.S. lawsuit against the tobacco companies in which the Department of Justice sought to recover costs for smoking-related diseases in government-run health programs (Veterans, Medicare, Medicaid). She found that the major tobacco companies violated civil racketeering laws, stating, "The evidence in this case clearly establishes that Defendants have not ceased engaging in unlawful activity. Their continuing conduct misleads consumers in order to maximize Defendant's revenues by recruiting new smokers (the majority of whom are under the age of 18) preventing current smokers from quitting, and thereby sustaining the industry." She stated that

> this case was about an industry that survives and profits from selling a highly addictive product which causes diseases that lead to a staggering number of deaths per year, an immeasurable amount of human suffering and economic loss, and a profound burden on our national health care system. Defendants have known these facts for at least 50 years or more. Despite that knowledge, they have consistently, repeatedly, and with enormous skill and sophistication, denied these facts to the public, to the Government, and to the public health community. In short, Defendants marketed and sold their lethal products with zeal, with deception, with a single-minded focus on their financial success, and without regard for the human tragedy or social costs that success exacted.[66]

Although public health agencies sought $130 billion to fund smoking cessation programs, the U.S. Justice Department reduced this in 2005 to $10 billion, and the U.S. Circuit Court of Appeals did not allow any financial remedy. Instead the Final Judgment and Remedies Order stated that the tobacco companies were prohibited from racketeering in the future and the making of false, misleading, or deceptive statements concerning cigarettes and their health risks. It also banned terms. including *low-tar, light, ultra light, mild,* or *natural,* required corrective statements concerning the health risks of smoking and secondhand smoke and their deceptive practices through newspaper and television advertising, their websites, and as part of their cigarette packaging and made tobacco companies report marketing data annually to the government.

In 1992 the EPA declared ETS a Class A human lung carcinogen. In 1994 the Occupational Safety and Health Administration released a proposed rule on indoor air quality that would broadly limit nonsmokers' exposure to tobacco smoke in the workplace.

Global Smoking Today

In 2008, 17% of students ages 13 to 15 years world-wide report current tobacco use. Approximately 82,000 to 99,000 children, roughly half living in Asia, start smoking every day. Young people spend more than $1.26 billion on tobacco.

Minors can buy cigarettes illegally 67% of the time, and 88% of the time they buy cigarettes via vending machines. Moreover, many children use smokeless tobacco products such as snuff and chewing tobacco. Of the 6 million Americans who use smokeless tobacco, as many as 1 in 4 are under the age of 19 years. Educating children about tobacco is important, since only half of high school students who smoke report that more than one pack per day constitutes a serious health risk. More than 90% of 6-year-olds know Joe Camel smokes, and 46% of 8- to 13-year-olds see tobacco advertising on billboards.

Today developing countries have 70% of the global share of smoking. Nearly half of the world's 1.3 billion smokers live in China, India, and Indonesia. U.S. tobacco companies provide 20% of the 6 trillion cigarettes smoked in the world each year. Certainly, despite the fact that local, state, and federal anti-tobacco laws have reduced smoking by 20% since 1998, U.S. tobacco companies increased their exports by 260%. In 1997, Congress passed the Doggett Amendment, which banned the use of government monies from the Commerce, Justice, and State Departments to promote the sale or export of tobacco overseas or to seek the removal of any nondiscriminatory foreign country restrictions on tobacco marketing. Early in 1998, after considerable delay, the Clinton administration issued a directive to U.S. embassies to implement the law. Although a positive step forward, this weak amendment is subject to annual renewal, does not cover all federal agencies, and leaves compliance responsibility in the hands of agencies (such as the U.S. Trade Representative) that have historically been oblivious or antagonistic to public health concerns.

The Framework Convention on Tobacco Control provides international legal documentation for all countries to regulate tobacco. It passed the World Health Assembly in Geneva in 2003. The negotiation of this treaty spanned two U.S. administrations that had diametrically opposed views on the tobacco industry, with the administration of President George W. Bush opposing mandatory taxes and ten additional measures. The United States signed the treaty in 2004, but it hasn't been sent to the Senate for ratification. The treaty requires all nations to ban tobacco advertising, promotion, and sponsorship.[67] It requires that countries implement tobacco control measures, such as large graphic health warnings, bans on such misleading terms such as *light* and *low-tar,* and bans or restrictions on tobacco marketing. One hundred and seventy two nations have ratified the treaty. A 10% price increase reduces consumption by about 4% in high-income countries and 8% in developing countries. Taxation also raises revenue, which can be used for effective tobacco prevention and cessation programs. The World Bank proposes that taxes should account for two-thirds to four-fifths of the retail price of cigarettes.

Summary

Cigarette smoking is a major public health problem that causes chronic lung diseases, lung and other cancers, and cardiovascular diseases. On June 22, 2009, President Obama signed the Family Smoking Prevention and Tobacco Control Act into law, giving the Food and Drug Administration authority to regulate the manufacture, distribution, and sale of tobacco products to protect the public health. By June 2010 the FDA's Center for Tobacco Products implemented three important provisions of the law: new warning labels must take up 20% of the packages and advertisements for all smokeless tobacco products; tobacco companies no longer will be allowed to call their products "light" or "low," and the youth access and advertising rule, first proposed in 1996 and restricting the way the tobacco industry can advertise and sell cigarettes and smokeless tobacco products, will finally go into effect.

Key Terms

Active smokers

Environmental tobacco smoke

Mainstream smoke

Passive smokers

Secondhand smokers

Sidestream smoke

Discussion Questions

1. List some of the diseases linked to smoking.
2. What are some of the health effects of passive smoking or secondhand smoke?
3. What are some methods to help people quit smoking?
4. How has smoking been regulated by the governments in the United States?
5. What groups are tobacco companies targeting in today's world?

The author thanks Stephen S. Hecht, Ph.D., and Jonathan M. Samet, M.D., for permission to use parts of the Cigarette Smoking chapter published in *Environmental and Occupational Medicine*, 4th ed., by Lippincott, Williams and Wilkins.

CHAPTER 6

CHILDREN'S ENVIRONMENTAL HEALTH

Mercury and Lead

Leonardo Trasande

LEARNING OBJECTIVES

- To understand the unique vulnerability of children to environmental hazards
- To become familiar with the regulatory efforts to protect children
- To understand how mercury, lead, and outdoor air pollution affect children's health and how the government regulates these substances
- To become familiar with the goals of the National Children's Study and the future protection of children

Public concern about environmental health threats to children has intensified in recent years and has caused scientists, politicians, regulators, and public health officials to take notice. The issue is whether young children, infants, and fetuses are at an increased health risk from environmental chemicals, because they have a heightened susceptibility to such compounds and/or because they have higher relative exposures to environmental chemicals than do adults. From a public health perspective, this is a legitimate concern. And because both as a society and as individuals we place great value on providing a safe environment for children, we need to determine whether this concern is scientifically valid. The vulnerability of children to environmental chemicals was first identified at the beginning of the twentieth century when physicians began to report severe lead poisoning in children who were chewing paint from crib railings and walls and verandas of houses.[1,2] Despite acknowledgment by the National Lead Company that lead was toxic, a policy debate would ensue for over a half century until the U.S. Environmental Protection Agency (EPA) would promulgate a phase-out of lead from gasoline that occurred from 1975 to 1986, and the Consumer Product Safety Commission would ban lead in paint in 1977.[3] Delays in policy protections of children from other chemicals in the environment have followed a similar pattern, with a presumption of safety given to chemicals and the burden of proof on scientists, families, and children before regulations are implemented to limit children's exposure to chemical hazards.

The first section of this chapter provides an overview of the physiologic and other reasons for children's unique vulnerability to environmental chemicals. Subsequent sections present the general framework in which chemicals are regulated and assessed for their potential toxicity for children and provide specific policy updates with regard to mercury, lead, and outdoor air pollutants. A final section describes the hope presented by the National Children's Study to produce proactive policy on behalf of children to prevent the health effects of environmental hazards.

The Unique Vulnerability of Children

The biological basis for the unique vulnerability of children to environmental chemicals is best codified in a 1993 National Academy of Sciences (NAS) report, "Pesticides in the Diets of Infants and Children":

- One important reason why children are so vulnerable to environmental chemicals is that they have disproportionately heavy exposures. Pound per pound of body weight, children drink more water, eat more food, and breathe more air than adults, and they take proportionately more of the toxins in water, food, and air into their bodies. Young children's exposure is magnified further by their normal behaviors—their play close to the floor and their hand-to-mouth activity, which pediatricians call "normal oral exploratory behavior."

- A second reason for children's great susceptibility to chemical toxins is that children do not metabolize, detoxify, and excrete many toxins in the same way as adults; thus the chemicals can reside much longer in children's bloodstreams and cause more damage.

- A third reason is that children are undergoing rapid growth and development, and those very complex developmental processes are easily disrupted.

- Finally, children have more future years of life than most adults and thus have more time to develop chronic diseases that may be triggered by early environmental exposures.

- Over the past thirty years, chronic diseases of environmental origin have become epidemic in American children and are the diseases of greatest current concern. These include:

   ○ Asthma, which has more than doubled in frequency since 1980 and has become the leading cause of pediatric hospitalization and school absenteeism[4]

   ○ Birth defects, which are now the leading cause of infant death[5,6]

   ○ Neurodevelopmental disorders, autism, dyslexia, mental retardation, and attention deficit/hyperactivity disorder (ADHD)—which affect 5%–10% of the 4 million babies born each year in the United States[7]

   ○ Leukemia and brain cancer in children and testicular cancer in adolescents, whose incidence rates have increased since the 1970s, despite declining rates of mortality[8,9,10]

Increases in these chronic conditions have occurred simultaneously with the widespread use of chemicals in the environment. Today there are more than 80,000 synthetic chemicals, most of them developed only since the 1950s.[11] These chemicals include plastics, pesticides, motor fuels, building materials, antibiotics, chemotherapeutic agents, flame retardants, and synthetic hormones. Children are especially at risk of exposure to the 2,800 synthetic chemicals that are produced in quantities of one million tons or more per year.[12] These high-production-volume (HPV) chemicals are the synthetic materials dispersed most widely in the environment—in air, food, water, and consumer products in homes, schools, and communities. In recent national surveys, quantifiable levels of a number of HPV chemicals have been detected in the bodies of most Americans.[13]

Increasing evidence links common chemical exposures in childhood with these chronic conditions. Numerous pollutants in the indoor environment have been shown to be triggers for childhood asthma—secondhand tobacco smoke, mold and mites, cockroach droppings, animal dander, and certain pesticides.[14,15] Ambient pollutants—airborne fine particulates, ozone, oxides of nitrogen, and diesel exhaust—also have been shown to increase incidence of asthma and to trigger asthmatic attacks.[16] Ionizing radiation, benzene, 1,3-butadiene, and pesticides have been etiologically associated with childhood malignancies.[17,18] Additionally, a recent National Academy of Sciences (NAS) study suggested that at least 28% of developmental disabilities in children may be caused by environmental factors acting alone or in concert with genetic susceptibility.[19]

Federal regulation of environmental chemicals has proven successful in the reduction of childhood disease and disability.[20] Reductions in exposure associated with the elimination from lead in gasoline in the United States resulted in IQs among preschool-aged children in the 1990s that were 2.2–4.7 points higher than they would have been if those children had a distribution of blood lead levels found among children in the 1970s.[21] Local policy can also dramatically influence children's exposure to environmental chemicals and result in reductions in childhood morbidity. Restrictions instituted by the city of Atlanta on vehicular travel during the 1996 Olympic Games were associated with significant reductions in ambient ozone and in asthma acute care events.[22]

Mercury as a Case Study

Mercury is used in a number of scientific research applications, in amalgam material for dental restoration, and in lighting. Mercury can be emitted into the atmosphere by natural sources (volcanic eruptions) and industrial sources (coal-fired power plants). Mercury exposure can be toxic, with effects such as tremors, impaired cognitive skills, and sleep disturbance in workers with chronic exposure to mercury vapor even at low concentrations. Acute exposure to mercury vapor has been shown to result in profound central nervous system effects, including psychotic reactions characterized by delirium and hallucinations. Although scientific evidence about the environmental hazards of mercury in children as well as adults has been known for a long time, regulatory policy has been lagging. The development of regulation of mercury emissions of coal-fired power plants remains a striking example. Anthropogenic emissions now account for approximately 70% of the 5,500 metric tons of mercury that are released into the Earth's atmosphere each year. The leading sources of these emissions in the

United States are coal-fired power plants, chlorine plants, and incinerators. Elemental mercury, once emitted, readily aerosolizes, and once airborne deposits into soil and water. It is transformed within microorganisms into methylmercury and is subsequently consumed by fish, which are in turn eaten by larger fish. Methylmercury reaches very high concentrations in predatory fish, such as swordfish, tuna, king mackerel, and shark. Consumption of contaminated fish is the major route of human exposure to methylmercury.

Methylmercury toxicity was first recognized in the 1950s in Minamata, Japan, when consumption of fish by pregnant women resulted in at least thirty cases of cerebral palsy in children. Exposed women were themselves affected minimally, if at all.[23] A similar episode occurred in 1972 in Iraq, when use of a methylmercury fungicide led to poisoning in thousands of people.[24] Studies in New Zealand,[25,26] the Faroe Islands,[27,28] and the Seychelles Islands[29] have followed cohorts to assess the impact of fetal methylmercury exposure. In a review of these three studies, the National Academy of Sciences found strong evidence for neurotoxicity, even at relatively low exposure.[30] Since the NAS report, an American cohort has associated elevated hair mercury levels with decreases in cognition among infants. The association persisted even after controlling for fish consumption by mothers in the data analyses.[31]

In January 2003, the issue of early life exposure to methylmercury became the topic of intense debate after the Environmental Protection Agency announced a proposal to reverse strict controls on emissions of mercury from coal-fired power plants. This proposed "Clear Skies Act" would have slowed recent progress in controlling mercury emission rates from electric generation facilities and would allow these releases to remain as high as twenty-six tons per year through 2010.[32,33] By contrast, existing protections under the Clean Air Act would limit mercury emissions from coal-fired power plants to five tons per year by 2008.[33] EPA's technical analyses in support of Clear Skies failed to incorporate or quantify consideration of the health impacts resulting from increased mercury emissions.[34] After legislative momentum for this proposal faded, EPA promulgated an almost identical Utility Mercury Reductions Rule, which again failed to examine impacts on health.

To inform the policy discussion, a series of analyses were performed to quantify the health and economic costs of prenatal methylmercury toxicity. The first of these analyses found that between 316,588 and 637,233 babies are born each year in the United States with cord blood mercury levels $>5.8\ \mu g/L$. These infants suffer mercury-related losses of cognitive function ranging from 0.2 to 5.13 IQ points. The authors calculated that this loss of cognitive function results in an aggregate economic cost in each annual birth cohort of $8.7 billion annually (range: $0.7–$13.9 billion, 2000 dollars). Of this cost, $1.3 billion (range:

$51 million–$2.0 billion) is attributable to mercury emitted from American coal-fired power plants.[35]

A second analysis quantified the increase in the number of children with mental retardation associated with methylmercury toxicity. This analysis was predicated on the reality that, as methylmercury exposure shifts the distribution of IQ in an exposed population downward, the number of children with an IQ score below 70 (as mental retardation, or MR, is conventionally defined) is increased. This analysis found that downward shifts in IQ resulting from prenatal exposure to methylmercury of anthropogenic origin are associated with 1,566 excess cases of MR annually, or 3.2% of MR cases in the United States. The costs of caring for these children amount to $2.0 billion per year. After incorporating uncertainties in the relationship of IQ loss with increases in blood mercury levels and applying a range for the true cord/maternal mercury ratio, the authors estimated that between 115 and 2,675 excess cases of MR, or 0.2%–5.4% of MR cases in the United States are associated with methylmercury toxicity. Applying a sensitivity analysis, the true cost of caring for children with methylmercury-associated MR was found to range between $28 million and $3.3 billion.[36]

As a result of these and other findings, the EPA's Clean Air Mercury Rule was widely criticized as dangerous to the public's health, and the American Academy of Pediatrics, the American Public Health Association, and a number of leading medical and public health organizations joined thirteen states in a lawsuit that would force the EPA to implement more stringent mercury emissions standards. In their efforts to block the EPA's Clean Air Mercury Rule, they cited the evidence we have provided in the peer-reviewed literature of the health and economic consequences of methylmercury toxicity.[37]

Though these analyses did not ultimately lead to changes in the EPA rule, they were used in the multistate lawsuit against EPA. On February 8, 2008, the U.S. Court of Appeals for the D.C. Circuit ruled that the EPA violated the Clean Air Act by adopting a cap and trade rule that allowed oil and coal-fired plants to purchase credits to cover excessive emissions rather than install pollution controls. In spite of this victory, it was unclear whether the evidence supporting the prenatal methylmercury toxicity would be incorporated in revised regulatory proposals for mercury emissions from coal-fired power plants.

Lead as a Case Study

Despite great progress in elimination of lead from gasoline and paint, recent reports have documented the significant and persistent prevalence of lead-based paint hazards in American homes. An estimated 4.1 million homes in the United

States (25% of U.S. homes with children ages <6 years) have a lead-based paint hazard. Lead-based paint hazards were especially prevalent in housing constructed before 1978, and more than 30% of housing units with lead-based paint contained hazards even when the paint was in good condition.[38]

In 2000, the Secretary of Health and Human Services announced a national goal of ending childhood lead poisoning by 2010.[39] As part of the federal strategy to meet this goal, the President's Task Force on Environmental Health Risks and Safety Risks to Children predicted that a $230 million per year investment over ten years would eliminate lead poisoning in low-income children (<130% of the Federal Poverty Level) under six years of age living in housing built before 1960.[40] Despite this recommendation, funding of HUD's Lead Hazard Control Grant Program has only increased since Fiscal Year 2000 from $60 million to $140 million in fiscal year 2003.[41] It now appears unlikely that the federal government will eliminate lead poisoning in the near future.

Since the task force performed its analysis, a series of studies has also suggested the adverse impact of lead levels in children below 10 µg/dL, the current Centers for Disease Control and Prevention (CDC) definition of an elevated blood level.[42,43] This has not been met with further reductions in the action level set by CDC. As more evidence arrived,[44] further controversy brewed,[45] in part because of the effort to purge members of the Childhood Lead Poisoning Prevention Federal Advisory Committee by the George W. Bush administration to achieve its policy goals.[46]

Whatever the action level set by CDC, efforts must be redoubled to eradicate lead-based paint and other hazards. The economic benefits of lead poisoning prevention are indeed very great, as the elimination of lead in gasoline produced economic benefits on the order of $110–$319 billion annually in enhanced lifetime productivity.[21] As other chemicals of concern emerge, scientific advisory committees cannot have their recommendations ignored or thwarted by political or economic interests.

Outdoor Air Pollution as a Case Study

Asthma prevalence more than doubled in incidence between 1980 and 1996, with prevalence reaching very high rates in urban communities, such as 19% in Hartford, Connecticut, and 25% in the Harlem section of New York City. While more recent U.S. data suggests that there is no longer an increasing trend, only limited decreases in U.S. asthma hospitalization and death rates have been attained despite intensive efforts to optimize outpatient management. A major reason for this quandary is the presence of outdoor air pollutants that are known to worsen and in some cases trigger the development of asthma. In one espe-cially enlightening study, Gent et al. compared 130 children who used mainte-nance medications for asthma with 141 children with asthma who did not use medications. In the group using maintenance medication, each 50 ppb increase in 1-hour average ozone was associated with an increased likelihood of wheezing (by 35%) and chest tightness (by 47%). The authors directly addressed possible confounding effects of other air pollutants and did not find any when they in-cluded fine particles in their analysis.[47] As described earlier in this chapter, the natural experiment produced by traffic restrictions during the 1996 Atlanta Olympics produced decreases in ozone levels that explained decreases in acute care asthma outcomes in children.[48]

Despite proven health concerns about ozone and other air pollutants and benefits of prevention, 122 million people in the United States live in areas exceeding the EPA's ozone standard.[49] A 2004 American Academy of Pediatrics policy statement, "Ambient Air Pollution: Health Hazards to Children," recom-mended that National Ambient Air Quality Standards for PM_{10}, $PM_{2.5}$, O_3, and NO_2 be revised in light of recent studies that suggest that children are not ade-quately protected by current regulations.[50]

In the relative absence of federal regulations, states have interceded to enact regulations that limit significant point sources of outdoor air pollutants. California has instituted model regulations for other states and the federal gov-ernment in its diesel emissions requirements, instituting a cap on particulate matter emissions beginning in model year 2004. Several years later, the federal government implemented similar regulations including requiring ultra-low-sulfur diesel fuel and capping particulate matter emissions from heavy-duty engines. To limit exposures in the school setting, four states have implemented legislation or regulation that limits the time allowed for school bus idling and/ or requires a minimum distance for the parking of buses near school buildings. Additionally, ten states have implemented retrofit programs for school buses.[51] While federal regulation and legislation can produce greater uniformity in prevention of childhood disease and disability across states, state policy inter-ventions can be very effective in limiting exposures until national policy accel-erates and reflects scientific and public health concerns.

The National Children's Study

In response to rising rates of chronic childhood conditions and increasing con-cerns about environmental factors contributing to these conditions, the U.S. Congress, through the Children's Health Act of 2000, authorized the National

Institute of Child Health and Human Development (NICHD) "to conduct a national longitudinal study of environmental influences (including physical, chemical, biological and psychosocial) on children's health and development."[52] The National Institute of Environmental Health Sciences (NIEHS), the CDC, and the EPA have joined the NICHD in planning this study, now named the **National Children's Study (NCS),** a longitudinal study of 100,000 U.S. children to identify the preventable and environmental causes of chronic disease in childhood.

NCS is an ambitious, observational, longitudinal study of 100,000 U.S. children that is intended to identify the preventable and environmental causes of chronic disease in childhood. Participants will be recruited before conception or early pregnancy and their children will be followed through age 21. Families who are enrolled in the study will participate in a minimum of fifteen in-person visits with research teams across stages of development (that is, before conception; three times during pregnancy; at birth; at 1, 6, 12, and 18 months of age in early childhood; at 3, 5, 7, 9, and 12 years of age in childhood; and at 16 and 20 years of age in adolescence). Seven of these visits will be in the participants' homes, and eight will be in clinical settings, including the infants' places of delivery. Data will be remotely collected via telephone, computer, or mail-in questionnaires every three months through the age of 5 and annually thereafter. Biological samples from the mother and child to measure body burdens of environmental chemicals and environmental samples such as air, water, dirt, and dust from the child's home environment will be collected over the course of the study. Individual parent, child, and family psychosocial domains to be assessed include family composition, family conflict, mother and/or father's physical and mental health history, mother and/or father's current emotional and cognitive adjustment, parent–child interaction, and quality of the caretaking environment.[53]

Six of the chronic diseases that the study plans to examine—obesity, injury, asthma, diabetes, schizophrenia, and autism—cost America $642 billion per year. If the NCS were to produce a reduction of only 1% in incidence of these diseases, the annual savings would amount to $6.4 billion, far more than the $2.7 billion price tag of the study over twenty-five years.

Regulatory Policy and Children

Despite strong and emerging scientific evidence about environmental hazards to children's health, regulatory policy has lagged behind. The current **Toxic Substances Control Act (TSCA),** the main legislation that regulates approval of chemicals for their widespread distribution into the environment, makes the presumption that, even in the absence of toxicological testing data, chemicals cause no injury to health until injury is irrefutably proven. Chemicals are reviewed by the EPA for a ninety-day period prior to approval without any requirement for toxicity testing. Most chemicals are approved without the most basic testing for their potential to cause toxicity in animals or in humans. In large part, these deficits derive from the absence of revisions to TSCA since its becoming law in 1976.[54]

In response to the findings of the NAS report (Section 6.2), the U.S. Congress unanimously passed into law the **Food Quality Protection Act (FQPA) of 1996**. In contrast to TSCA, this legislation specifically directs EPA to use an additional tenfold safety factor in assessing the risks to infants and children to take into account the potential for pre- and postnatal toxicity, particularly when the toxicology and exposure databases are judged to be incomplete. The statute also authorizes EPA to replace this default tenfold "FQPA safety factor" with a different factor only if, based on reliable data, the resulting margin would be adequate to protect infants and children.[55] While implementation of FQPA remains an ongoing challenge, and some regulatory thresholds have still not been set, this legislation represents a watershed moment in the recognition of the unique vulnerability of children with regard to environmental hazards. Before the U.S. Environmental Protection Agency phase-out of diazinon and chlorpyrifos, which resulted from FQPA, these two pesticides were frequently detected in the cord blood of New York City children and associated with decrements in birth weight and length. After these phase-outs, the pesticides and the association with predictors of cognitive potential were no longer detected.[56]

Another watershed moment was President Bill Clinton's **Executive Order 13045**, which established a President's Task Force on Environmental Health Risks and Safety Risks to Children. It was co-chaired by the Secretary of the Department of Health and Human Services and the Administrator of the Environmental Protection Agency. The task force was specifically directed to develop measures to protect children from environmental hazards[57] and played a critical role in efforts to fund eradication of lead-based paint hazards from homes. These efforts worked toward achieving the Surgeon General's Healthy People 2010 goal of eradicating childhood lead poisoning.[3] The task force played a critical role in informing the design of the National Children's Study.[58]

Summary

Children have unique vulnerabilities to environmental toxicants stemming from in utero exposure to mothers, exposure as neonates and young children, and extending into adolescence. As examples, heavy metals such as mercury and lead have abilities to affect mental development and attained IQ. The National Children's Study will follow 100,000 children prospectively to analyze environmental and genetic contributions to diseases such as obesity and autism.

Key Terms

Executive Order 13045

Food Quality Protection Act of 1996

National Children's Study

Toxic Substances Control Act

Discussion Questions

1. Why are children uniquely vulnerable to environmental hazards?
2. Outline the history of protection of children against environmental hazards.
3. How do mercury, lead, and outdoor air pollution affect children's health?
4. How are mercury, lead, and outdoor air pollution regulated by the government?
5. What are the goals of the National Children's Study?

The author thanks the Environmental Health Perspectives (ref. 35) for permission to reproduce parts of the article.

CHAPTER 7

THE ROLE OF COMMUNITY ADVOCACY GROUPS IN ENVIRONMENTAL PROTECTION

Example of September 11, 2001

Catherine McVay Hughes
Kimberly Flynn
Craig Hall
Joan Reibman

LEARNING OBJECTIVES

- To understand how community and labor-based organizations allied to press government agencies for a comprehensive emergency response to the environment during the aftermath of the September 11, 2001, attacks on the World Trade Center
- To be able to discuss the Community Advisory Committee (CAC) that resulted from the World Trade Center disaster

The terrorist attacks on the World Trade Center (WTC) in New York City on September 11, 2001, resulted in one of the worst environmental disasters ever to hit a major American city. This chapter illustrates the ways many diverse community and labor-based organizations, from across Lower Manhattan and beyond, allied with each other to press government agencies and officials at the federal, state, and local levels for a comprehensive emergency response to the environmental aftermath of the 9/11 attacks. Key lessons were learned in the following eight years of struggle. (These lessons are summarized at the end of the chapter.) Many affected groups united in the call for a federally funded **World Trade Center (WTC) Environmental Health Center (EHC)** to provide specialized health care for all residents, students, and area workers whose health was harmed by WTC exposures. In 2007, the groups formed the **Community Advisory Committee (CAC) to the WTC EHC** at New York City Health & Hospitals Corporation at Bellevue Hospital, which now has expanded to two additional clinics. It is the CAC's mission to draw on the expertise and experiences of its members to advise the WTC EHC and ensure that the evolving WTC-related health care needs of the affected communities are met, now and in the future. The CAC serves as a brain trust with a sophisticated real-world set of lessons learned that should inform a community advocacy framework for future disasters. This chapter illuminates the perspective of these community-based advocacy organizations.

Communication of information from government agencies is critical for residents, students, school parents, and office workers to help them understand the health risks of being exposed to the WTC toxic dust and smoke that pervaded the area surrounding the World Trade Center, indoors and out, after the disaster. 9/11 resulted in massive displacements, disruption of basic services, factory and small business closures, and job loss in Lower Manhattan, with ripple effects well beyond the area hit with the heaviest damage. Attempts to address the multiplicity of disaster-related needs of neighborhoods posed unprecedented challenges to those who lived and worked there, including community advocates and activists.

When residents, workers, parents, and advocates sought government help, they confronted an array of agencies on the federal, state, and local levels that had been tasked with a variety of disaster-related functions. Typically, agencies disavowed their disaster duties and passed the buck to other agencies. On the environmental health front, the Environmental Protection

THE WORLD TRADE CENTER ENVIRONMENTAL HEALTH CENTER COMMUNITY ADVISORY COMMITTEE

The World Trade Center Environmental Health Center (WTC EHC) Community Advisory Committee (CAC) includes, but is not limited to, the following list of organizations:

- 105 Duane Street Residents
- 125 Cedar Street Residents
- 9/11 Environmental Action
- Beyond Ground Zero Network
- Civil Service Employees Association
- Communications Workers of America District 1
- Concerned Stuyvesant Community
- AFSCME District Council 37
- Ecuadorian International Center
- Good Old Lower East Side, Inc. (GOLES)
- Henry Street Settlement
- Lin Sing Association
- Independence Plaza North Tenants Association (IPN)
- Manhattan Community Board 1
- Manhattan Community Board 2
- Manhattan Community Board 3
- New York from the Ground Up
- New York Committee for Occupational Safety & Health (NYCOSH)
- New York State Public Employees Federation Division 199
- New York State Laborers' Union
- Organization of Staff Analysts (OSA)
- Rebuild.Downtown.Our.Town
- Rebuild with a Spotlight on the Poor
- South Bridge Tower Residents Coalition
- Stuyvesant High School Parents Association
- University Settlement
- World Trade Center Residents Coalition (WTCRC)

Agency (EPA) simply asserted, without evidence, that the air was safe, with Mayor Rudy Giuliani and other agencies following suit.[1]

In response to this failure of government to protect the public, the community and some labor-based organizations engaged in on-the-ground organizing efforts to compel the government to disclose the WTC hazards and to educate their affected constituencies about the dangers in the dust and smoke. For the first six months after 9/11, different groups framed a spectrum of different environmental health demands: WTC health care for those already experiencing symptoms; reparations for those whose health and ability to work would be permanently damaged; and a science-based effective cleanup of WTC contamination from people's homes, schools, and workplaces that would prevent further harm from chronic exposures, to name the most notable tasks.

Since 2003, these groups have advocated for the health of the affected communities. They have demanded corrective action from agencies still entrenched in denials of the health risks and later health impacts. The individuals and organizations that comprise the WTC EHC CAC have attempted to hold accountable, among others, the EPA, the Federal Emergency Management Administration (FEMA), the New York City Department of Health and Mental Hygiene (NYCDOHMH), the New York City Office of Emergency Management (NYCOEM), and the Lower Manhattan Development Corporation (LMDC). At times, even their best efforts were enough only to prevent the government or its agencies from acting with even greater negligence. However, WTC EHC CAC believe they have made important gains that construct a foundation for future efforts to improve the protections of the public in the event of disasters.

Early on, the community questioned the safety of the air quality indoors and outdoors and the adequacy of the government response. For many members of the CAC, the most productive partnership with a government agency has been work with WTC EHC. Provided following are snapshots of critical moments in their struggle. A more extensive timeline appears at the end of the chapter.

The Disaster

On September 11, 2001, terrorists attacked the United States by hijacking four airplanes and crashing two of them into the two 110-story World Trade Center towers, leading to the towers' collapse, destroying the WTC complex, killing nearly 2,800 individuals, and severely damaging many other skyscrapers. (See Figure 7.1.) Everything inside the WTC towers (thousands of computers containing lead and mercury; florescent lights containing mercury; and plastics of every kind, just to name a few materials) was broken apart and became part of the dust cloud that resulted from the towers' fall.

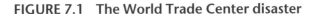

FIGURE 7.1   The World Trade Center disaster

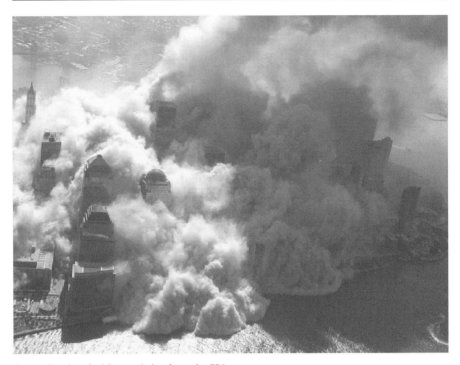

Source: Reprinted with permission from the EPA.

Indeed, the destruction of the towers resulted in the unprecedented massive release of hundreds of tons of asbestos, fiberglass, lead, highly alkaline concrete dust, polycyclic aromatic hydrocarbons (PAHs), and many other toxic substances. The massive clouds from the collapse chased people down the streets, blocking out the sun and choking those caught in the clouds. Moreover, the dust infiltrated buildings over a wide geographic area, forcing tiny particulates at very high speed into every possible point of entry, including closed windows and ventilation systems. WTC debris traveled as far as Brooklyn and New Jersey, and WTC fires could be smelled there for months. The destruction would leave 16 acres of burning rubble, quickly named "the pile." Ground Zero became the focal point for the cleanup and later the rescue; and cleanup workers were called "responders," and those exposed to the dust as residents and workers in the area "survivors."

In the absence of any agency-coordinated evacuation, downtown residents, office workers, and students were left to fend for themselves. While many fled the area, many others stayed in the immediate vicinity. Cellular communications failed first, followed by land lines, Internet, electricity, water, and gas. As early as September 12, some residents and office workers were forced to return to indoor spaces that were virtual moonscapes, with heavy dust coatings on every surface. Many suffered eye and throat irritation, nosebleeds, and WTC cough. Fires burned and smoldered, releasing pollutants carried by the wind, creating a powerful odor that could be smelled for many miles. Chaos reigned. Access to basic services was disrupted.

Two days after 9/11, as residents confronted the environmental conditions in their homes and workplaces, ABC News reported, "Despite fires and a pungent odor at the wreckage of the World Trade Center, most tests for contaminants in New York's air have not triggered alarm, health officials say. U.S. Environmental Protection Agency spokeswoman said Wednesday that EPA officials 'really don't detect any real danger' in air and dust tests. And New York Mayor Rudolph Giuliani echoed the sentiments this morning. . . . "[2]

On September 18, then-EPA Administrator Christine Todd Whitman gave a White House–mandated assurance that the "air was safe to breathe." With these reassurances, people moved back to normal activities and were thus exposed to dangerous materials. Certainly, owners and tenants were forced back when federal and city agencies reopened contaminated buildings as insurance firms stopped payments to landlords, tenants, and residents. Some tenant–landlord struggles erupted in lawsuits when landlords sued tenants who moved out, often at the advice of their doctors and pediatricians. Local area vacancy rates exceeded 45%. Some Battery Park City–based residents formed the 9/11 Tenants Association, which later expanded to become the WTC Residents Coalition. The same process unfolded in other buildings to the north and east. For many months after 9/11, the 16 acres of WTC dust and debris was transported in loosely covered or open trucks and past several schools, then was dumped onto a hazardous debris barge in a residential area next to the air intakes for Stuyvesant High School. Fires continued to burn through March 2002; even after the major fires were out, smaller fires flared as debris removal exposed them to oxygen.

In early spring, groups of residents and school parents, beleaguered by their separate struggles with unresponsive agencies, began to recognize the need to pull affected constituencies together into a united front.

Snapshot 2002: WTC Environmental Summit

On April 12, 2002, seven months after 9/11, as the EPA continued to resist demands that it address WTC contamination in indoor commercial and residential spaces, U.S. Rep. Jerrold Nadler (D-NY) released his "White Paper: Lower Manhattan Air Quality," calling on the EPA "to redeem itself and to make Lower Manhattan truly safe."

Shortly thereafter, representatives of WTC residents, tenants, and environmental and parent groups organized an environmental summit meeting to define a new, united approach to ridding their neighborhoods and schools of toxic contamination. After being briefed by Rep. Nadler and Hugh Kaufman, at that time the EPA's National Ombudsman's Office Chief Investigator, on the EPA's legal responsibilities under the National Contingency Plan—a blueprint for the federal government for responding to both oil spills and hazardous substance releases—more than forty organizations (including New York Committee for Occupational Safety & Health, Natural Resources Defense Council, and the WTC Residential Coalition) voted to abandon the strategy of fighting for landlord cleanup. Instead, they agreed to move forward together, demanding that the EPA take the lead role in a comprehensive indoor test and cleanup program for all affected areas.

This was followed shortly by a conference called "Beyond September 11—Environmental and Public Health Policy: A Working Conference" on May 9, 2002. It was organized by the New York Committee for Occupational Safety and Health (NYCOSH) and the City University of New York and was co-sponsored by thirty-eight grassroots organizations. More than 200 participants representing more than eighty labor, community, faith-based, environmental, immigrant, tenant, and public health organizations attended.[3]

Ironically, that evening, the Children's Allergy, Immunology and Respiratory (AIR) Foundation was honoring EPA Administrator Christie Todd Whitman for her commitment to asthma prevention with its Gift of Breath Award "for raising awareness of the environment as a possible first line of defense against asthma." Outside the event, 9/11 Environmental Action held a protest attended by some fifty affected residents, school parents, and worker safety advocates from NYCOSH.

In the fall of 2001, the **Beyond Ground Zero (BGZ) Network** was formed from community-based organizations working together to address severe health and economic impact resulting from 9/11 on Lower Manhattan's low-income communities. In 2002, the National Mobilization Against Sweatshops (NMASS) and the Chinese Staff and Workers' Association (CSWA) partnered with the Asian American Legal Defense and Education Fund (AALDEF), the Commission of the Public's Health System (CPHS), and the Community Development Project of the Urban Justice Center (UJC). This network brought together a unique combination of legal and political, public health, participatory research experience, and worker's rights and compensation expertise.[4]

In 2002, BGZ began surveying their target population, which consisted of the immigrants and the poorest residents and workers in Chinatown and the Lower East Side. BGZ found that thousands of people were still coping with health issues that resulted from 9/11 and that there was no access to health care or assistance. BGZ began to mobilize people on a larger scale to address unmet health care needs through a series of events. They organized two major town hall meetings in May 2002—one of which was attended by 2,000 people at PS 124 in Chinatown. These meetings led to BGZ's 7,000-person march from the Lower East Side to Foley Square in Chinatown on June 5, 2002. The fight for health care for residents and people affected by 9/11 was then taken to Washington, D.C. On July 31, 2002, BGZ sponsored the "March for Our Health, March for Our Lives" for which 1,000 people rallied.

Meanwhile, as a result of the advocacy of labor unions and some elected officials, in the spring of 2002 Congress provided initial limited funding for a one-time screening for responders under the WTC Worker and Volunteer Medical Screening Program, coordinated by the Mount Sinai Medical Center. At this time, however, there was still no recognition of need or funding for the WTC health needs of those living and working in the vicinity of Ground Zero and beyond.

Snapshot 2003: EPA Inspector General Releases Reports

Near the two-year anniversary of 9/11, the U.S. EPA Office of Inspector General (OIG) released two reports that confirmed what many had suspected. The August 21, 2003, "Evaluation Report: EPA's Response to the World Trade Center Collapse: Challenges, Successes, and Areas for Improvement" concluded:

> EPA's early public statements following the collapse of the WTC towers reassured the public regarding the safety of the air outside the Ground Zero area.[1] However, when EPA made a September 18 announcement that the air was "safe" to breathe, it did not have sufficient data and analyses to make such a blanket statement. At that time, air monitoring data was lacking for several pollutants of concern, including particulate matter and polychlorinated biphenyls (PCBs). Furthermore, The White House Council on Environmental Quality influenced, through the collaboration process, the information that EPA communicated to the public through its early press releases when it convinced EPA to add reassuring statements and delete cautionary ones. An EPA draft risk evaluation completed over a year after the attacks concluded that, after the first few days, ambient air levels were unlikely to cause short-term or long-term health effects to the general population. However, because of numerous uncertainties—including the extent of the public's exposure and lack of health-based benchmarks—a definitive answer to whether that the air was safe to breathe may not be settled for years to come.

A month later the EPA OIG released another evaluation report called the "Evaluation Report: Survey of Air Quality Information Related to the World Trade Center Collapse" on September 26, 2003.[5] This report found that "overall, the majority of respondents wanted more information regarding outdoor and indoor air quality, wanted this information in a more timely manner, and did not believe the information they received."

Snapshot 2003–2004: Gains on Rebuilding Environmental Protections

With increased awareness about air quality after 9/11, the need to make Lower Manhattan livable, and with consistent public pressure at community board meetings and public hearings during the initial years of the rebuilding process, some gains were made on environmental protections.

In November 2001, a state–city authority called the **Lower Manhattan Development Corporation (LMDC)** was created to help in the planning and coordinating process of rebuilding Lower Manhattan. LMDC was funded through a community development block grant from the U.S. Department of Housing and Urban Development (HUD). In 2003, LMDC adopted an environmental framework for the rebuilding of the WTC site. It consisted of four components:

(1) Green Design, Green Construction, and Sustainability Principles;
(2) Construction of Environmental Protection Plan
(3) Public Involvement and Government Entities Coordination Plan;
(4) Baseline Assessment of Resources & Coordinated Cumulative Effects Analysis.[6]

As a result, every WTC office tower, Santiago Calatrava's WTC Transportation Hub (the design evokes the image of a bird in flight and will deliver natural light to the train platform 60 feet below), and the 9/11 Memorial & Museum were aiming for the Leadership in Energy and Environmental Design (LEED) gold rating. The U.S. Green Building Council has a building certificate program that encourages a sustainable building rating system that recognizes projects that implement best environmental and health performance. LEED professional credentials and exams are administered by a Green Building Certification Institute. LMDC is tracking the sustainability of the entire 16-acre WTC site, the largest commercial sustainable site in the country.

With increased public concern about air quality, it was necessary to reduce the impact of diesel engines during the rebuilding process. A private public initiative called the "7 WTC Diesel Emissions Reduction Project," with developer

Silverstein Properties working with their contractors to use less polluting ultra-low-sulfur diesel fuel (ULSD) and best available technology retrofits for off-road diesel construction equipment to reduce emission pollutants in 2002, was successful. This pilot study, along with the community, led to Local Law 77 Use of Ultra Low Sulfur Diesel Fuel by Nonroad Vehicles, which Mayor Michael Bloomberg signed into law on December 22, 2003. It extended ULSD use and retrofits to all of Lower Manhattan and public work contracts. This was a win-win for both the workers and the surrounding community.

With the support of business leaders and the community, a new state and city agency called the **Lower Manhattan Construction Command Center (LMCCC)** was created in November 2004. LMCCC was to coordinate the massive redevelopment of the WTC site and surrounding area, involving more than $30 billion and consisting of sixty ongoing construction projects in less than one square mile in a short period of time by city, state, and federal agencies, private developers, and utilities. In addition, LMCCC was to oversee the implementation of the Environmental Performance Commitments (EPC), which include the oversight, monitoring, and mitigation of air, noise, and, vibration. At the request of Community Board 1, the air quality monitoring data was posted on a public access website in real time so that timely intervention could be made, if necessary. As a result of engineering controls in Lower Manhattan, the background levels of particulate matter (2.5 and 10) were below that of 9/11 using EPA's benchmark for National Air Quality Standards. The EPC framework could be considered for large-scale, complicated construction projects in dense urban environments.[7]

An example of community input in emergency response was the creation of the **Community Emergency Response Team (CERT)** in the summer of 2003 in Battery Park City (BPC), the area just west of the WTC site. The BPC CERT was formed as a direct result of 9/11 and its aftermath. It was the first CERT created on the east coast and in April 2005 was followed by the Tribeca CERT, which covered the area north of the WTC site. The community realized that after a major disaster such as 9/11, police, fire, and EMT workers were stretched to the breaking point. The BPC CERT drew from doctors, police, firefighters, and experienced CERT trainers to train local area residents in emergency rescue and medical care techniques. They were taught fire suppression, crowd control, search and rescue, and emergency medical treatment. A high percentage of the members undertook and were certified as Red Cross First Aiders. Later, sea search and rescue was added, with the addition of BPC's own rescue boat. A number of individuals from the group volunteered to help in the aftermath of Hurricane Katrina in New Orleans in 2005. CERT teams definitely have a role, but they need to be cognizant of their abilities in complementing existing first responders during an emergency and knowing when to exit the area.

Snapshot 2004: Bellevue WTC Health Impacts Clinic and EPA WTC Expert Technical Review Panel

Dr. Joan Reibman, NYU School of Medicine academic pulmonary physician at Bellevue Hospital Center, had worked with the NYS Department of Health on a WTC Residents Respiratory Health Study to assess the incidence of new-onset asthma and other respiratory symptoms after 9/11 and the persistence of symptoms. In May 2002, Asthma Moms organized the first Asthma Day in the WTC area. Dr. Reibman agreed to come into the streets to try to answer the medical questions of traumatized and sometimes angry community residents. Although BGZ had been meeting with Dr. Reibman over the years, BGZ, armed with the health survey data, reached out to Bellevue Hospital in 2004. Bellevue Hospital and the BGZ partnership worked to create the Bellevue WTC Health Impacts Clinic for BGZ residents and workers. This was the first program that treated nonresponders for WTC-related illnesses. A unique feature of the program was volunteers who did outreach through door-to-door surveys, town hall meetings, and the formation of a local community center. In 2005 BGZ and Bellevue were funded from the Red Cross September 11 Recovery Grant.[4]

In March 2004, Sen. Hillary Clinton of New York had forced the EPA to convene this scientific advisory panel to review EPA's response. The purpose of the panel was "to obtain greater input on ongoing efforts to monitor the situation for workers and residents impacted by the collapse of the World Trade Center. An expert technical review panel, convened by EPA, was formed to help facilitate the Agency's use of available exposure and health surveillance databases and registries to characterize any remaining exposures and risks, identify unmet public health needs, and recommend any steps to further minimize the risks associated with the aftermath of the World Trade Center attacks." Only after public pressure did the EPA include a community liaison as an ex-officio panel member. Although WTC community and labor representatives were meeting periodically, this twenty-one-month process formalized the World Trade Center Community Labor Coalition. It became a unified force that was much more powerful than its separate groups. Many of these groups now have representatives on the WTC EHC CAC.

After several panel meetings and public pressure, EPA allowed a labor representative in July 2004, in addition to the community liaison, to be seated on the panel. One key community gain came that same day: the 125 Cedar Street Residents, whose building sits directly across the street from the heavily contaminated Deutsche Bank building, delivered a PowerPoint presentation, raising key concerns and emphasizing the need for EPA to exercise oversight of all aspects of the building's demolition. At that time, WTC damaged buildings could still be demolished without environmental oversight or appropriate precautions, as if no contamination was present.

EPA shut down the EPA WTC Expert Technical Panel after its twelfth meeting in December 13, 2005. This was after EPA released its final Test and Clean Program, which was underfunded and inadequate. This technically and scientifically flawed program would repeat the most serious limitations and deficiencies of the 2002 program as delineated by the inspector general. The deficiencies included defining a limited geographic area, not addressing buildings as an integrated system, omitting mechanical ventilation systems, and excluding workplaces, schools, small businesses, and firehouses. Although there was an original split at the beginning of the panel process in March 2004 between public-focused committee members and the scientific agency members, it eventually aligned against the EPA. The EPA again proceeded with its limited test program, which resulted in limited participation. Although the panel process was a frustrating one, it did provide enough public pressure that the EPA took a leadership role in the deconstruction of several large WTC-contaminated buildings, including 130 Liberty Street (Deutsche Bank) in December 2004.

The community labor presentation requested that the EPA follow the "Precautionary Principle" during the EPA WTC Expert Technical Panel Process (2004): If the precautionary principle was initially followed, much of the exposure of the WTC toxins could have been limited and the first responders and community could have taken the necessary precautions, which would have limited liability, medical, and legal costs.

Snapshot 2006: WTC Bellevue Environmental Health Center Announced

Public pressure for health care for the WTC residents, students, and office workers who were affected by 9/11 was mounting as the five-year anniversary approached. One public town hall event and an announcement by Mayor Bloomberg marked a major turning point in the recognition of 9/11 health impacts to the community. On September 5, 2006, Mayor Bloomberg and Health and Hospitals Corporation President Alan Aviles announced the establishment of the WTC Environmental Health Center at Bellevue

Hospital Center. It would expand medical and mental health treatment to nonresponders exposed to the toxic dust and fumes at the WTC. This timely financial commitment was critical, since the private Red Cross funding for the limited WTC-related health services for the BGZ community was coming to an end in 2006. It had taken five years for the first public funds to be allocated to provide outreach and treat residents, office workers, students, and other affected people. Since then, the WTC EHC expanded to Gouverneur and Elmhurst Hospitals.

The following day, on September 6, 2006, 9/11 Environmental Action sponsored a town hall forum: "Affected but Neglected: the Impact of 9/11 on Community Health and a Call for Federal Action." More than 300 residents, office workers, parents, and students filled St. Paul's Chapel, located across the street from the WTC site. Findings were presented by doctors from the two centers for excellence (Bellevue and Mount Sinai, respectively) that treated both nonresponder and responder populations and by the New York Committee on Occupational Safety and Health. The moderator was Juan Gonzalez, who more than any other reporter had written early on about WTC air quality and 9/11 health impacts for the *New York Daily News*. Still, after five years, many people had questions. Consequently, after the formal presentations, there was a very long line at the microphone to ask questions of the medical and scientific experts.

Snapshot 2009: Community Advisory Committee

The Community Advisory Committee (CAC) of the WTC EHC of the New York City Health and Hospitals Corporation (HHC) developed out of the fluid collaborative process over the years to tackle environmental health issues arising after 9/11. The CAC illustrated how community collaboration can play a major role in developing and delivering effective medical services to diverse populations, often requiring unique outreach in numerous languages, from Chinese to Polish. In addition, the CAC has taken an integral role in advising WTC EHC scientists on proposed research of WTC environmental health impacts to the community. The WTC EHC CAC has operated on the community-based participatory research model and has shown what genuine partnership can accomplish—unlike the community's long experience in the EPA WTC Expert Technical Panel Process. The WTC EHC CAC is an arena for direct, meaningful input on the part of the participating organizations and individual members. For example, as it became apparent that children were suffering from serious and lasting WTC health consequences, the community began to press for a pediatric division at the WTC EHC. In October 2007, it was announced that a pediatrician would join the Bellevue clinic staff.

Summary and Lessons Learned

We present here a short list of lessons learned of interest not only to environmental advocates, but also to policymakers.

1. *Push for prevention first.* The first rule of environmental health is to prevent further harm by preventing further exposures. Government health and environmental authorities must issue proper risk communications, must provide the proper safety equipment, such as respirators, and must enforce their use. In the case of the WTC disaster, EPA should have conducted representative testing and comprehensive cleanup, indoors and out, in all affected neighborhoods, as prescribed by the National Contingency Plan.

2. *Apply the "Precautionary Principle."* This means that the public should be protected from harm when there is plausible risk, although a direct relationship between cause and effect may not be definitively concluded, and that decision-making process be democratic and include the potentially affected party. For example, in the WTC environmental disaster, where emerging illnesses were not instantaneous, the burden of proof should fall on the party advocating an action—or in this case, inaction—instead of the exposed community. The community called upon the EPA to follow the Precautionary Principle during the EPA WTC Expert Technical Panel Process (2004).

3. *Recognize and support the public's right-to-know.* Environmental struggles are often first and foremost battles over the truth about health risks. The community's first step is to press for the public release of all relevant data and information.

4. *Recognize and support the public's right to have input.* The community has a right to have meaningful input into the formulation of government policies that affect the public's health. An open, transparent public process is the foundation for community involvement and input and the appropriate arena for community engagement at every stage in environmental health decision making—from designing studies, to designing testing, cleanup or mitigation programs, to planning and preparedness for disasters. Public process can also serve as the "court of public opinion," especially when the media are

present, and thus can be an effective means to educate and mobilize the broader public.

5. *Educate for engagement.* Although most students are required to take a civics class sometime in the course of their education, the real nuts and bolts of civic engagement are not taught. Consumer advocate Ralph Nader, who pioneered the Freedom of Information Act, was right to call for a "university requirement of civil practice aimed at bolstering the ability of ordinary citizens to protect and advance their interests." Nader has observed that although universities excel at the production of knowledge, they lag when it comes to putting it into practice.[3] It is not enough for people to know their rights; they also need to understand how the wheels of government turn, and especially how the community can gain traction for its demands. Much of the success of the community has relied on its ability to seize every opportunity for civic engagement, whether that was with the community boards, the New York City Council, the EPA WTC Expert Technical Panel, or the affected community representatives to the U.S. Congress. Institutionalized resistance to community calls for more protective policies exist at every level of government.

Key Terms

Beyond Ground Zero (BGZ) Network

Community Advisory Committee (CAC) to the WTC EHC

Community Emergency Response Team (CERT)

Lower Manhattan Construction Command Center (LMCCC)

Lower Manhattan Development Corporation (LMDC)

World Trade Center (WTC) Environmental Health Center (EHC)

Discussion Questions

1. Summarize the role played by community groups in advocating for environmental protections after 9/11.
2. Summarize the government response to post–9/11 health risks.
3. Summarize the lessons learned about community groups and their ability to advocate for environmental health protections.

WTC ENVIRONMENTAL HEALTH HISTORY TIMELINE

2001

September 11: Terrorists hijacked two airplanes (American Airlines Flight 11 and United Airlines Flight 175) and attacked the United States by crashing them into the World Trade Center (WTC) Towers 1 and 2, leading to their collapse and destruction of the WTC complex (including WTC Tower 7), killing nearly 2,800 individuals, and severely damaging many other skyscrapers.

September 14: "OSHA, EPA, Update Asbestos Data. Continue to reassure public of contamination fears . . . The U.S. Environmental Protection Agency and the Department of Labor's Occupational Safety and Health Administration today announced that the majority of air and dust samples monitored in New York's financial district do not indicate levels of concern for asbestos. The new samples confirm previous reports that ambient air quality meets OSHA standards and consequently is not a case for public concern. New OSHA data also indicates that indoor air quality in downtown buildings will meet standards."[1,3]

Initial days after 9/11: International Union of Operating Engineers and Transport Workers Union Local 100 began to test the air at Ground Zero and many unions (including AFSCME District Council 37, TWU Local 100, Public Employee Federation, Civil Service Employees Association, Communications Workers of America, Association of Legal Aid Attorneys, Professional Staff Congress) working in buildings in Lower Manhattan to determine what their members might be exposed to; NYCOSH worked closely with the unions and community, immigrant and tenant organizations and issued the first WTC fact sheets and conducted outdoor and indoor sampling; Tenant groups (BPC, Independence Plaza North, 105 Duane Street, and 125 Cedar Street) and parent associations at seven neighboring public schools began to organize around environmental health issues.

September 17: The New York Stock Exchange on Wall Street reopened for first time after 9/11 after being closed for four business days; NYCDOH responds to the WTC disaster with "Recommendations for People Re-Occupying Commercial Buildings and Residents Re-Entering Their Homes" . . . "*How should I clean the dust in my apartment when I move back in?* The best way to remove dust is to use a wet rag or wet mop. Sweeping with a dry broom is not recommended because it can make dust airborne again. Where dust is thick, you can directly wet the dust with water, and remove it with wet rags and mops."

October 11: First Community Forum on 9/11 Health took place at PACE University.

October: NYCOSH meetings foster first discussion among diverse labor unions of health consequences of WTC environmental exposures.

Fall: Beyond Ground Zero (BGZ) Network was formed.

December 18: "Residents Rally Over Air Quality in Lower Manhattan . . . More than 100 downtown residents gathered on the steps of City Hall Tuesday night to protest what they say is unsafe air quality in Lower Manhattan. Many of the protesters say the air downtown is still making residents, students, and workers sick. They want city officials to relocate the removal of debris away from large housing complexes . . . ."[3]

2002

January 24: "Some Concerns Remain as High Schools Closest to Ground Zero Prepare to Reopen."[3]

January 25: "Parents concerned about the conditions of an elementary school just blocks from Ground Zero were in court Friday. School officials insist PS 89 is safe, but parents aren't ready to take their word for it."[5]

April 12: U.S. Rep. Jerrold Nadler released white paper, "Lower Manhattan Air Quality."

April 20: Environmental Health Summit with Lower Manhattan community, tenant, environmental, and school groups and Rep. Jerrold Nadler agreed to demand that EPA perform a comprehensive sampling and cleanup.

Spring: Congress agreed to provide initial limited funding for the WTC Worker and Volunteer Medical Screening Program, based initially at Mount Sinai Medical Center (later growing to five additional clinics) after much union campaigning.[1]

May 7: First Mobile Asthma Program for Annual World Asthma Day for NYC WTC Downtown Residents and Workers sponsored by Asthma Moms, Bellevue Hospital Center-Asthma Clinic, NYU, and American Lung Association of New York.

May 8: EPA to clean WTC apartments to "reassure" residents after much public pressure; a reversal of EPA's earlier position that EPA is not responsible for indoor conditions that resulted from 9/11; 9/11EA and NYCOSH met with EPA to try to strengthen the limited program with little success.

May 9: NYCOSH/City University of New York conference "Beyond September 11: Environmental and Public Health Policy, A Working Conference" co-sponsored by thirty-eight grassroots organizations and attended by more than 200 participants representing labor, community, faith-based, environmental, and public health organizations.

May 5 and 19: Major town hall meetings called by BGZ; included 2,000 people in PS 124 in Chinatown to mobilize people to address unmet health care needs.

June 5: Major march with about 7,000 people from the Lower East Side to Foley Square, Chinatown organized by BGZ.

July 31: 1,000 people rallied in Washington, D.C, for "March for Our Health, March for Our Lives" sponsored by BGZ for health care for residents and people affected by 9/11.

July: EPA began cleanup "pilot program in an unoccupied building at 110 Liberty St. to test eight techniques for removing indoor dust and debris. Air and dust will be tested for a wide range of pollutants before and after the cleaning."[8]

July: WTC Health Registry created by Agency for Toxic Substances and Disease Registry and NYCDOH to monitor the health of those directly exposed to the WTC disaster; initial funds from FEMA.

2003

March 26: The New York City Department of Environmental Protection (DEP) completed work removing the dust and debris that accumulated on the roofs, windows, and facades of downtown buildings following the WTC collapse. At the project's close, DEP crews had cleaned the exteriors of 221 buildings, totaling more than 3.6 million square feet.

May 6: Second Annual World Asthma Day for NYC WTC Downtown Residents and Workers held in Tribeca and Chinatown; participants included Asthma Moms, NYU, Bellevue Hospital Center Asthma Clinic, American Lung Association of New York, and AALDEF.

September 23: Environmental Protection Agency, Office of Inspector General releases "Evaluation Report: Survey of Air Quality Information Related to the World Trade Center Collapse": "Overall, the majority of respondents wanted more information regarding outdoor and indoor air quality, in a timely manner, and did not believe the information they received. The survey results suggest disconnect between government statements about air quality and respondents' perceptions of possible health risks from breathing the air in Lower Manhattan. The majority of respondents reported that they thought breathing outdoor and indoor air in Lower Manhattan in the weeks following the WTC collapse could expose them to short- and long-term health effects. Further, data indicated that contamination from the collapse of the WTC towers spread into the homes of respondents located beyond the perimeter of the zone designated as eligible for the EPA-led testing and cleaning program."[5]

December 15: New York City Council approves bill to curb diesel emissions, which makes NYC a national leader in fight against environmental triggers of asthma.

2004

March 10: Lawsuit (*Benzman v. Whitman*) filed by Lower Manhattan residents, office workers, business owners, parents, and students against Christie Todd Whitman (head of EPA on 9/11) and the EPA for issuing false safety assurances and failing to comply with the federally mandated requirement to clean up buildings contaminated by the 9/11 terrorist attacks.

March 24: "Gold Standard" for Remediation of WTC Contaminations published.[8]

March 31: First meeting held of the WTC Expert Technical Review Panel: "To obtain greater input on ongoing efforts to monitor the situation for workers and residents impacted by the collapse of the World Trade Center, an expert technical review panel, convened by EPA, was formed to help facilitate the

Agency's use of available exposure and health surveillance databases and registries to characterize any remaining exposures and risks, identify unmet public health needs, and recommend any steps to further minimize the risks associated with the aftermath of the World Trade Center attacks." After pressure, the panel included a community liaison as an ex-officio panel member.[9] Although WTC community and labor representatives were meeting periodically, this panel process formalized the World Trade Center Community Labor Coalition.

May 18: Manhattan Community Board 1 (CB1) unanimously passed resolution on the WTC Memorial and Redevelopment Plan Final Generic Environmental Impacts Statement reiterating its concern about the cumulative impact (including air quality) of the various redevelopment and reconstruction projects and request a Lower Manhattan Construction Coordination Group.

July 26: EPA WTC Expert Technical Review Panel was allowed to include a labor representative in addition to the community liaison to be on the panel and present; 125 Cedar Street Residents presented "Environmental Concerns Raised by the Deutschebank Demolition."

September 8: General Accountability Office (GAO) released report "September 11 Health Effects in the Aftermath of the World Trade Center Attack"; describes continuing health impact based on evidence that thousands of people involved in rescue, recovery, cleanup, as well as those who lived and worked in the WTC vicinity.[10]

October 19: CB1 unanimously passed resolution calling upon the EPA to publicly commit itself to seven principles—including that EPA will conduct with appropriate input from the community, comprehensive indoor environmental testing for multiple contaminant for both residences and workplaces, and include mechanical ventilation systems; subsequently passed.

December: EPA took leadership role in the deconstruction of several large WTC contaminated buildings, including 130 Liberty Street (Deutsche Bank).

2005

January: Demolition of first WTC contaminated building (4 Albany) under EPA oversight began.

November 29: EPA released a final Test and Clean Program that was underfunded, inadequate, and technically and scientifically flawed and repeated the most serious limitations and deficiencies of the 2002 program as delineated by the inspector general—including reverting to the limited geographic area and excluding workplaces, schools, small businesses, and firehouses and not addressing buildings as an integrated system and omitting mechanical ventilation systems.

December 13: Twelfth and final WTC Expert Technical Review Panel; EPA disbanded panel. EPA to clean apartments although second plan rejected by residents and panel members.

2006

February 2: Federal District Court Judge Deborah Batts issued a ruling allowing *Benzman v. Whitman,* the lawsuit filed by Lower Manhattan residents, office workers, business owners, parents, and students against Christie Todd Whitman and the EPA, to proceed on the grounds, noting that "no reasonable person would have thought that telling thousands of people that it was safe to return to lower Manhattan, while knowing that such return could pose long-term health risks and other dire consequences, was conduct sanctioned by our laws."

February: New York congressional delegation convinced Bush administrator to appoint Dr. John Howard, director of the National Institute for Occupational Safety and Health (NIOSH), as 9/11 Health Coordinator; CB1 passed resolution strongly supporting the bipartisan call for the appointment of a September 11 Federal Health Czar to coordinate the federal government's response to short- and long-term adverse health effects resulting from 9/11.

April 6: More human remains found near WTC: 74 bone fragments found on roof of 130 Liberty Street, which is to be demolished.

April 7: Centers for Disease Control and Prevention released report detailing widespread prevalence of respiratory and psychological illness among survivors; Rep. Nadler states, "The study confirms what community leaders and medical professionals have asserted for years that the World Trade Center dust poses a grave and long-term threat to public health."

April: Rank-and-file activists and local officers formed the 90 Church Street Labor Coalition to ensure comprehensive remediation and future safety. The coalition fought for three major health and safety improvements: well-sealed double windows; an above standard HVAC filtration system; and a regular program of air testing. The coalition had a major health and safety victory after a rigorous two-year campaign, when agency managements agreed to install interior windows throughout a building located across from the WTC that was severely contaminated on 9/11. 90 Church Street housed more than 2,000 employees of the U.S. Postal Service and the New York City Housing Authority. On 9/11, 90 Church Street was breached, fires were started, and the sprinkler system discharged. Toxic substances, including lead, asbestos, mercury, dioxin, and mold, permeated the building. It took nearly three years to resolve insurance disputes and decontaminate and renovate the building. Almost everything within 90 Church Street, except for major structural elements and some Sheetrock, had to be discarded. Returning federal and city workers united with incoming state workers in an unprecedented health and safety campaign. After a long campaign and extensive negotiations by CSEA and PEF representatives, interior windows were installed on all state (Department of Health and Department of Public Service) floors (4, 13, 14, 15) before they moved to 90 Church Street in early 2005. They then worked cooperatively with federal workers to obtain the same windows for New York City Housing Authority and U.S. Postal Service workers in the building. The coalition credits its success to union solidarity enhanced by the support of community health and safety and environmental organizations (including NYCOSH, 9/11 EA, CB1, and the Sierra Club) and assistance from elected officials. The windows were completely installed by the end of 2006/early 2007. There is no more powerful weapon in the labor arsenal than real solidarity.

August: NYCDOHMH released first "Clinical Guidelines for Adults Exposed to the World Trade Center Disaster."[11]

September 5: Mayor Bloomberg and HHC President Aviles announced establishment and January 2007 opening of the WTC Environmental Health Center at Bellevue Hospital Center.

September 6: Town hall forum held on the impact of 9/11 on community health and a call for federal action, St. Paul's Chapel.

September 8: "World Trade Center Will Be Green" press conference announced that WTC site will be built to a standard 20% more efficient than the New York Energy Conservation Construction Code.

October 22: Workers uncovered more remains at WTC in manholes and utility areas that were overlooked in previous years.

2007

January 3: More human remains were found—tiny fragments about 1 to 2 inches long, in addition to four other bones, and more than 200 other remains since October 2006—were found during excavation of a street-level service road at Ground Zero.

January 11: New York City Council held hearing on U.S. EPA's Cleanup of WTC Dust Contamination in Residences and Offices in Lower Manhattan, specifically EPA's December 2006 Test and Clean Program.

April 17: CB1 unanimously passed a resolution calling on NYCDOHMH to develop WTC physical and mental health guidelines for children who lived or attended school in the WTC area (more than 25,000 on 9/11).

June 20: "World Trade Center: Preliminary Observations on EPA's Second Program—Statement of John B. Stephenson, Director Natural Resources and Environment to Address Indoor Contamination.". . . "EPA has taken some actions to incorporate recommendations from the Inspector General and expert panel members into its second program, but its decision not to incorporate other recommendations may limit the overall effectiveness of this program."

August 18: Tragic seven-alarm high-rise fire at 130 Liberty Street (Deutsche Bank) killed two firefighters, Robert Beddia and Joseph Graffagnino.

September: "World Trade Center: EPA's Most Recent Test and Clean Program Raises Concerns That Need to Be Addressed to Better Prepare for Indoor Contamination Following Disasters—Report to Congressional Requesters" released by U.S. Government Accountability Office.[12,13]

September: 9/11 health care vigils conducted by many Lower Manhattan organizations at Foley Square, Chinatown.

2008

February 21: Manhattan Borough President Scott Stringer announced the creation of the Manhattan Borough Construction Watch in response to several tragic construction accidents, including the 130 Liberty Street fire.

April 13: 9/11 Health forum on continuing health problems were organized by many coalitions including BGZ & 9/11 EA.

April 22: Second Circuit Court of Appeals hearing *Benzman v. Whitman* issued its decision rejecting efforts to hold Christine Todd Whitman, and by extension any government official, personally liable for false safety assurances about Lower Manhattan's air quality in the days after 9/11, thus setting a dangerous precedent for future disasters.

June 20: WTC Health Registry study showed importance to continue tracking 9/11–related pediatric health effects; still no pediatric guidelines have been released by NYCDOH.[14]

July: U.S. EPA released "Breathing Clean by Building Green: Clean Diesel Construction" video, which highlights retrofit technologies that have been used in significant projects such as in Lower Manhattan to reduce diesel emissions from construction equipment to protect public health when organizations collaborate.

July: New York City Construction, Demolition & Abatement Working Group released "Strengthening the Safety, Oversight and Coordination of Construction, Demolition and Abatement Operations: Report and Recommendations to Mayor Michael R. Bloomberg" in response to the August 18, 2007, tragic fire at 130 Liberty Street; it strengthened interagency practices between the Department of Buildings (DOB), Fire Department of New York (FDNY), and Department of Environmental Protection (DEP).

July: Bush administration alerted Dr. Howard that he would not be reappointed to a second term as the federal government's 9/11 health coordinator, although he had earned the respect of government, labor, and community leaders.

September: World Trade Center Medical Working Group of New York City released "2008 Annual Report on 9/11 Health." . . . "More than 40,000 rescue and recovery workers have been screened nationally, primarily at New

York City's three WTC Centers of Excellence. Of these, more than 10,500 have received federally funded treatment for physical health conditions including respiratory problems, asthma and gastroesophageal reflux disease, and more than 5,500 have been treated for mental health conditions such as post-traumatic stress disorder (thousands of others have been treated with private funding). In addition, nearly 2,700 Lower Manhattan residents and area workers—including those who worked in Lower Manhattan, though they may live elsewhere—have sought treatment for these same conditions from New York City's Health and Hospitals Corporation. Some of these people have recovered, but others have not."

September 7: 9/11 health care vigils conducted by many Lower Manhattan organizations at Foley Square, Chinatown.

October 2: WTC EHC received its first federal funding ($30 million over the next three years) for screening, monitoring, and treatment of Lower Manhattan area workers, residents, and students.

December 4: Mayor Bloomberg announced launch of the Notify NYC pilot program to deliver emergency public information by e-mail, text messages, and reverse-911 alerts in four New York City community districts, including Lower Manhattan, which strongly advocated for its creation.

December 22: Manhattan District Attorney Robert M. Morgenthau announces 130 Liberty Street indictments (Deutsche Bank Building): "But the work has been protracted, tortuous, deadly and—it now seems—criminally negligent . . . manslaughter charges were filed against three construction supervisors and the John Galt Corporation, saying, 'Everybody who could have screwed up, screwed up here.' Galt, virtually a shell corporation, was in charge of the demolition on Aug. 18, 2007, when two firefighters were killed and two more injured in a fire at the building. Though New York City was not named in the indictment, the Bloomberg administration acknowledged 'the failures of our agencies to inspect and detect the conditions that contributed to the deaths.'"

2009

January 23: Medical examiner attributes second sarcoidosis-related death to WTC collapse: Leon Heyward, an investigator for Department of Consumer Affairs, was working in Lower Manhattan on 9/11. More cases of sarcoidosis and granulomatous lung disease have now been reported among those exposed to World Trade Center dust.

February 24: New York congressional delegation, labor union leaders, 9/11 responders, and Lower Manhattan residents urged reappointment of Federal 9/11 health coordinator, Dr. John Howard.

February 24: CB1 unanimously passed resolution expressing its dismay that NYC-DOHMH has yet to provide health guidelines to assist in the diagnosis and treatment of children and adolescents exposed to the World Trade Center disaster.

March 11: House investigative report found that officials from the Agency for Toxic Substances and Disease Registry (ATSDR) "deny, delay, minimize, trivialize or ignore legitimate health concerns."[15] Although this report was not about 9/11, it should be noted that ATSDR is responsible for protecting the public near toxic sites which some consider the 9/11 WTC site fell in.

2010–2011

James Zadroga 9/11 Health and Compensation Act of 2010 passed, funded, and contracts awarded for clinical and data coordinating centers for WTC Environmental Health Center (Bellevue), New York University, Mt. Sinai, Queens College, and the Fire Department of New York (FDNY). Research contracts were awarded to study distal airways disease at New York University, cardiovascular disease at Mt. Sinai, and cancer at FDNY

We thank those public servants who represented our district: Congressman Jerrold Nadler and his chief of staff Amy Rutkin, New York State Assembly Member Linda B. Rosenthal; former New York Sen. Hillary Rodham Clinton and staff Chris Falvo; and Case Button; New York Sen. Charles Schumer; Congresswoman Carolyn Maloney; New York State Speaker Sheldon Silver; Manhattan Borough President Scott Stringer, who appoints the members of all Manhattan Community Boards (including 1, 2, and 3, which are the closest to the WTC site); former New York City Council Member Alan Gerson; EPA National Ombudsman Robert J. Martin and EPA Chief Investigator Hugh Kaufman; and Dr. John Howard. In addition, we thank the media that documented the past 7 1/2 years: *Downtown Express* (editor Josh Rogers, Julie Shapiro, Rhonda Kaysen, and Elizabeth O'Brien); the *TribecaTrib* (editor Carl Glassman and Etta Sanders), the *Battery Park Broadsheet* (Robert Simko); and the *New York Daily News* (Greg Smith and Juan Gonzalez). Special thanks to Micki Siegel de Hernandez, Dave Newman, Rob Spencer, Stan Mark, Paul Stein, Paul Bartlett, Jo Polett, and Kathleen Moore.

CHAPTER 8

THE MEDICAL RESPONSE TO AN ENVIRONMENTAL DISASTER

Lessons from the World Trade Center Attacks

Caralee Caplan-Shaw
Angeliki Kazeros
Sam Parsia
Joan Reibman

LEARNING OBJECTIVES

- To understand how the government responded to environmental health risks immediately after the World Trade Center disaster
- To become familiar with how the government disseminated information and dictated cleanup of affected areas
- To understand exposure risk research and funding related to the WTC disaster
- To become familiar with the long-term health effects of exposure to WTC disaster materials

The September 11, 2001, terrorist attacks on the World Trade Center (WTC) in New York City resulted in collapse of the towers, generated a thick plume of dust and fumes that wafted across Lower Manhattan and Brooklyn, ignited fires that smoldered for months, and deposited more than one million tons of debris in one of the most densely populated and vitally important commercial districts in the world. In addition to the event's devastating personal, emotional, political, and economic consequences for New York City and the nation, the tragedy was an unprecedented and unanticipated environmental disaster. The scale of the environmental impact—both in terms of quantity and complexity of pollutants released and the size and diversity of populations at risk for adverse health effects—made the emergency response in the immediate aftermath of the attack exceedingly difficult.

Balancing the need for search and rescue operations, a criminal investigation of the cause of the disaster, restoring function to the financial district, and ensuring the safety of the residents and workers in the area was a complex task that fell upon multiple local and federal agencies. Criticism of the actions of the Environmental Protection Agency (EPA), **National Institute for Occupational Safety and Health (NIOSH)**, Occupational Safety and Health Administration (OSHA), the New York State Department of Environmental Conservation (DEC), and the many other government agencies present during the aftermath has been intense. It has become common knowledge that personal protective equipment was underutilized by rescue and recovery and cleanup workers. Many people focus on the air quality assessment by the EPA and the famous statement made by its director at the time, Christie Todd Whitman: "The air is safe to breathe, and the water is safe to drink." Reassured by the words of a well-known public figure, many area workers and residents returned to their homes and businesses with a sense that the danger had passed. Subsequently, the shortcomings of the agencies responsible for advising residents and workers on how to clean the debris may have needlessly increased the exposure and health risks of these individuals.

Certainly, the magnitude of the situation could never have been anticipated by any of these agencies, and, in fact, it could be suggested that each individual agency was able to achieve its particular mission with some success given the circumstances. Unfortunately, the actions of each agency were overlaid by political concerns and were never synthesized into a global assessment of the situation at Ground Zero (GZ) to guide health regulations and protect responders, workers, and the public. Furthermore, one might imagine that public health departments might have stepped in early on; however, the reality is that health departments have expertise in the domains of preventive medicine and infectious diseases, but little to no experience in acute environmental exposures. The lack of a single authority, coupled with an enormous amount of political pressure to allow life in Lower Manhattan to resume, is likely the real reason that many warning signals of potential health threats were ignored.

This chapter focuses on the role of the medical and scientific community in the days, months, and years after 9/11 in elucidating the characteristics and toxicity of WTC dust and in caring for individuals with adverse health effects related to 9/11 exposures. We describe the accumulated knowledge on the characteristics and toxicity of WTC dust. We then follow a loose chronology to tell the story of how our understanding of WTC health effects emerged from single centers and grew through partnerships among medical, government, philanthropic, and community organizations. Finally, we discuss lessons learned from the WTC experience for future disasters and for environmental health in general.

This chapter was completed before the signing of H.R. 847, the "James Zadroga 9/11 Health and Compensation Act of 2010" on January 6, 2011, by President Barack H. Obama. This law, a result of continued efforts by rescue and recovery workers, community members, medical personnel, organized labor, and persistent congressional and senate members, puts into place a screening, monitoring and treatment program for adverse medical and mental health effects for rescue and recovery workers as well as community members. The hopes for this compromise bill are that funding will now be in place for continued health monitoring and treatment of populations at risk for adverse health outcomes. The fears are that onerous reporting requirements, rigid restrictions, and interesting additions (the government requires the name of each patient to ensure that they are not on the terrorist watch list), will provide barriers to care. Regardless, the signing of this bill, nearly ten years after the event, represents the culmination of combined efforts from diverse groups to move the federal government to provide an appropriate health response to an environmental disaster with wide ramifications.

Immediate Response to Environmental Exposure

Governmental agencies provided early reassurance about the components of the WTC dust as reports came in from an assortment of federally monitored sites.[1] Residents, rescue workers, and local workers were told that it was safe to go back to work one week after the event. The EPA did not declare Ground Zero a hazardous waste site or a Superfund site, thus allowing for reduced protection requirements for workers and diminishing the pressure for building owners to remediate their buildings. In addition, the EPA denied that it had legal responsibility for assessing or addressing indoor environmental contamination, thus leaving the task in the hands of New York City agencies. Ultimately, no governmental agency took responsibility for indoor spaces. Indoor environmental testing and remediation of common spaces was up to the building owners, and commercial and residential tenants were left to contend with their private spaces. Technical advice provided by the federal and city government agencies was incomplete and incorrect; none of the agencies sought outside help from academic or private sources with expertise in the areas in which they were lacking information. In 2002, almost one year after the event, the EPA began a "Test and Clean Program" that was nonmandatory and limited to residences.[1,2] This program, targeted to a limited area, allowed for either testing or cleaning followed by testing. Only 18% of eligible apartments were either cleaned or tested, and no commercial or institutional buildings in Lower Manhattan were included.[2]

Analysis of World Trade Center Dust

As it rapidly became evident that the risks imparted by the 9/11 event would require immediate and extensive study, the **National Institutes of Environmental Health Science (NIEHS)** expanded funding of four existing Environmental Health Science Core Centers (New York University; Columbia University; University of Medicine/Dentistry in New Jersey, R. W. Johnson Medical School, [RWJ-UMDNJ]; and Johns Hopkins Center in Urban Environmental Health) to perform exposure assessments, characterize debris, and monitor health effects. These research centers, funded for toxicologic and environmental studies in adult and pediatric populations, had a wealth of expertise in toxicology and epidemiologic studies. Additional funding was rapidly provided to these centers to expand their mandate, and investigators with a range of expertise were recruited to develop and implement studies using air sampling, toxicologic assessment, and human outcomes. These centers, working as an NIEHS consortium distinct from governmental agencies, subsequently provided a wealth of information about specific hazards posed by the dust and helped describe some of the resultant symptoms and syndromes that became widely recognized in affected populations.

Prediction of health effects was exceedingly complex for many reasons. There was a tremendous diversity of materials contained in the office buildings that made up the WTC site. By some estimates, the buildings contained 300–400 tons of asbestos, 50,000 personal computers containing lead and mercury,

300 mainframe computers, hundreds of miles of wire and cable containing polyvinyl chloride and copper, thousands of mercury-containing fluorescent lights, unknown tons of plastics, which would produce dioxins and furans when burned, thousands of chairs and other office furniture containing polybrominated biphenyls, several storage tanks containing petroleum products, and 130,000 gallons of transformer oil.[3] The combustion of this colossal mass of material at the extreme temperatures and force generated by the impact, fires, and subsequent collapse made the situation at Ground Zero even more unprecedented. Members of the NIEHS consortium collected dust samples from the area in the days after the attacks. Within three days of the event, air sampling sites were set up within close proximity to Ground Zero for daily particulate matter (PM) sampling, and bulk samples of settled debris were obtained from several indoor and outdoor sites for subsequent analysis.[4] An air sample provided from an ongoing sampling study within Manhattan was donated as well.[4] These samples provided some of the most comprehensive information on the characteristics that have become widely known, namely that the dust had a characteristic alkaline pH, was mainly composed of pulverized building and construction materials, with some contamination by agents such as lead, asbestos, glass fibers, and **polycyclic aromatic hydrocarbons(PAH)**.[4] Despite the success the investigators had in collecting samples and data on the environmental impact of the event, they encountered several delays and limitations in what they could achieve in the postdisaster environment. There were difficulties in accessing the site, damage to the local infrastructure (electricity), inadequate numbers of sampling devices and trained personnel, and devices that were overwhelmed by excess particulates in the presence of the initial plume.[5]

Despite limitations, much information has been derived from the NIEHS consortium studies. These studies revealed that more than 90% of the particles in the bulk samples tested were >10 microns in diameter, and many were fibers with widths <5 microns and >10 microns.[6,7] While these large particles are generally trapped and cleared by the upper respiratory tract, the massive amount of material had the potential to overcome normal respiratory protective mechanisms, and a study from the consortium demonstrated that these large fibers lodged in human lungs.[8] One area of particular concern was the small particulates of the dust (those particles smaller than 2.5 microns, $PM_{2.5}$), which have the ability to travel to the sensitive distal airways of the lung and evade mucociliary and cough mechanisms of clearance. Although $PM_{2.5}$ represented a small percentage of the particulate mass (10%), the quantity of particulate matter released was so massive that $PM_{2.5}$ levels in the air at the GZ perimeter were very high, typically above the EPA level of concern of $40ug/m^3$, with occasional increases to 100–400 ug/m^3, according to monitors available after September 21.[9] Characterization of the PM$_{2.5}$ revealed an alkaline pH similar to that of unfractionated dust, with subtle differences in the other substances analyzed (sulfate, PAH).[10] It has been well understood that high levels of non–WTC PM$_{2.5}$ are associated with adverse cardiovascular and respiratory health effects. As a result, there was concern that the WTC dust would represent a particular health risk. Using samples provided by the NIEHS consortium, the investigators at the EPA demonstrated a biologic effect of WTC PM$_{2.5}$ in a mouse model. They showed that airway hyperresponsiveness (AHR) could be induced with exposure,[11] providing proof of concept to the human studies that were being reported at the time.

Members of the NIEHS consortium and the EPA analyzed the PAH content of the dust. As combustion of different types of fuel produce different types of PAH, the types present in the materials collected could be traced back to the airplanes used in the attacks. Dust collected in the days after the event by the NIEHS consortium was compared to those collected several weeks later and were found to have similar types of PAH, indicating that the fires that remained burning at the site were an ongoing source of toxic products of incomplete combustion of jet fuel.[4] Surface dust that had accumulated in indoor areas was also examined and showed a profile of PAH types similar to that collected outdoors in the initial days after the attacks, suggesting a greater likelihood that this dust was a result of the attacks rather than dust that had been present before the attacks took place.[12] It was estimated that 100–1,000 tons of PAH had settled over a localized area. Variations in the levels of individual PAH were identified in indoor bulk samples; these differences were thought to have resulted from the wide variety of unburned and partially burned hydrocarbons from the materials in the collapsed buildings as well as differences in penetration of the outdoor dusts.[13,14]

These findings were a counterpoint to those of the EPA, which had collected samples from the air filters. Analysis of these samples showed that although concentrations of mutagenic and carcinogenic PAH were among the highest reported for outdoor sources on the first days, they rapidly diminished over the subsequent 100 days, after which diesel sources predominated.[15] The EPA concluded that the transient elevation in PAH posed a very small cancer risk among non-occupationally exposed residents of New York City. The human data to support this assertion has yet to be collected. There was little to no communication among the interested public health parties in regard to sampling, analyses (although these took time), publication, or dissemination of results to the public.

Role of the Medical Community in Identifying Adverse Health Effects in Diverse Populations

The Fire Department of New York

Within minutes of the terrorist attacks on the WTC, the Fire Department of New York City (FDNY) operated a continuous rescue and recovery effort at the WTC site involving approximately 11,000 firefighters until May 2002. During the collapse, 343 FDNY rescue workers died and, during the next 24 hours, an additional 240 FDNY rescue workers sought emergency medical treatment, mostly for eye and respiratory tract irritation. Three FDNY rescue workers required hospitalization for life-threatening inhalational injuries.[16] The FDNY had a well-established medical program for routine monitoring and treatment of its members. FDNY members were required to undergo and pass yearly medical evaluations that included lung function testing. The medical officers of the FDNY Bureau of Health Services responded to the rescue and recovery effort at the WTC site by providing rapid emergency medical services. These physicians, many of whom were caught in the initial dust cloud themselves, were the first to report on adverse health effects related to WTC dust and fume exposure in September 2002.

Studies of the firefighter population provide unique insights into the potential adverse health effects of WTC dust and fume exposure for several reasons. First, the firefighters generally had intense exposure to WTC dust and fumes, with short-term intense exposure on the day of the attack and many with sustained daily exposure on the burning pile of rubble over the subsequent months. Second, case ascertainment is complete because all FDNY rescue workers must report to FDNY Bureau of Health Services for regular evaluations if they present to hospitals or treatment centers while on duty, require on- or off-duty medical leave, file workers' compensation, or require retirement disability. Furthermore, firefighters are overall a healthier group than the general population because of the extensive medical screening they undergo to determine employment eligibility. Finally, the firefighter population is the only one reported on to date for which pre–9/11 clinical and pulmonary function data are consistently available.

Within weeks of the terrorist attacks, the Centers for Disease Control and Prevention (CDC) awarded $4.8 million to the FDNY to screen its members for health problems as a result of their early and intense exposure to hazardous conditions at Ground Zero. In the same year, the federal government, in recognition of the high casualties experienced by FDNY and the impact of the WTC disaster on nearly every member of the department, provided $132 million for treatment and mental health evaluation for FDNY members and to provide crisis counseling in New York City and ten surrounding counties for more than two years after the disaster. These funds were distributed through Project Liberty, which was created by the New York State Office of Mental Health with support from the Federal Emergency Management Agency with a Crisis Counseling Regular Services Grant. The rapid federal response was in response to the New York congressional delegation funding requests, especially because of a special personal interest by Sen. Hillary Rodham Clinton (D-NY).

The work of the medical community of the FDNY allowed the first identification of adverse respiratory and other health effects in those that responded to the WTC crisis.[17] Prezant and colleagues described "World Trade Center cough" (**WTC cough**), defined as cough serious enough to require medical leave for four weeks, and bronchial hyper-responsiveness in FDNY firefighters.[18] Within 24 hours after exposure, all 332 firefighters with WTC cough reported a cough productive of black to grayish sputum infiltrated with "pebbles or particles." In the first six months after 9/11, WTC cough occurred in 128 of 1,636 firefighters with high-level exposure (8%), 187 of 6,958 FDNY with moderate level of exposure (3%), and 17 of 1,320 with low level of exposure (1%). Ninety-five percent had symptoms of dyspnea, 87% had gastroesophageal reflux symptoms, and 54% had nasal congestion. Bronchial hyper-responsiveness was common in firefighters with WTC cough and in those with high- or intermediate-level exposure. The use of respiratory protection was not associated with a significantly decreased risk of lower airway symptoms, decreased pulmonary function, or airway hyper-reactivity, probably because of the hypervigilant rescue efforts during the first two weeks after the collapse of the towers, with only intermittent use of respirators.

Prezant and colleagues showed that these firefighters were not only symptomatic but that their symptoms were associated with a significant decline in lung function. Mean lung function remained within normal limits; however, forced vital capacity (FVC) and forced expiratory volume in one second (FEV_1) showed a drop of at least 0.5 liters in 58% and 54% of firefighters respectively before and after 9/11.[18] Of the seventy-eight firefighters with normal findings on plain chest radiography, high resolution inspiratory and expiratory CT scans were obtained, and air trapping was seen in more than 50% and bronchial wall thickening in 30% of the firefighters. Over the six-month follow-up period, practically all of the firefighters with upper airway symptoms were medically cleared to return to work; only 34% of those with predominantly lower respiratory tract symptoms were allowed to return to duty.[18]

Studies of the firefighters documented the presence of WTC particles and an inflammatory response in the lungs immediately after exposure as well as persistence of these particles and inflammation years after the event. Analysis of bronchoalveolar lavage fluid from a firefighter who worked on the WTC pile on September 24, 2001, and presented with respiratory failure as a result of acute eosinophilic pneumonia revealed fly ash, degraded glass fibers, chrysotile, amosite, silicates, chromium, and asbestos within an inflammatory milieu.[8] Subsequently, sputum obtained from thirty-eight highly WTC exposed FDNY firefighters two years after the event demonstrated ongoing inflammation (increased neutrophils, eosinophils, and matrix metalloproteinase levels) in the presence of particles with a size distribution and composition that was different from unexposed controls and consistent with WTC exposure.[19]

In an effort to elucidate further the relationship between WTC exposure intensity and respiratory symptoms, the FDNY Bureau of Health Services collaborated with the National Institute for Occupational Safety and Health to evaluate symptoms, lung function, and use of personal protective equipment in firefighters.[20] In this study utilizing a stratified random sample of 362 firefighters, firefighters were categorized as high exposure if they were present the morning of the collapse, intermediate exposure if they arrived in the afternoon of the day of the collapse or the next day, or low exposure if they arrived 48 hours after the collapse. The firefighters reported that 19% did not wear respirators during the first two weeks, 50% only rarely, and approximately 70% wore a half-face respirator or disposable mask by the end of the second week. In early October 2001, respiratory symptoms (cough, shortness of breath, wheeze, chest pain) were reported by almost 80% in high- and intermediate-exposure groups, by 46% in low-exposure, and by 9% among unexposed. When compared to lung function performed in the previous year, spirometry performed immediately after WTC exposure showed mean declines of 268 mL and 264 mL for FVC and FEV_1, respectively. Both declined significantly in the high- and intermediate-exposure groups with a striking dose–response, and respiratory symptoms were significantly correlated with lung function decline.

Subsequent studies of FDNY approached the question of persistence of symptoms, whether those who developed new symptoms had a delayed or more chronic asthma-like picture, and whether the symptoms were severe enough to cause disability. In a representative sample of 179 rescue worker firefighters, bronchial hyper-reactivity at one, three, or six months was associated with exposure intensity and airflow obstruction.[21] High-exposure FDNY were nearly 7 times more likely to have bronchial hyper-reactivity than those who had intermediate exposure, and initial hyper-reactivity predicted persistent hyper-reactivity at six months. Among 12,079 FDNY followed prospectively,

WTC–dust exposed FDNY rescue workers experienced a significant decline in adjusted average FEV_1 during the year after the attacks (372 ml) equivalent to twelve years of aging-related decline in lung function.[22] Again, a clear exposure intensity–response gradient was seen, with the most highly exposed individuals faring the worst. The FDNY studies went on to describe a higher incidence of sarcoid-like granulomatous pulmonary disease in FDNY rescue workers[23] as well as significant mental health effects. The FDNY established a lung function referral and treatment program for its members.

The WTC Workers Medical Screening Program

In addition to the 11,000 FDNY workers involved in rescue and recovery, an estimated 40,000 non–FDNY workers were involved in the cleanup of Ground Zero and the Staten Island landfill during the days, weeks, and months after September 11, 2001. These workers included a variety of first responders: police, construction workers, ironworkers, laborers, and public sector workers.[24,25]

The Mount Sinai Irving J. Selikoff Center for Occupational and Environmental Medicine, a university-based, New York State Department of Health (NYS DOH)–supported occupational health center, began evaluating these workers within weeks of the event. Officials from the National Institute for Occupational Safety and Health began regular conference calls to enhance communication among the health care workers providing care for the responders. Numerous labor organizations concerned about the health of their constituents and physicians at Mount Sinai Medical Center began advocating among nationally elected officials and representatives about the need for a monitoring program. These efforts resulted in the award of federal funding in April 2002 for the establishment of a medical monitoring program for WTC rescue and recovery workers. The WTC Worker and Volunteer Medical Screening Program was established at Mount Sinai, with additional clinic sites at State University of New York-Stony Brook, Queens College, UMDNJ-RWJ New Jersey Medical School, and New York University-Bellevue Hospital, all of whom were members of a pre-existing infrastructure of the New York State Occupational Health Clinic Network.

The design of this program began in April 2002 and implementation started three months later.[26] Numerous challenges were faced in the design of the program, including the limited data on exposures and potential health consequences, the absence of a systematic roster of responders, and the potential diverse needs of the responders.[27] Although some of the clinical screening evaluations were based on asbestos screening, the clinical screening examination was expanded to include an exposure questionnaire, physical and mental health questionnaires, a standardized physical examination, spirometry, complete blood count, chemistries, and chest radiograph.[26] After an initial baseline evaluation, individuals were given appropriate referrals for further care if needed and were educated about potential hazards at the WTC and other work sites.

These initial funds were intended for medical and mental health screening of individuals involved in rescue, recovery, and debris removal but not for treatment of these individuals. Moreover, funds were never available on a long-term basis but rather were provided as congressional appropriations, thus requiring continued advocacy efforts and precluding long-term planning. Continuing funds for the program and support for a longitudinal monitoring program were provided in 2003 when Sen. Hillary Clinton and Representatives Caroline Maloney (D), Jerrold Nadler (D), and Vito Fossella (R) promoted the first congressional appropriations of $90 million for the FDNY and workers' responder program, now called the WTC Worker and Volunteer Screening and Monitoring Program. Private philanthropy supported a program for treatment of some of the responders; this program was expanded in 2005 with the provision of increased funding from the American Red Cross Liberty Disaster Relief fund. In 2006, NIOSH funds were increased to include treatment, and the program was renamed the WTC Worker and Volunteer Monitoring and Treatment Program.

Of the first 9,442 responders examined in the WTC Worker and Volunteer Monitoring Program between 2002 and 2004, 69% reported new or worsened respiratory symptoms while performing WTC work, and these persisted until the time of examination in 59% of them.[25] Sixty percent of these workers reported having been in the initial dust cloud on 9/11. Upper respiratory symptoms, cough, dyspnea, chest tightness, and wheeze were the most common symptoms. There was a significant association between the presence of a low FVC and the time of arrival at the site, with a higher prevalence of abnormality in those who arrived earlier. In a study of longitudinal lung function consisting of baseline and follow-up spirometry in 3,160 workers, 20% had a low FVC on the first examination and 16% on the second.[28] Eight percent had obstruction at both examinations. The decline in FEV_1 was 13 mL/year, but 131 individuals lost greater than 300 mL of FVC annually. No special associations were noted for this rapid decline group, and respiratory symptoms at first examination were not predictive of lung function decline. Radiographic imaging using CT scans in a subgroup of workers revealed air trapping, consistent with that described in the FDNY study.[29] Data from this worker cohort also provided descriptions of gastroesophageal reflux symptoms[30] as well as information on social and mental health issues. Of more than 10,000 workers surveyed, 11% had symptoms consistent with post-traumatic stress disorder (PTSD), a rate higher than that seen in the general population.[31] Many had concurrent depression and anxiety.

In summary, the collaboration between labor forces and an existing occupational program allowed for the rapid implementation of a comprehensive medical program as well as the ability to advocate at the federal level for funding for this program. The expansion from a screening and monitoring program to a program offering medical treatment required continued advocacy but became an invaluable resource for those without adequate health insurance and allowed for the development of expertise among medical practitioners.

Local Residents, Workers, and Children

Residents

At the community level, no organized group represented residents at the time of the 9/11 attack. After 9/11 there were some minor efforts to combat community health risks. For example, EPA counseled that tenants use "appropriate" equipment but failed to specify respirators.[32] Additionally, the New York City Department of Health and Mental Hygiene (NYCDOHMH) distributed leaflets recommending cleaning techniques, such as shampooing carpets, using wet rags and mops and HEPA vacuum cleaners.[33] Community physicians were less well equipped to deal with exposure complications than were occupational physicians. This was because community physicians had fewer sources for information and no clear recommendations for their patients. Those who listened to the results of monitoring provided by the EPA and the NYCDOHMH tried to alleviate the fears of their patients. Others recommended that patients move, if only temporarily.

These problems were especially acute given the number of people affected by the disaster. Indeed, estimates suggest that approximately 300,000 nonresponders were at risk for exposure from the WTC disaster.[34] This population included the daily workforce (estimated at greater than 250,000), grade school students (8,000), students in local colleges (45,000), and the more than 60,000 residents living south of Canal Street.[34,35] The local residential, working, and school population had potential for multiple exposures to WTC dust, fumes, and gasses. Some were caught in the initial debris as the buildings were hit. Many were caught in the initial dust clouds as the multiple buildings collapsed, and some wandered for hours in the debris immediately after the collapse. Those who lived on the west side of Manhattan were evacuated for days to months after the event: 19,000 families were displaced and forced to find temporary lodging, some for more than one year.[36] These individuals were especially at risk because there was no systematic way in which affected apartments were cleaned. Some hired cleanup agencies, most of which were staffed with unskilled workers; others cleaned on their own. Cleaning of ventilation systems was inconsistent. Although funding was available for replacement of furniture and carpeting for some, the distribution of this funding was haphazard, and recommendations regarding under what circumstances furniture ought to be replaced were not available.

Workers

Individuals who worked in the area were also put at risk. Although businesses in Lower Manhattan closed immediately after the event, nearly all offices reopened one week later. Workers returned with patriotic enthusiasm to offices that had undergone varied degrees of cleaning. Again, in the absence of formal recommendations, some were cleaned with vigilance, and others were cleaned partially, with ventilation systems ignored.

Schools, too, experienced problems that led to exposure. On 9/11, the local schools dealt with the emergency in a variety of ways. Some opened their doors and told the children to run. Others shut the children in the building, only letting them out after the towers had collapsed. All closed for weeks to months. The cleanup activities of these schools were varied and depended on advocacy from parent-led organizations. Continued fumes and dust generated by the ongoing fires and the re-suspension of dust from the WTC site required continued cleaning activities, none of which were formally recommended by governmental agencies. Anecdotes of respiratory complaints emerged within days.

In response to these various hazards to the community, members of the New York State Department of Health and physicians at New York University began a collaboration to design a study to investigate respiratory health effects in local residents. Funding for this project was provided by the Centers for Disease Control. Together they met with community members of local tenants' organizations, community boards, newly formed environmental groups, and local advocacy groups. The WTC Residents Respiratory Health Study was designed, implemented, and completed within the first year and a half after 9/11. This study included sampling of residents within a 1-mile radius of Ground Zero (exposed population) as well as those in a control group. The exposed population was oversampled, because at the time the study was the only survey of residents, and the plan was to develop this group as a longitudinal cohort. Questionnaires in English, Spanish, and Chinese were mailed; however, with the dysfunction of postal service due to the disruption of the attack and the concurrent anthrax scare, questionnaires were subsequently hand-delivered, building by building, door to door.

This study resulted in the first documentation of the presence of health effects in a local population of residents exposed to deconstructed, pulverized, and incinerated buildings.[37] Among the more than 2,800 residents who answered the questionnaire, there was a greater than threefold increase in the presence of new-onset persistent respiratory symptoms compared to the control population. More than 6 times as many exposed individuals had new-onset wheezing compared to the control population. Furthermore, higher rates of new-onset upper respiratory symptoms were associated with unplanned medical visits and increased use of rescue inhaler medications.[38] Adverse home conditions, such as the presence of physical damage, dust, and odors, were related to new-onset respiratory symptoms, with the greatest risk observed in individuals who reported an increased duration or frequency of dust or odors in their homes, suggesting a dose–response.[39] Although the study was completed and the manuscript written within the first two years of the event, these studies were delayed in publication as they wound their way through governmental and peer review. The results were borne out in other studies, which suggested increased asthma rates in the community and increased asthma-related clinic visits among asthmatic children living near the WTC site after 9/11.[40,41]

Children

As in many toxic environmental exposures, developing fetuses and young children are generally more susceptible to adverse effects due to the vulnerability of developing organ systems, the neurologic system in particular. Because Lower Manhattan had become an increasingly popular neighborhood for young families, the number of children and pregnant women in the area was substantial. In addition, there were many pregnant women in the workforce. The NIEHS Environmental Center at Mount Sinai Hospital examined a cohort of 187 pregnant women with exposures via residence or occupation stratified by an exposure index that took into account distance from the site and direction of debris dispersal based on PM measurements in the area. Although no statistically significant differences in the formation of DNA adducts related to PAH exposure, PCBs, or dioxins were detected, women who had samples collected shortly after the event had elevated PAH-related DNA adducts compared to those who submitted samples several months after the event. In addition, reduced intrauterine growth was reported.[42,43]

The Columbia Center for Children's Environmental Health at Columbia University's Mailman School of Public Health embarked on several studies to determine phenotypic effects the exposure may have had on birth and developmental outcomes. Initial review of birth records from three downtown Manhattan hospitals showed significantly lower birth weight and length among babies born at term to WTC–exposed women than to unexposed women. Women who were in their first trimester of pregnancy at the time of the attacks were found to have a small but significantly shorter period of gestation (-3.6 days) and newborns with smaller head circumference when compared to women exposed at later stages of pregnancy.[44] No difference in mercury levels in cord blood could be found between WTC–exposed and control subjects. There was an increase in DNA adducts, suggesting a cancer-related risk, although the adduct level was less than amounts found in cities with higher pollution levels in Poland and China.[45,46] The difference in DNA adducts present in the WTC area compared to other areas of NYC correlated with smaller birth size as well as with standardized measurements of child development.[45,47] Long-term developmental consequences remain an ongoing area of concern and research. Unfortunately, no funding has been available to continue longitudinal study of the first children studied at Mount Sinai Hospital. The WTC EHC screening and treatment program has expanded to include children who were residents or students in the area during the attack. The DOHMH has provided medical guidelines about the detection or treatment of WTC-related illness in children.

WTC Environmental Health Center

Local residents and workers with WTC-related illness sought care in a variety of locations. Because of the high profile generated from the **WTC Residents Respiratory Study** and Bellevue Hospital's ability, as a local public hospital, to treat uninsured patients, some sought care at the Bellevue Hospital Asthma Clinic. Failing to acquire a governmental program, the Beyond Ground Zero (BGZ) Network approached the administration at Bellevue Hospital and, with the physicians running the asthma program, began a pilot program to treat residents with presumed WTC-related illness. This program expanded in 2005, when it received three years of funding (approximately $2 million) from the American Red Cross Liberty Disaster Relief fund to develop the first treatment program for local residents and workers with WTC exposure and symptoms. A community advisory committee was organized to help define the populations most in need, to provide outreach for the program, and to provide guidance around services that were needed. The committee expanded to include a wide range of affected persons, including residents, local workers, small business owners, students, and labor representatives. Advocacy from these community organizations resulted in an additional five years of funding provided by the City of New York for an expanded and ongoing treatment program for adults and initiation of a pediatric program. In 2008, after advocacy from governmental representatives, including then-senators Clinton and Schumer and congressional representatives Maloney, Nadler, and Fossella, as well as continued pressure from the City of New York and community groups, money was provided to the Centers for Disease Control and a three-year grant was awarded by NIOSH for a "nonresponder" program to provide expanded medical and mental health treatment services for community members with presumed WTC-related illness.

The World Trade Center Environmental Health Center (WTC EHC) was developed as a comprehensive medical and mental health treatment program based on requests from community representatives. Although recruitment for the program continues, more than 5,000 individuals have enrolled for treatment in the program. These members have predominantly respiratory complaints of dyspnea, cough, and wheeze that began after 9/11 and persist nearly eight years after the event.[48] Lung function abnormalities have been detected in some, while others have hyper-reactive airways. Many have concurrent gastrointestinal symptoms, and there is a very high rate of PTSD, depression, and anxiety. The need for the program has been challenged, and the question has been raised repeatedly about causality and attribution. Due to the absence of pre-existing medical data in this community, and the absence of a program providing screening and evaluation in the immediate aftermath of the event, causality can only be presumed based on standard criteria.[48]

Although the medical consequences of the attack were not clearly evident until several weeks after the event, the potential for significant mental health issues was recognized and acted upon immediately. Many of the large corporations in the financial district hired on-site counselors to help their employees cope with the trauma and fear that resulted from the attacks, and multiple governmental and nongovernmental relief agencies provided mental health services on a walk-in basis (Project Liberty). Within weeks, a formal survey of a broad area of the city was undertaken by the New York Academy of Medicine in conjunction with New York University, Columbia University, and the National Crime Victims' Research and Treatment Center of the Medical University of South Carolina. Data from 1,008 respondents were obtained, and the prevalence of symptoms consistent with PTSD or depression were 7.5% and 9.7% respectively, which is approximately twice the rate given in historical estimates. Extrapolation of these estimates to the geographic range sampled (area of Manhattan below 110th Street) suggests that there were 67,000 individuals with PTSD symptoms and 87,000 with depression during the month the survey was conducted between mid-October to November 2001.[49] A follow-up survey performed by a different group of investigators three to six months after the attacks indicated that while the number of those with symptoms had decreased, a relatively small percentage (11.9%) had sought psychiatric services or were taking medications for anxiety, depression, or psychotic conditions, despite the increased treatment capacity that had been put in place.[50]

The WTC Health Registry

In 2003, the New York City Department of Health and Mental Hygiene in conjunction with federal, state, and private agencies launched a program to collect data on the physical and mental health issues in the exposed populations. This was named the **WTC Health Registry (WTCHR)** (www.wtcregistry.org). This $20 million joint research program developed by the federal Agency for Toxic Substance and Disease registry and the New York City DOHMH had a goal of monitoring of the health of people directly exposed. It would also create and propose guidelines for future disasters. Initially met with hostility by local community members and labor because of their lack of inclusion in the development of the project, an advisory panel was subsequently developed that included these advocacy groups. To date, the WTCHR is the largest effort in U.S. history to study health effects of a disaster and has enrolled more than 71,000 exposed people. The goal is to monitor the cohort for at least a twenty-year period; however the funding for the program depends on federal agencies.

The WTCHR began voluntary enrollment in 2003–2004. People who lived, worked, or were involved in rescue and recovery efforts were invited to complete a confidential baseline health survey, which included their location on 9/11, their experience on that day and in the aftermath, and any symptoms they developed after their exposure. In 2006, the first adult survey in the registry was completed; the data revealed that 67% of survivors of collapsed or damaged buildings reported new or worsening respiratory symptoms, including cough, shortness of breath, wheezing, or sinus irritation. Nearly 3% ($n = 1,967$) reported a new asthma diagnosis after 9/11, suggesting a 2–3 times higher rate than would be expected in the general population.[34] Mental health outcomes were monitored; 16% of adult enrollees screened positive for current PTSD, with 8% having serious psychological distress.[34,51] Health findings among children in the registry ($n = 3184$) demonstrated that WTC exposure increased the likelihood of a new asthma diagnosis, with twice the likelihood of the diagnosis if the children were caught in the dust cloud.[52] In addition, 6% of children under 5 years of age had a reported diagnosis of asthma after 9/11, a rate twice that reported in the Northeast for the same age group. The data demonstrate that the registry enrollees were heavily exposed to physical and psychological risks and that these exposures correlate with symptoms.[51] There were limitations of the WTC Registry, including the delay in implementation of the survey allowing for recall bias, the lack of a control population, making it difficult to calculate the expected background incidence of diseases, and the possibility of selection bias. These limitations notwithstanding, the WTCHR is an essential resource for understanding the long-term health effects of the 9/11 attacks among adults and children.

Several subgroups of the registry population, including rescue and recovery workers, residents, and local workers, have submitted to in-depth evaluations to determine health effects in specific populations. So far, although methodologically different from the studies at the clinical centers, the results of the registry studies have been consistent with the findings in the FDNY and labor studies. Review of registry data on 25,748 rescue, recovery, and cleanup workers revealed a risk of asthma twelvefold higher than the expected background three-year risk in the general population (3.6% versus 0.3%).[53] Significant risk factors for worse health outcomes were earlier arrival at the site, longer duration of work, exposure to the dust cloud, and working on the pile at the WTC site.

Further in-depth studies have looked at mental health issues, particularly in rescue and recovery workers and volunteers. In an analysis of 28,962 WTCHR rescue and recovery workers interviewed two to three years after the disaster, the prevalence of PTSD was 12.4% and ranged from 6.2% for police officers and 21.2% for unaffiliated volunteers.[54] The highest rate of PTSD was documented in construction workers and engineers, volunteers, and sanitation workers, suggesting that performing tasks not relevant to one's occupation poses a distinct risk, a finding relevant for future disasters. When Lower Manhattan residents ($n = 11{,}039$) who resided within 1 mile of the WTC site were evaluated for psychological stress two to three years after 9/11, an estimated 12.6% rate of probable PTSD was found and was associated with older age, female gender, Hispanic ethnicity, and low socioeconomic status.[55] This rate was estimated to be 3 times higher than would be expected had the WTC attack not occurred and has raised awareness that psychological symptoms may persist eight years after the event.

Lessons Learned

The events of 9/11 and their aftermath were tragic and resulted in the worst environmental disaster in the history of New York City. The response of the medical community highlights both the strengths of the community and its weaknesses, and some lessons have been reviewed elsewhere.[27,56] In an environmental catastrophe, who is responsible for the medical response? What is the chain of command? Scores of medical personnel ran to the WTC site and offered their help during the immediate crisis, and all hospitals were on emergency standby during the first few days; however, there was no coordination for the medical response to subsequent environmental issues. The lack of expertise of the local governmental agencies in toxicologic or environmental health monitoring became apparent early on and could have been remedied by collaborations with experts in the field; these collaborations were slow to develop, although they have strengthened in the subsequent years. Furthermore, when decisions about public health were made by governmental entities concerned with economic and security issues as well, the inherent conflict of interest may put communities at risk. Thus, rapid independent input from private as well as academic medical and scientific communities is needed in the setting of environmental disasters.

These same medical and academic communities need to learn to work with one another for the public good. There is a conflict between the need for rapid information and the snail's pace at which the medical community develops and presents its data. Data cannot be presented to the press, the fastest route of communication, until it has been published in a peer-reviewed journal. But the peer review and publication process can take months, if not years, and depends on reviewers and editors who may have lost interest in the subject. In addition, the reality of medical communities is that they function as independent and competitive groups, each vying for funding for its own institution. Collaboration is often limited because of this competition. The academic and medical response to the WTC crisis used some pre-existing structures to overcome some of these limitations. The presence of a network of NIEHS centers provided a forum for communication and the ability to share resources that led to some of the most comprehensive toxicologic analyses. The presence of pre-existing occupational health centers allowed for the development of a network of programs that comprised the WTC Workers Monitoring and Treatment Program. The absence of any such network in place for the nonresponder community highlights this need.

Finally, there is a difference between toxicologic studies and health responses. Toxicologic studies monitor levels of chemicals, but the human response to these chemicals requires human studies. Some of the chemical compounds in the WTC dust might have been expected to have been present; others, because of the extreme pressure and heat, were difficult to identify and remain unknown. The true levels of exposure will never be known. Assumptions derived from studies of healthy humans may not hold true for a diverse population with individuals who may have greater susceptibility for adverse health effects (children, the elderly, and individuals with comorbid conditions). Thus, all populations, not only the most highly exposed but also those with a potentially lower exposure but greater susceptibility, need to be monitored. In addition, if there is no knowledge about the response to a compound or mixture of compounds, or if the level of exposure is not measurable, as in those persons exposed to the dust cloud, an assumption of the absence of an adverse health effect should only be made after study results are available. The finding of adverse WTC health effects in every population studied suggests the need for greater vigilance in future disasters. The criticism of all studies on the basis of recall bias or lack of control populations should be a reminder that these studies ought to have been implemented more rapidly. Two years later is too late.

Summary

Perhaps the most important lesson to be learned from the medical response to the WTC events is the importance of partnership among the affected populations and academic and government agencies. The medical response for the FDNY had an advantage in that it was already in place on 9/11 as part of an ongoing medical program. In contrast, it was the organized efforts of politically skilled labor organizations that established a health program for their constituencies. And it was the loud, unrelenting, often angry efforts of diverse grass-roots community organizations that eventually won a health program for their disparate communities. Rather than disregard lay anecdotes and stories, physicians and scientists should consider these reports as the most sensitive and earliest indication of a need for a medical and scientific response. The WTC environmental disaster of respiratory exposures to alkaline dust with adsorbed PAH, metals, and other compounds is now being repeated in the aftermath of the BP Gulf oil spill, where workers are exposed to high levels of crude oil and its volatiles and dispersants, cleanup workers are exposed to oil and tar balls that wash up on beaches, and community residents are exposed to oil and volatile hydrocarbons as well as the mental stress associated with lost income.

Key Terms

National Institute for Occupational
  Safety and Health (NIOSH)

National Institutes of Environmental
  Health Science (NIEHS)

Polycyclic aromatic hydrocarbons
  (PAH)

The World Trade Center Environmental
  Health Center (WTC EHC)

WTC cough

WTC Health Registry (WTCHR)

WTC Residents Respiratory Study

Discussion Questions

1. What was the government's immediate response to the health risks of the WTC disaster?
2. What information did the government disseminate about the health risks of the disaster?
3. How was the cleanup of WTC materials organized?
4. What were the results of the exposure risk research surrounding those affected?
5. What are some of the long-term health effects of exposure to WTC disaster materials?

CHAPTER 9

CHLOROFLUOROCARBONS AND THE DEVELOPMENT OF THE OZONE HOLE

LEARNING OBJECTIVES

- To understand what CFCs are and how they have contributed to destruction of the ozone layer in Antarctica
- To become knowledgeable about the ozone layer and how it is being depleted
- To become familiar with the Montreal Protocol and to discuss its effectiveness
- To understand the connections among the ozone layer, UV radiation, and biological health

Chlorofluorocarbons (CFCs), along with other chlorine- and bromine-containing compounds, have been implicated in the accelerated depletion of ozone in the Earth's stratosphere. CFCs were developed in the early 1930s and are used in a variety of industrial, commercial, and household applications Production and use of chlorofluorocarbons experienced nearly uninterrupted growth as demand for products requiring their use continued to rise. It wasn't until the early 1970s that the link between CFCs and **ozone depletion** was made. Molina and Rowland published in *Nature* in 1974 that stratospheric ozone could be depleted as a consequence of the release of chlorofluorocarbons to the environment.[1] Observations of the ozone layer itself showed that depletion was indeed occurring; the most dramatic loss was discovered over Antarctica by the British Antarctic Survey in 1984. Ozone depletion epitomizes the global environmental problems humans face: it is an unintended consequence of human activity. The way it was solved is a success story contributed to by many, including scientists, technologists, economic and legal experts, environmentalists, and policymakers.[2]

Chlorofluorocarbons

In the 1930s, Thomas Midgley[3] invented CFCs during a search for nontoxic substances that could be used as coolants in home refrigerators. Because of their chemical inertness and stability, the CFCs were considered to be "miracle" compounds. These substances are nontoxic, nonflammable, and nonreactive with other chemical compounds. These desirable safety characteristics, along with their stable thermodynamic properties, make them ideal for many applications—as coolants for commercial and home refrigeration units, aerosol propellants, electronic cleaning solvents, and blowing agents. All this activity doubled the worldwide use of CFCs every six to seven years with an annual industrial usage of about one million tons, with more than 20 billion pounds produced worldwide since the 1930s. Although chemical inertness has previously been regarded as a beneficial property of CFCs, scientists now recognize that this same property has created a global-scale problem. It has enabled CFCs to reach the stratosphere, where they decompose, releasing chlorine atoms that affect the ozone layer.

Ozone Layer

Ozone is a gas that is present naturally in the Earth's atmosphere. Ozone was discovered by the Swiss chemist C. F. Schöenbein in 1840 while observing an electrical discharge; he noted its distinctively pungent odor and named it "ozone," which means "smell" in Greek. An ozone (O_3) molecule is made from three oxygen atoms, instead of the two of a normal oxygen molecule (O_2), which makes up 21% of the air we breathe. The average concentration of ozone in the atmosphere is about 30 parts per million by volume (ppmv), although most of it ($\sim$90%) is contained in the stratosphere, where it is present at levels of several parts per million by volume. Even though it occurs in such small quantities, ozone plays a vital role in supporting life on Earth. It is continuously being made by the action of solar radiation on molecular oxygen, predominantly in the upper stratosphere and at low latitudes. Unfortunately, ozone is also continuously being destroyed throughout the atmosphere by a variety of chemical processes. The basic ozone formation/destruction mechanism consists of the following reactions, which were first suggested by Chapman[4,5] in the 1930s:

$$O_2 + h\nu \rightarrow O + O \qquad [1]$$

$$O + O_2 \rightarrow O_3 \qquad [2]$$

$$O_3 + h\nu \rightarrow O + O_2 \qquad [3]$$

$$O + O_3 \rightarrow O_2 + O_2 \qquad [4]$$

Molecular oxygen absorbs solar radiation at wavelengths $\sim$200 nm and releases oxygen atoms (reaction 1), which rapidly combine with oxygen molecules to form ozone (reaction 2). In reactions 1 and 3, $h\nu$ denotes a solar photon. Ozone absorbs solar radiation very efficiently at wavelengths $\sim$200 to 300 nm and is destroyed by this absorption process (reaction 3), but the oxygen atoms produced by this reaction readily regenerate the ozone molecule by reaction 2. Thus, the net effect of reactions 2 and 3 is the conversion of solar energy to heat without the destruction of ozone. This process leads to an increase of temperature with altitude, which is the feature that gives rise to the stratosphere; the inverted temperature profile in this layer is responsible for its large stability toward vertical movements. In contrast, in the lowest layer—the troposphere—temperature decreases with altitude, and winds disperse atmospheric trace components very efficiently on a global scale, on a time scale of months within each hemisphere and about a year or two between the two hemispheres.

Most of the time, oxygen atoms make ozone (as in reaction 2), but occasionally they destroy ozone (as in reaction 4). However, the calculated ozone concentration based on Chapman's mechanism was considerably higher than the observed amount; thus, there must be other reactions that contribute to the reduction of the ozone concentration. In the early 1970s Crutzen[6] and Johnston independently suggested that trace amounts of nitrogen oxides (NO_x)—formed in the stratosphere through the decay of chemically stable nitrous oxide (N_2O), which originates from soil-borne microorganisms, control the ozone abundance through a catalytic cycle consisting of the following reactions:

$$NO + O_3 \rightarrow NO_2 + O_2 \tag{5}$$

$$NO_2 + O \rightarrow NO + O_2 \tag{6}$$

$$\frac{O_3 + h\nu \rightarrow O + O_2}{Net : 2\,O_3 \rightarrow 3\,O_2} \tag{3}$$

The species NO and NO_2 are still present after these three reactions have occurred, but two molecules of ozone have been destroyed. These species have an odd number of electrons; they are free radicals and are chemically very reactive. Although the concentration of NO and NO_2 is small (several ppbv), each radical pair can destroy thousands of ozone molecules before being temporarily removed, mainly by reaction with hydroxyl (OH) radical to form nitric acid:

$$OH + NO_2 \rightarrow HNO_3 \tag{7}$$

Ozone is also present in the troposphere; some of it is generated there by photochemical reactions, and some is transported from the stratosphere. The ingredients for its photochemical formation are NO_x, hydrocarbon fragments, and solar radiation; thus, NO_x plays a dual role, destroying or generating O_3 depending on the altitude. Ozone is a key component of urban smog, where it is present in amounts that are relatively small on a global scale but very significant on a local scale because of the human health effects. The description of these chemical equations was regarded as a paramount achievement, and their authors were rewarded with the Nobel Prize in Chemistry in 1995.

Chlorine atoms are also very efficient catalysts for ozone destruction and may participate in a very similar catalytic cycle:

$$Cl + O_3 \rightarrow ClO + O_2 \tag{8}$$

$$ClO + O \rightarrow Cl + O_2 \tag{9}$$

$$\frac{O_3 + h\nu \rightarrow O + O_2}{Net : 2\,O_3 \rightarrow 3\,O_2} \tag{3}$$

However, only small amounts of chlorine compounds of natural origin exist in the stratosphere: the only important source is methyl chloride (CH_3Cl), which is present at a level of less than one ppbv. This species is produced at the Earth's surface by biological activity and also to some extent by biomass burning; most of the CH_3Cl is destroyed in the troposphere, but a small percentage of it reaches the stratosphere. There are large natural sources of inorganic chlorine compounds at the Earth's surface, for example, NaCl and HCl from the oceans; however, these compounds are water soluble and are removed very efficiently from the atmosphere by clouds and rainfall long before they reach the stratosphere.

Conversely, the CFCs are practically insoluble in water and thus are not removed by rainfall. Furthermore, they are inert toward the OH radical; reaction with this radical to form water is the process that initiates the oxidation of hydrocarbons in the lower atmosphere, which eventually leads to CO_2 and water. Thus, the CFCs are not removed by the common atmospheric cleansing mechanisms that operate in the lower atmosphere. Because CFC molecules are transparent from 230 nm through the visible wavelengths, they are effectively protected below 25 km by the stratospheric ozone layer that shields the Earth's surface from ultraviolet (UV) light. Instead, they rise into the stratosphere, where they are eventually destroyed by the short-wavelength ($\sim$200 nm) solar UV radiation. A CFC molecule takes on average fifteen years to go from the ground level up to the stratosphere, where it can stay for about a century, destroying up to 100,000 ozone molecules during that time. (See Figure 9.1.)

FIGURE 9.1   Regions of the atmosphere

REGIONS OF THE ATMOSPHERE

UV/visible sunlight

MESOSPHERE

infrared radiation

STRATOSPHERE

0°F

~50 km
(50 miles)

TROPOSPHERE

ozone layer

Mt Everest
~9 km
(5.5 miles)

~8 km
(5 miles)

−80°F

infrared radiation

~9 - 12 km
(5.5 - 7.5 miles)

60°F

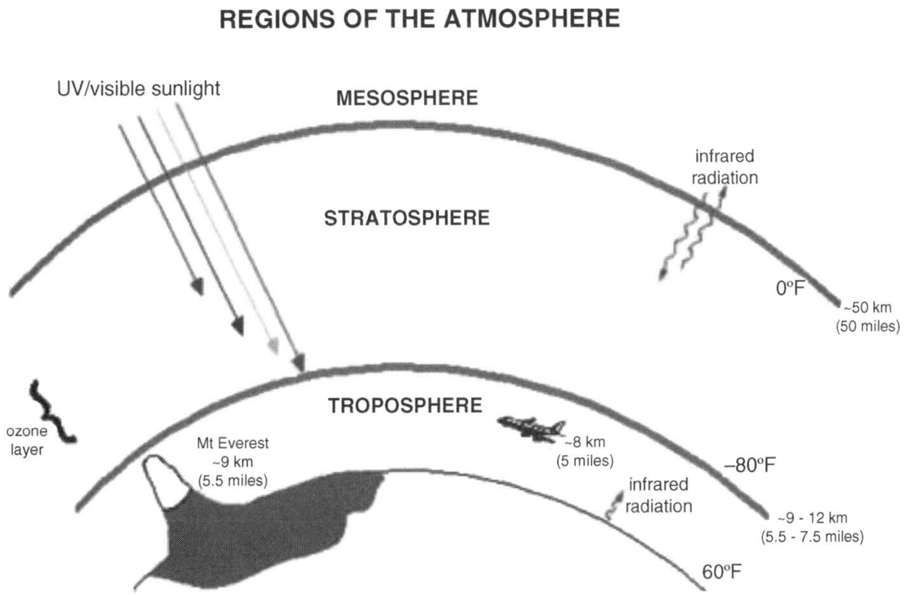

Source: National Oceanic and Atmospheric Administration.

In 1973, using the newly developed electron capture detector, Lovelock and coworkers[7] were able to detect measurable levels of CFCs in the atmosphere over the South and North Atlantic. Rowland and Molina[1] decided to investigate the ultimate atmospheric fate of these wonder compounds. After carrying out a systematic search of chemical and physical processes that might destroy the CFCs in the lower atmosphere, they concluded that the only significant sink (*sink* being defined as a source of the reduced ozone and where this occurred and what was the mechanism of this) was solar ultraviolet photolysis in the middle stratosphere (~25–30 km).

The destruction of CFCs by solar radiation leads to the release of chlorine atoms, which participate in ozone destruction cycles: these atoms attack ozone within a few seconds (as in reaction 10) and are regenerated on a time scale of minutes (as in reaction 11).[8] These cycles may be temporarily interrupted, for example, by reaction of chlorine monoxide (ClO) with HO_2 or NO_2 to produce hypochlorous acid (HOCl) or chlorine nitrate ($ClONO_2$), respectively; or by reaction of the Cl atom with methane (CH_4) to produce the relatively stable hydrogen chloride (HCl):

$$ClO + HO_2 \rightarrow HOCl + O_2 \qquad [10]$$

$$ClO + NO_2 \rightarrow ClONO_2 \qquad [11]$$

$$Cl + CH_4 \rightarrow HCl + CH_3 \qquad [12]$$

The chlorine-containing product species HCl, $ClONO_2$, and HOCl function as temporary inert reservoirs: they are not directly involved in ozone depletion, but they are eventually broken down by reaction with other free radicals or by absorption of solar radiation, thus returning chlorine to its catalytically active free radical form.[9] At low latitudes and in the upper stratosphere, where the formation of ozone is fastest, a few percentage of the chlorine radicals are in this active form; most of the chlorine is in the inert reservoir form, with HCl the most abundant species.[10] The temporary chlorine reservoirs remain in the stratosphere for several years before returning to the troposphere, where they are rapidly removed by rain or clouds. There are two reasons for this long stratospheric residence time: (1) transport is very slow in the vertical direction, because of the inverted temperature profile; and (2) there is no rain in the stratosphere, and clouds do not normally form there, thus preventing the rapid removal of water-soluble compounds such as the chlorine reservoir species. This is due to the fact that a large fraction of the water vapor present at lower altitudes condenses on its way up into the stratosphere, making it very dry. A schematic representation of these processes is presented in Figure 9.2.[2]

FIGURE 9.2   Ozone in the atmosphere

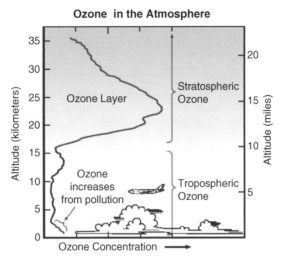

Note: Most ozone (about 90%) is found in the stratosphere, a region that begins about 10–16 kilometers (6–10 miles) above the Earth's surface and extends up about 50 km (31 miles) altitude. Ten percent is found in the troposphere, which is the lowest region of the atmosphere.
Source: National Oceanic and Atmospheric Administration.

   Besides chlorine, bromine also plays an important role in stratospheric chemistry. There are industrial sources of brominated hydrocarbons as well as natural ones; the most important of them are the halons and methyl bromide (CH_3Br). Methyl bromide is a common agricultural fumigant. The halons are fully halogenated hydrocarbons, produced industrially as fire extinguishers; examples are CF_3Br and CF_2ClBr. These sources release bromine to the stratosphere at parts per trillion volume (pptv) levels, compared with parts per billion volume (ppbv) for chlorine. On the other hand, bromine atoms are about 50 times more efficient than chlorine atoms for ozone destruction on an atom-per-atom basis;[11] a large fraction of the bromine compounds is present as free radicals, because the temporary reservoirs are less stable and are formed at considerably slower rates than the corresponding chlorine reservoirs. In contrast, fluorine atoms abstract hydrogen atoms very rapidly from methane and from water vapor, forming the very stable hydrogen fluoride (HF) molecule, which serves as a permanent inert fluorine reservoir. Hence, fluorine-free radicals are extremely scarce and the effect of fluorine on stratospheric ozone is negligible.[12]

Polar Ozone Chemistry

It is important to understand unique features of the polar regions that impact on ozone chemistry before one can understand how an ozone hole can form and what this means in the context of human-made anthropogenic pollution in our planet in modern times. The polar stratosphere is unique in several ways. First of all, ozone is not generated there, because the short-wavelength solar radiation that is absorbed by molecular oxygen is scarce, as a consequence of the solar inclination (large solar zenith angles). In addition, the total ozone column abundance (meaning stratospheric ozone 10–50 km. See Figure 9.2) at high latitudes is large because ozone is transported toward the poles from higher altitudes and lower latitudes. Furthermore, the prevailing temperatures over the stratosphere above the poles in the winter and spring months are the lowest throughout the atmosphere, particularly over Antarctica. Thus, ozone is expected to be rather stable over the poles if one considers only gas phase chemical and photochemical processes, because regeneration of ozone-destroying free radicals from the reservoir species would occur only very slowly at those temperatures.[2]

Another important feature of the polar stratosphere is the seasonal presence of **polar stratospheric clouds (PSCs).** PSCs are clouds in the winter polar stratosphere at altitudes of 15,000–25,000 meters. They are implicated in the formation of ozone holes because they support chemical reactions that produce active chlorine that catalyzes ozone destruction, and also because they remove gaseous nitric acid, perturbing nitrogen and chlorine cycles in a way which increases ozone destruction. As mentioned previously, the stratosphere is very dry—water is present only at a level of a few ppmv, a level comparable to that of ozone itself. Over the poles, a somewhat larger amount of water is present, resulting from the oxidation of methane. Furthermore, the temperature can drop to below −85°C over Antarctica in the winter and spring months, leading to the formation of ice clouds, which are known as type II PSCs. The presence of trace amounts of nitric and sulfuric acids enables the formation of polar stratospheric clouds a few degrees above the frost point (which is the temperature at which ice can condense from the gas phase); these acids can form cloud particles consisting of crystalline hydrates, known as type I PSCs.

Solomon et al.[13] first suggested that PSCs could play a major role in the depletion of ozone over Antarctica by promoting the release of photolytically active chlorine from its reservoir species. This occurs mainly by the following reaction:

$$HCl + ClONO_2 \rightarrow Cl_2 + HNO_3 \qquad [13]$$

Laboratory studies have shown that this reaction occurs very slowly, if at all, in the gas phase;[14] however, in the presence of ice surfaces, it proceeds with remarkable efficiency.[15] HCl is taken up very efficiently by liquid water, forming hydrochloric acid as it dissolves. However, HCl is only barely soluble in the ice matrix; when dilute hydrochloric acid solutions freeze, almost pure water ice forms, as the ice crystals reject impurities. Experimental observations[15] and theoretical calculations[16] indicate that HCl solvates readily on the ice surface and forms hydrochloric acid. Compared to the crystal, the ice surface is disordered—it behaves more like a liquid than a solid—thus explaining the high affinity of ice for HCl. As a consequence, chlorine activation reactions on the surfaces of ice crystals proceed through ionic mechanisms analogous to those in aqueous solutions.[2]

The presence of PSCs also leads to the removal of nitrogen oxides (NO_x) from the gas phase; the source for these free radicals in the polar stratosphere is nitric acid, which condenses in the cloud particles. Furthermore, some of the particles consist of large enough ice crystals to fall out of the stratosphere, permanently removing the nitric acid, a process referred to as **denitrification**. This process has important consequences: the nitrogen oxides normally interfere with the catalytic ozone loss reactions involving chlorine oxides, mainly by scavenging chlorine monoxide to form chlorine nitrate, as in reaction 11.[17] In the absence of nitrogen oxides, chlorine radicals destroy ozone much more rapidly.

Field Measurements of Atmospheric Trace Species

Various fundamental aspects of the CFC-ozone depletion hypothesis were verified in the late 1970s and early 1980s, following the initial publication of the Molina-Rowland article.[1] Measurements of the atmospheric concentrations of the CFCs indicated that they accumulated in the lower atmosphere and that they reached the stratosphere in the amounts predicted. Chlorine atoms and ClO radicals were found in the stratosphere, together with other species such as HCl, $ClONO_2$, HOCl, O, NO, NO_2, OH, HO_2, and so on, with observed concentrations in reasonable agreement with the model predictions. On the other hand, a decrease in stratospheric ozone levels was not observable at that time because of the large natural variability of this species. However, the ozone levels in the Antarctic stratosphere dropped dramatically in the spring months starting in the early 1980s, as first reported by Farman and coworkers[18] in 1985. Subsequently it became evident that ozone was being depleted in the Northern Hemisphere as well, particularly at high latitudes and in the winter and spring months. Later on, it became possible to show by examination of the ozone records that significant

FIGURE 9.3   Southern Hemisphere ozone hole area, 2008

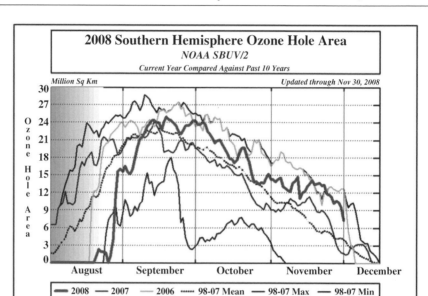

Note: Current year compared against past ten years.
Source: National Oceanic and Atmospheric Administration.

changes have also taken place in the lower stratosphere at mid-latitudes.[11] Furthermore, satellite measurements have directly confirmed conclusions that the bulk of the chlorine present in the stratosphere is of human origin.[19]

The depletion of ozone over Antarctica—the ozone hole—was not predicted by the atmospheric sciences community.[2] However, the cause of this depletion became very clear in subsequent years: laboratory experiments, field measurements over Antarctica, and model calculations showed unambiguously that the ozone hole could indeed be traced to the industrial CFCs.

The next phase of research was to map the extent of the ozone hole by using various scientific techniques. Farman et al.[18] conducted their measurements of rapid ozone loss in the stratosphere over Antarctica from the ground using a spectrophotometer; their findings were subsequently confirmed by satellite data from the total ozone mapping spectrometer (TOMS),[20] which measures ozone by a similar principle, namely by monitoring at two wavelengths the attenuation of solar radiation that has been back-scattered from the atmosphere below the ozone layer. More recent measurements from satellites and high-altitude balloons indicate that the extent of ozone depletion over Antarctica in the spring months continued to increase after 1985. (See Figure 9.3 for recent data.)

Several expeditions were launched in the years following the initial discovery of the ozone hole to measure trace species in the stratosphere over Antarctica; for example, NASA used ER-2 high-altitude aircraft. The results provided strong evidence for the occurrence of the chemical reactions described above, and hence for the crucial role played by industrial chlorine in the depletion of ozone.[21] At the time that ozone is strongly depleted in the polar stratosphere (during the spring), a large fraction of the chlorine is present as a free radical. Anderson et al.[22] measured ppbv levels of chlorine monoxide, which were strongly inversely correlated with ozone loss monitored by Proffitt et al.[23] An analysis of these measurements indicated that the chlorine peroxide cycle accounted for about three-fourths of the observed ozone loss, with the bromine cycle accounting for the rest.[22] Furthermore, NO_x levels were found to be very low and nitric acid was shown to be present in the cloud particles. These data provided more support for the CFC hypothesis leading to ozone loss and the ozone hole over the Antarctic. (See Figure 9.4.)

FIGURE 9.4   Largest Antarctic ozone hole ever recorded, September 2006

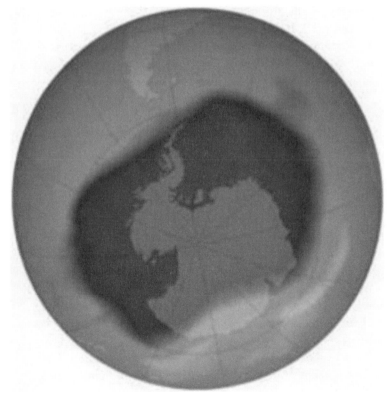

Source: National Oceanic and Atmospheric Administration.

Atmospheric field measurements have also been conducted in the Arctic stratosphere,[24] indicating that a large fraction of the chlorine is also activated there. Nevertheless, ozone depletion is less severe over the Arctic and is not as localized, because the temperatures are not as low as over Antarctica; the active chlorine does not remain in contact with ozone long enough and at low enough temperatures to destroy it before the stratospheric air over the Arctic mixes with warmer air from lower latitudes. On the other hand, as expected, cold winters lead to significant ozone depletion—30% or more—over large areas, as was the case over northern Europe in 1995–1996. Furthermore, as mentioned earlier, ozone is also being depleted to some extent at mid-latitudes.

Ozone Depletion and UV-B Radiation

Depletion of stratospheric ozone leads to increases in the level of solar UV radiation reaching the Earth's surface, predominantly at wavelengths ~290 to 320 nm, the so-called UV-B radiation. At shorter wavelengths, atmospheric ozone absorbs essentially all the solar photons (UV-C, 200–290 nm), and at longer wavelengths (UV-A, 320–400 nm) the absorption is negligible. UV-B radiation is partially shielded by clouds, dust, and air pollution. However, with a clear sky, each 1% reduction in the total ozone column results in an increase of about 1.3% in the intensity of UV-B at ground level. This increase is well documented by direct measurements under the Antarctic ozone hole, where the UV-B levels can exceed the maximum summer values measured at San Diego, California.[25] At other latitudes, where ozone depletion is less severe, the UV radiation increases are correspondingly smaller and more difficult to establish because of the lack of direct long-term measurements.

Biologic Effects of Ultraviolet Radiation

Ozone depletion leads to increased UV-B radiation, which in turn leads to potential risks in humans, plants, and aquatic ecosystems. Acute skin damage in humans is one such risk. Other potential risks of increased UV-B radiation on human health include increases in the morbidity and incidence of skin cancer, eye diseases, and infectious diseases.[26] The environmental and health effects of stratospheric ozone depletion have been summarized in several assessment reports.[27,28] Investigations of human epidemiology, as well as animal experiments, have established that UV-B radiation is a key risk factor for development of nonmelanoma skin cancer in light-skinned populations.[29] The two main types of this cancer are basal cell carcinoma and squamous cell carcinoma; it is estimated that a sustained 1% decrease in stratospheric ozone would result in an increase of about 2% in the incidence of these types of cancers.[30] A conservative estimate is that an additional 2,100 to 15,000 cases of nonmelanoma skin cancers would occur in the United States per year for each 1% reduction in ozone, with proportionately much larger effects for greater amounts of ozone reduction. In Punta Arenas, Chile, reduced O_3 and increased UV-B levels have resulted in a 56% increase in melanoma and a 46% increase in nonmelanoma skin cancer over seven years, and a significant increase in sunburns during the spring over the past five years.[31] During the past twenty springs, they have experienced 143 days with more than 25% ozone loss. Significant increases of UV-B were observed under ozone hole conditions, especially around 300 nm, the most carcinogenic wavelengths.

For cutaneous melanoma the situation is less clear; nonetheless, there are indications that the risk increases with sunlight exposure. The mechanism responsible for the UV damage may well be due to p53 mutations caused by UV radiation. In the presence of functional p53, during sunburn there is an increase in apoptosis, which can eliminate damaged cells. However, if one of the p53 alleles is damaged by UV, then it may be more difficult for that cell to undergo apoptosis.

In addition to affecting the skin, UV radiation can also harm the eyes and the immune system. Numerous experiments have shown that the cornea and lens of the eye can be damaged by UV-B radiation and that chronic exposure to this radiation is associated with the risk of cataract of the cortical and posterior subcapsular forms. In addition, studies in human subjects show that exposure to UV-B radiation can suppress the induction of some immune responses, and experiments in animals indicate that such exposure decreases the immune response to skin cancers and some infectious agents. The reason is that the immune system has some components that are present in the skin, which makes it susceptible to the effects of UV-B radiation.

Terrestrial plants can also be affected by UV-B radiation, although the response varies to a large extent among different species. In addition to stunting plant growth, the changes induced by UV radiation can be indirect, affecting, for example, the timing of developmental phases or the allocation of biomass to the different parts of the plant.[33] Aquatic ecosystems can also be damaged by UV-B radiation; for example, there is evidence for impaired larval development and decreased reproductive capacity in some amphibians, shrimp, and fish. As the O_3 layer thinned by as much as 50%, UV-B radiation increased and UV-B inhibition of photosynthesis occurred that could adversely affect the productivity of natural phytoplankton communities in Antarctic waters.[34]

The phytophlankton communities are also adversely affected by global warming, causing a reverberation up the food chain threatening the integrity of penguin colonies.

Policy and the Montreal Protocol

The National Academy of Sciences is called upon to issue reports on scientific challenges and in a 1976 report, stated that the atmospheric sequence outlined by Molina and Rowland was essentially correct.[35] The United States and some other countries responded in late 1970s by banning the sale of aerosol spray cans containing CFCs; this caused a temporary pause in the growing demands for CFCs. However, worldwide use of the chemicals continued, and the production rate began to rise again.

In September 1987, an international agreement limiting the production of CFCs was approved under the auspices of the United Nations Environment Programme (UNEP). This agreement, the **Montreal Protocol on Substances That Deplete the Ozone Layer**, initially called for a reduction of only 50% in the manufacture of CFCs by the end of the twentieth century. In view of the strength of the scientific evidence that emerged in the following years, the initial provisions were strengthened through the London and the Copenhagen amendments to the protocol in 1990 and 1992, respectively. The production of CFCs in industrialized countries was phased out at the end of 1995, and other compounds such as the halons, methyl bromide, carbon tetrachloride, and methyl chloroform (CH_3CCl_3) were also regulated. Carbon tetrachloride was phased out in 2000 and methyl chloroform in 2002. One hundred and sixty countries ultimately signed the Montreal Protocol after the initial twenty-two countries and the United States signed in 1987. The Montreal Protocol was codified in U.S. law under the 1990 Clean Air Act amendments.

Developing countries were allowed to continue CFC production until 2010, to facilitate their transition to the newer CFC-free technologies. An important feature of the Montreal Protocol was the establishment of a funding mechanism to help these countries meet the costs of complying with the protocol and with its subsequent amendments. It involved the creation of the Multilateral Fund, financed by the industrialized countries; the implementing agencies include UNEP, the United Nations Industrial Organization (UNIDO), the United Nations Development Programme (UNDP), and the World Bank. This fund has spent $2 billion on 5,250 projects in 139 developing countries. China emerged as the largest emitter of ozone-depleting substances, and multilateral fund projects executed by the World Bank phased out CFCs in mobile air conditioning and commercial refrigeration and reduced halons from 30,060 tons in 1998 to 1,000 tons by 2008.

Analyzing the Effectiveness of the Montreal Protocol

Overall, the provisions of the Montreal Protocol have been successfully enforced. Chlorine levels have already peaked; in fact, atmospheric measurements indicate that the abundance of chlorine contained in the CFCs and other chlorocarbons is already declining in response to the Montreal Protocol regulations.[36] On the other hand, because of the long residence times of the CFCs in the atmosphere, relatively high chlorine levels in the stratosphere— with the consequent ozone depletion—are expected to continue well into the twenty-first century.[2]

A significant fraction of the former CFC usage is being dealt with by conservation and recycling. Furthermore, roughly one-quarter of the former use of CFCs is being temporarily replaced by hydrochlorofluorocarbons (HCFCs)—compounds that have similar physical properties to the CFCs but that are less stable in the atmosphere. A large fraction of the HCFCs released industrially react in the lower atmosphere with the OH radical before reaching the stratosphere, forming water and an organic free radical that rapidly photo-oxidizes to yield water-soluble products, which are then removed from the atmosphere mainly by rainfall. Some hydrofluorocarbons (HFCs), which do not contain chlorine atoms, are also being used as CFC replacements, for example, HFC-134a (CF_3–CH_2F), for automobile air conditioning. About half of the CFC usage has been replaced by not-in-kind compounds; for example, CFC-113—used extensively as a solvent to clean electronic components—has been phased out by CFC-free cleaning technologies such as soap and water or terpene-based solvents; there are also new technologies to manufacture clean electronic boards.

There are problems with using HCFCs, however. In fact, three of the twelve HCFCs can break down into trifluoroacetic acid (TFA) found in wetlands. TFA is produced in the atmosphere through interaction with OH radicals with three HCFCs: HCFC -123, -124, and HFC-134a. TFA is resistant to degradation processes such as photolysis and hydrolysis, and is virtually unmetabolizable by most plants and animals. TFA may be a hazard in urban environments due to high levels of OH radical in the air pollution. Furthermore, TFA is highly mobile in xylem tissue of plants and has been demonstrated to bioaccumulate by at least a factor of 30 in vascular plants. As a result, the solution to CFCs may have unintended consequences. In response to these issues, the Clean Air Act amendments of 1990, which added the provisions of the Montreal Protocol to U.S. law, also proposed a phase-out of the HCFCs by 2030 under Stratospheric Ozone and Global Climate Protection.

Atmospheric measurements show that the total combined effective abundance of ozone-depleting compounds continues to decline slowly from the peak that occurred around 1993. As predicted, total chlorine is declining, while bromine from industrial halons was still increasing slightly at the beginning of the twenty-first century. However, the atmospheric abundances of HCFCs continue to increase.

Throughout the last decade of the twenty century and the first years of the twenty-first century, Antarctic ozone depletion in the springtime (the ozone hole) has been quite large. By 2015 the Antarctic O_3 hole (AOH) will be reduced by one million km^2 out of 25 million km^2; recovery will occur by 2024, being almost complete by 2050 and reach 1980 levels by 2068. Similarly, winter/spring ozone loss in the Arctic is highly variable as a consequence of changes in meteorological conditions in the stratosphere from one winter to another; in some recent cold Arctic winters, ozone losses have reached 30%. By the middle of the twenty-first century, the amounts of halogens in the stratosphere are expected to be similar to those present in 1980, prior to the onset of the ozone hole. However, the influence of climate change could accelerate or delay ozone recovery.

Ozone Depletion and Climate Change

The understanding of the interaction between ozone depletion and climate change has been strengthened in recent years. Because ozone is a greenhouse gas, ozone change and climate change are linked in important ways.[37] Austin et al. noted that the stratosphere is expected to become cooler due to both CO_2 increases and long-term ozone decreases.[37] This should increase the likelihood of PSCs forming over the Arctic because the saturation vapor pressure of gas-phase water and nitric acid are strong exponential functions of temperature. With extensive PSCs, increased chlorine- and bromine-driven ozone destruction can be expected over the Arctic region. Ozone-depleting substances, such as the CFCs and halons, also contribute to climate change. Certain changes in Earth's climate could affect the future of the ozone layer. Stratospheric ozone is influenced by changes in temperatures and winds in the stratosphere. While the Earth's surface is expected to warm in response to the positive radiative forcing from increases in carbon dioxide, the stratosphere is expected to cool. A cooler stratosphere would extend the time period over which PSCs are present in the polar region. This change might increase winter ozone depletion. As a result, it is likely that the recovery of the ozone layer following the decline in chlorine and bromine compounds reaching the stratosphere will be delayed by climate change, but the extent of the interaction is not yet well established.

Further challenges to the ozone layer come from methyl bromide. The sum of organic bromine from methyl bromide (CH_3Br) and halons has more than doubled in the atmosphere since the mid-1900s. This information has been inferred from measurements of the composition of Southern Hemisphere air archives and from samples of air bubbles trapped in compressed Antarctic snow (so-called firn air). The atmospheric lifetime of methyl bromide is estimated to be about 0.7 years, and the fraction of emissions derived from industrially produced methyl bromide is estimated to be 10–40%, based upon our understanding of source and sink magnitudes. This result strengthens the conclusion that the industrial production of methyl bromide needs to be further controlled, as stipulated by the Montreal Protocol, in order not to delay the recovery of the ozone layer.

Medihaler Impediments to Controlling Ozone Depletion

Another obstacle to the efforts to stop ozone depletion is the fact that more than 70 million patients with chronic obstructive pulmonary disease (COPD) and asthma use 450 million aerosols per year worldwide. Traditional CFC-based metered dose inhalers (MDIs) used a mixture of two propellants to achieve the required vapor pressure: CFC-11 was a vehicle for drug suspension, allowing filling into the can, and CFC-12 acted as the propellant. Major technological development of hydrofluoroalkane HFA 134a as a liquefied compressed gas and new MDIs with new metering valves and manufacturing techniques replaced the role of CFCs. Dry powder inhalants became widely used also. Albuterol was the last generic MDI and used 1,200 tons of CFCs to produce it per year. The Food and Drug Administration (FDA) approved two non–CFC albuterol MDIs: Proventil HFA-134a (1996) and Ventolin HFA-134a (2001); Proair HFA and Xopenex HFA have also been approved.

In response to these technological developments, Sen. Hillary Rodham Clinton wrote to the FDA in 2004 to urge the removal of CFCs from MDIs post-haste. In March 2005 the FDA issued a final rule that albuterol MDIs using CFCs must no longer be produced, marketed, or sold in the United States after December 31, 2008. Schering-Plough and its Warrick subsidiary announced in 2007 that it was phasing out production of CFC-propelled albuterol inhalers and would increase production of its CFC-free product, Proventil HFA.

Recently, the success of removing CFCs has been temporized by the realization that nitrous oxide (N_2O) is the dominant ozone-depleting substance emitted in the twenty-first century.[38] Nitrous oxide has anthropogenic sources from synthetic and organic fertilizers, production of nitrogen-fixing crops, fossil fuel, biomass and biofuel combustion, and application of livestock manure to croplands and pasture, although 70% is from natural sources. It has increased by 20% over the past two centuries and is transported to the stratosphere, where it breaks down to NOx and destroys O_3. It is mainly removed from the atmosphere through photolysis and combining with reactive oxygen species, but it persists for more than 120 years.

Summary

It is now clear that human activities can lead to serious environmental problems not just on a local but also on a global scale. One of the key steps in any rational approach to addressing global environmental issues is to promote internationalism—a widespread understanding that all of our human problems are interconnected. Regional and international cooperation will be essential to the solution of environmental problems. The formulation of the Montreal Protocol sets a very important precedent for addressing global environmental problems. It demonstrates how the different sectors of society—scientists, industry people, policymakers, and environmentalists—can work together and can be very productive by functioning in a collaborative mode rather than in an adversary mode.

Key Terms

Chlorofluorocarbons (CFCs)

Denitrification

Montreal Protocol on Substances That
   Deplete the Ozone Layer

Ozone

Ozone depletion

Polar stratospheric clouds (PSCs)

Discussion Questions

1. What are CFCs and how have they contributed to ozone depletion?
2. What is the ozone layer and how is it being depleted?

3. What are the effects of ozone depletion on UV radiation?
4. What are the effects of UV radiation on biological health?
5. What were the main tenets of the Montreal Protocol?
6. How effective was the Montreal Protocol in reducing ozone depletion?
7. What are some of the remaining challenges to stopping ozone depletion and how are they being addressed?

The author thanks Mario J. Molina and Luisa T. Molina for permission to use parts of the chapter "Chlorofluorocarbons and Destruction of the Ozone Layer" published in *Environmental and Occupational Medicine*, 4th ed., by Lippincott, Williams and Wilkins.

.

CHAPTER 10

GLOBAL WARMING SCIENCE AND CONSEQUENCES

LEARNING OBJECTIVES

- To understand the workings of the Intergovernmental Panel on Climate Change and its role in climate change research
- To become familiar with the current knowledge surrounding global warming and its sources
- To understand the environmental and human consequences of global warming

The National Oceanic and Atmospheric Administration (NOAA) collected data from 300 scientists from forty-eight countries to report in 2010 that the past decade was the warmest on record and that the Earth has been growing warmer over the past fifty years. Seven of 10 indicators were rising: air temperature over land, sea surface temperature, air temperature over oceans, sea level, ocean heat, humidity, and tropospheric temperature in the "active weather" layer of the atmosphere closest to the Earth's surface. Three indicators were declining: arctic sea ice, glaciers, and spring snow cover in the Northern Hemisphere.

Weather is what we experience locally over a short period of time; **climate** is the pattern of weather in a region or globally over an extended period of time. The commonly accepted theory that human or anthropogenic activities are contributing to **climate change** by altering the atmospheric composition of heat-trapping chemicals is known as **global warming**. Global warming is the major challenge facing our planet, our youth, and future generations. We need to end our dependence on fossil fuels and their attendant pollution and develop novel strategies to enjoy technology without the consequences of global climate change.

In 2007 former Vice President Al Gore shared the Nobel Peace Prize with Rajendra K. Pachauri, Chairman of the **Intergovernmental Panel on Climate Change (IPCC)**.[1,2] Al Gore, in his Nobel acceptance speech, stated:

> Major cities in North and South America, Asia and Australia are nearly out of water due to massive droughts and melting glaciers. Peoples on low-lying Pacific islands are planning evacuations of places they have long called home. Unprecedented wildfires have forced a half million people from their homes. . . . Stronger storms in the Pacific and Atlantic have threatened whole cities. Millions have been displaced by massive flooding in South Asia, Mexico, and 18 countries in Africa. As temperature extremes have increased, tens of thousands have lost their lives. We are recklessly burning and clearing our forests and driving more and more species into extinction. The very web of life on which we depend is being ripped and frayed. . . . After performing 10,000 equations by hand, Svante Arrhenius calculated that the earth's average temperature would increase by many degrees if we doubled the amount of CO_2 in the atmosphere. Seventy years later, my teacher, Roger Revelle, and his colleague, Dave Keeling, began to precisely document the increasing CO_2 levels day by day.

Finally, Al Gore said, "We have everything we need to begin solving this crisis, with the possible exception of the will to act. But in America, our will to take action is itself a renewable resource."

Global Warming Basic Science: Greenhouse Gases

Greenhouse gases (GHG), such as CO_2, CH_4, and NO_x, among many others, are responsible for the temperature of the Earth. They form a layer in the Earth's troposphere to reflect infrared radiation back to the surface, thus causing surface warming (greenhouse effect). The greenhouse gas layer in the troposphere allows visible light to penetrate and reach the surface where infrared is activated, heating the surface and rising to the troposphere. There the greenhouse gas layer reflects it back again to the Earth's surface, increasing heating. Approximately 30% of the visible light spectrum is reflected back into space, with another 20% absorbed in the troposphere before reaching the Earth, allowing the remaining 50% to reach the Earth's surface.

There are several types of greenhouse gases, with carbon dioxide being the most common and prevalent. Water vapor is a major greenhouse gas, but it varies on a daily basis as a component of weather and does not affect climate. It is removed by condensation and precipitation. CO_2 is the major greenhouse gas, results from burning fossil fuels, and is long-lived in the troposphere (approximately >80 years).[1] Estimates by James Hansen of the Goddard Space Institute, NASA, are that one-fourth of anthropogenic CO_2 may persist up to 500 years in the Earth's troposphere.[3] Methane is the second most important greenhouse gas and is 22 times more potent than CO_2 in reflecting infrared radiation back to Earth's surface.[1] The four other greenhouse gases include nitrous oxide, sulfur hexafluoride, perfluorocarbon, and hydrofluorocarbon (the latter three are like methane with >twentyfold greater ability to reflect infrared back to the surface). Carbon dioxide makes up 72% of the global greenhouse gases, with methane at 18% and nitrous oxide at 9%, but U.S. emissions are 84% CO_2, 7.4% methane, and 6.5% N_2O.

Natural sources of carbon dioxide are 20 times greater than anthropogenic but are balanced by natural sinks, including photosynthesis of carbon compounds by plants and marine plankton and oceans. Since 1990, we have known that a terrestrial carbon sink annually absorbs about one-third of global emissions from fossil fuels, and according to the median model, could annually absorb 5 billion metric tons of carbon by mid-century (compared to today's emissions of ~7 billion metric tons). As a result of this past historical balance, the atmospheric concentration of carbon dioxide remained between 260 and 280 parts per million (ppm) for the past 400,000–900,000 years. The excess anthropogenic emissions cited previously supports a recent increase in atmospheric concentrations of CO_2.

The main sources of greenhouse gases due to human activity include burning of fossil fuels and deforestation. Land use change (mainly deforestation in the tropics) accounts for up to one-third of total anthropogenic CO_2 emissions.

LIVERPOOL JOHN MOORES UNIVERSITY
LEARNING SERVICES

Calculations of the plant growth storage capacity for CO_2 are 113 billion tons of C (carbon) globally in 1900 that could increase to 171 billion tons by 2100; surface ozone pollution could stunt plant growth, and if controlled, more than 200 billion tons of C could be taken up by plants by 2100.[4] Livestock enteric fermentation and manure management, paddy rice farming, land use and wetland changes, pipeline losses, and covered landfill emissions lead to higher methane atmospheric concentrations. Methane levels have tripled since preindustrial times, although recently some tropical plants have been identified as in situ sources of methane release.[5] Fertilizers in agricultural activities are the main sources of nitrous oxide concentrations.

Annual sources of CO_2 by economic sector are electricity generation 34%, transportation 28%, industry 19%, agriculture 8%, commercial 6%, and residential 5%. Global fossil carbon emissions are more than 7 million metric tons per year, and global CO_2 emissions are nearly 4 times this amount, at approximately 28 million metric tons per year. This is an increase from 18 million metric tons of CO_2 in 1980. The concentration of CO_2 has increased by about 100 ppm (that is, from 280 ppm to 380 ppm); the first 50 ppm increase took place from the start of the Industrial Revolution to around 1973, and the next 50 ppm increase took place in about thirty-five years, from 1973 to 2008.[1] Greenhouse gas emissions due to human activities have grown by 70% from 1970 to 2004. The greenhouse gases differ in their **radiative forcing capability** (Watts/m^2) with CO_2 at 1.46, methane at 0.48, nitrous oxide at 0.15, and halocarbons at 0.34 indicating a difference in reflecting infrared reflection back to the surface of the Earth.[3,6,7]

Hansen calculates that the Earth is now absorbing 0.85 watts per square meter more energy from the sun than it is emitting to space.[6] CO_2 is the most abundant of these greenhouse gases. Since 2000, the 1.1% annual growth of CO_2 in the atmosphere has tripled to >3.5% per year, primarily due to developing countries' phenomenal growth and industrialization. Methane has not increased appreciably, and nitrous oxide has increased by 0.25% per year.

The United States has increased its greenhouse gas emissions 17.2% from 1990 to 2008, with 7.15 million metric tons of CO_2 emitted only to be surpassed by China at 7.2 million metric tons of CO_2. Relative to 2005, China's fossil CO_2 emissions increased in 2006 by 8.7%, while in the United States comparable CO_2 emissions increased in 2007 by 1.4%. The approximate per capita release of GHG is 24 tons in the United States, compared to 4 in China, 9 in Japan, 12 in Germany, 21 in Canada, and 11 in Great Britain. The historic range of CO_2 at 180–280 ppm maintains climate stability. By 2030 we may increase total CO_2 emissions to 42 million metric tons, and at this rate, we could reach 450 ppm CO_2 by 2050.[1]

A 1°C increase limit due to global warming would require a stabilization of CO_2 at ~440 ppm, but Hansen discusses the challenges of accomplishing this in the context of stabilizing methane and nitrous oxide that are indirect by-products of global warming, such as methane release from melting peat bogs due to anthropogenic CO_2 induced global warming.[7]

The average global annual temperature has risen from 14.5°C in 1886, when records began under the World Meteorological Organization, to 15.4°C in 1995. Warming toward the poles is exceeding the average. The average annual temperature in 2001 was 57.8°F, which was 0.9°F above the 1886–2000 long-term average. Eleven of the twelve hottest years on record have been observed since 1995, and 2008 was the ninth hottest. The summer of 2010 was the fourth hottest according to the Goddard Institute. (See Figure 10.1.) The IPCC Fourth Assessment Report declares, "Warming of the climate system is unequivocal, as is now evident from observations of increase in global average air and ocean temperatures, widespread melting of snow and ice, and rising global average sea level. Most of the observed increase in globally averaged temperatures since the mid-20th century is very likely due to the observed increase in anthropogenic greenhouse gas concentrations." They predicted that the global climate would be likely to warm 3°C plus or minus one degree if CO_2 concentrations reached twice the levels of 1750.

FIGURE 10.1   Global average temperature, 1850–2007

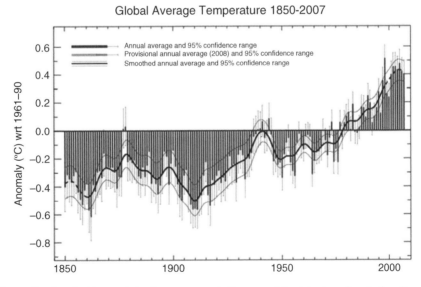

Source: Reprinted with permission from www.metoffice.gov.uk/hadobs, based on Brohan P. Journal of Geophysical Research 2006 26;111:D12106.

FIGURE 10.2 CO_2 concentration on Mauna Loa, Hawaii

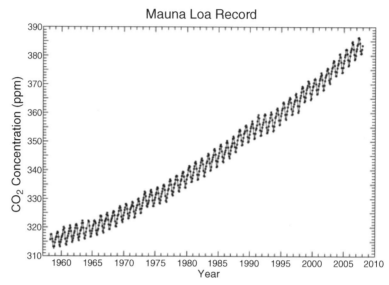

Source: Reprinted with permission from the Scripps Institution of Oceanography.

Charles David Keeling measured the concentration of CO_2 in the atmosphere on the summit of Mauna Loa in Hawaii in 1958 as part of the International Geophysical Year, and he was able to continue these measurements over the ensuing years with minimal grants and contributions.[8] What has emerged is an accurate record of CO_2 concentration beginning at 315.98 ppm in 1959, rising 19.4% to 377.38 ppm by 2004, and further increasing to 380 ppm by 2007. (See Figure 10.2.) Since 2000, Keeling also captured the acceleration in CO_2 concentration, and he observed an annual fluctuation in CO_2 in the Northern Hemisphere. When summer's leaves and vegetation utilized CO_2 for photosynthesis, there was a CO_2 decline followed by a concomitant increase in CO_2 in winter months as plants' leaves died off.

Calculations of dielectric conductivity, deuterium and ^{18}O can be used to determine temperature and CO_2 content in ice cores.[9] Samples of Antarctic Lake Vostok ice cores, dating as far back at 440,000 years, have been evaluated, and they show natural variation in temperature, with current temperatures at the highest level on record. In addition, when CO_2 concentration in these ice cores was measured, it ranged from 180 to 280 ppm over these millennia. The current level of 380 ppm exceeds the maxima of this ice record. Methane concentration was also measured; it ranged from 400 to 800 ppb compared to the

FIGURE 10.3 East Antarctica Ice Core data

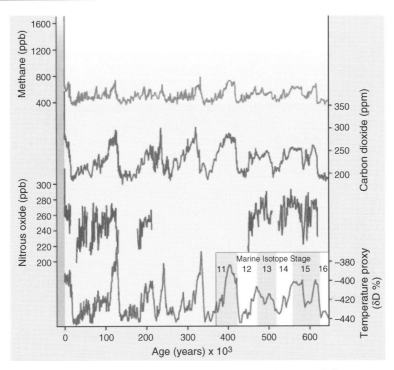

Note: Records from the European Project for Ice Coring in Antarctica Dome C show a strong 100,000-year periodicity for the past 650,000 years. At no time in the past 650,000 years is there evidence for levels of carbon dioxide or methane significantly higher than values just before the Industrial Revolution. There is covariation of carbon dioxide and methane cycles following essentially the same pattern as with climate (temperature record). Note that the highest peaks occur at the present (Age 0 time).
Source: Reprinted with permission from Brook EJ. Atmospheric Science. Tiny bubbles tell all. Science 2005; 310:1285–1287.

current level at >1700 ppb.[10] Deep ice cores have now been drilled in Antarctica Dome C to a depth corresponding to time that can be estimated back another 800,000 years, with confirmation of the more recent data from the first 440,000 years.[9,11] (Figure 10.3 illustrates the ice core data with periodicity in GHG over hundreds of thousands of years, with anthropogenic-driven peaks at the 0 point reflecting the human-made influence predominantly following World War II. Both the IPCC and the NASA/Goddard Institute/Columbia Center for Climate Systems Research conclude that the data since 1970 shows anthropogenic warming is likely to have had a discernible influence on many physical and biological systems.[12]

Black carbon from biomass and charcoal burning contributes to the greenhouse effect, and is concentrated in the Asian tropics, where solar irradiance is highest. Black carbon is transported over long distances, with transcontinental plumes of atmospheric brown clouds with vertical extents of 3 to 5 km. In the Himalayan region and the Kun Lun, solar heating from black carbon at high elevations may be important in the melting of snowpacks and glaciers.[13] Ramanathan and colleagues used unmanned aerial vehicles to measure solar irradiance directly due to Asian brown clouds over the Maldives 3 km aloft, calculating that black soot could account for an increase of 0.25°C per decade, close to actual measurements.[14] Black carbon has a short half-life of about a week in the atmosphere, and pollution mitigation strategies could have a major effect on reducing black carbon. Greenland ice cores show black carbon increasing sevenfold since 1850, with a maxima at 1910 and increasing levels after about 1951, resulting in an estimated surface climate forcing in early summer from black carbon in Arctic snow of about 3 watts per square meter.[15]

Environmental Consequences of Global Warming and Climate Change

Major environmental impacts of global warming will affect the glacial icefields in Greenland, the Alaskan and Canadian Arctic, Antarctica, glaciers on the Tibetan plateau, sea ice, and glaciers in the mountainous tropics. These are important for lower latitudes because of potential rise in sea level and potable water supplies for large cities and their agricultural/food needs. Global warming will also warm the oceans and cause a decline in pH, leading to coral bleaching. There will be changes in weather patterns with droughts increasing, increased rain in temperate regions, and changes in tropical storms.

Arctic Ice

There are many adverse consequences of global warming and climate change, beginning with the shrinking Arctic icepack (large areas of packed ice formed from seawater in the Earth's polar regions). The Arctic icepack declined $8.6 \pm 2.9\%$ per decade from 1979 to 2006, or about 100,000 km^2 per year.[16] Each year, the Arctic Ocean has a floating ice cover that ranges from about 16×10^6 km^2 in March to 7×10^6 km^2 at the end of the summer melt season in September. The September minima is getting lower each year, with 2005 at 5.56×10^6 km^2. This minima, which was 2.05 million square miles in 2005, had dropped astonishingly to 1.6 million square miles by September 2007. The U.S.

Navy nuclear submarines reported that the average ice thickness has declined from 3.1 meters to 1.8 meters, or 15% per decade from 1958 to 1997, although sparse sampling complicates interpretation. The Arctic ice has lost 24% of its volume in three decades; the chance of this occurring due to natural cycles is <0.1%. Indeed, the Northwest Passage along the northern Canadian coast to Alaska may be open for summer shipping in a few short years. The area of multi-year ice is also shrinking. Moreover, the polar icecap reflects 80% of the solar radiation, whereas open ocean only reflects 10% of solar energy (lower reflectivity), which tends to accelerate Arctic icepack melting.

Traverses by polar scientists evaluated the Northern Greenland ice sheet in 1953–1954 and again in 1995 and revealed significant thinning from 16.5 to 31 cm/year on the northwestern half. (See Figure 10.4). Greenland contains

FIGURE 10.4   Increase from 1979 (left) to 2007 (right) in the amount of the Greenland ice sheet melted in the summer

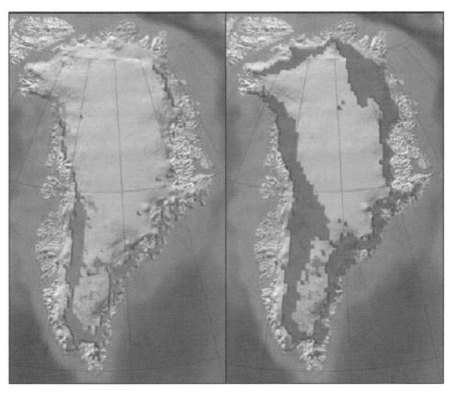

Source: Reprinted with permission from the National Aeronautics and Space Administration, Scientific Visualization Studio.

2.5 million cubic kilometers or 10% of the global ice mass. Melting has accelerated from 82 to 239 cubic kilometers per year; since 1979, summer melt, calculated from satellite observations over Greenland, increased from approximately 450,000 km^2 to more than 600,000 km^2.[17] Since 1997, warmer ocean waters were responsible for rapid thinning of the Jakobshavn Isbrae, a floating glacial ice tongue over a deep water fjord in western Greenland. Jakobshavn has doubled its melting speed in the past decade, and now discharges 11 cubic miles of icebergs per day, jamming its fjord.

NOTES FROM THE FIELD

In April 2008, along with the polar Inuit, I visited Siorapaluk by dogsled. I was able to interview Ikuo Oshima, a native Japanese hunter who has married and lived among the polar Inuit since 1973. Siorapaluk is the northernmost community on Earth. Ikuo said the ice has been breaking up every May during the past several years and that the ice has been getting more treacherous in recent years. In the 1980s the ice would last until August. He had experienced more slush and spots where the ice was too thin for a sled. He stated that the freeze-up is now getting delayed as well. In fact, he has hunted in boats in the darkness because the ice did not come until after Christmas. He was worried about the future of his culture, because it depended on hunting for its food and clothing. He was also concerned about finding enough cold and sun in the spring to dry and stretch the polar bear hides for making clothing. The polar Thule Inuit, with their unique culture and language, have only a thousand members remaining. Global warming may cause their demise. Under anthropogenic climate change, the Arctic sea ice and the Greenland ice sheet could be the closest to their tipping points.[18]

Alaska

Alaska spruce forests have their roots anchored into the frozen soil, and as the tundra melts, they lose their anchor and tilt in various directions, giving rise to the term "drunken forest." Due to the warming weather, spruce **bark beetles** are not killed by the extreme cold, and thousands of acres of spruce are infested. Bark beetles on Alaska's Kenai Peninsula have killed 3 million acres of spruce, covering nearly half of the peninsula. Drought weakens trees by drying the resin that drowns the beetles as they bore through the bark, while warming allows beetles to overwinter, expand into higher altitudes and latitudes, and sneak in an extra generation each year. Similar infestations have invaded the Mountain West of the United States, particularly Colorado near the continental divide.

The melting of the permafrost (soil at or below the freezing point of water [0°C] for two or more years) is a big problem as well. Up to a third of all soil C, 350–450 gigatons of C, could be released if permafrost were melted. Permafrost underlies 24% of the Earth and 80% of Alaska. The more rapid snowmelt reduces albedo, adding ~3 watts/m^2 of local heating, an amount roughly equivalent to a doubling of CO_2 levels in the global atmosphere. Global warming may also encourage more shrubs to grow in the tundra and boreal forest to grow farther northward. This may shift peatlands to a net C sink, although methane release may be significantly altering this balance.[19]

Throughout the Arctic, mining and oil companies use winter roads to transport large supplies by eighteen-wheeler trucks. The number of Alaska winter tundra travel days has been steadily declining due to global warming. Retreating ice also leaves Arctic communities more susceptible to ocean storms, winds over open water, and coastal erosion. Ice loss also affects Inuit traditional hunting practices and contributes to regional declines in polar bear health and abundance.

For several decades, ornithologist George Divoky has been studying the guillemots and their mating in the Arctic. These black pigeon-like Arctic birds feed on the edge of the Arctic icepack and migrate to Cooper Island, Arctic Alaska, for an eighty-day cycle of laying their eggs and fledging their chicks. From 1974 to 2001, Divoky noted that the birds arrived and laid their eggs five days earlier per decade. More recently he noted that there is decreased adult survival, more sibling aggression, and a gradual population drop due to the greater distance to fly to the retreating icepack for food. He observed a profound decrease in ^{13}C in guillemots' feathers from museum collections as their feeding range changed from the rich Bering Sea to the more parsimonious Beaufort and Chuckchi seas as the icepack receded northward.

Antarctica

The Antarctic Peninsula has experienced a several-degree warming compared to the rest of the continent. This has adversely affected the ice shelf, with increased break-ups and disappearance. Since 1989, near the northern end of Antarctica, there have been ice shelf break-ups near James Ross Island, culminating in the loss of the Larsen B Ice Shelf, published on the front page of the *New York Times* in March 20, 2002. In 2006, Antarctica lost three-quarters more ice than it did a decade earlier; the net ice loss was nearly 200 billion tons, comparable to Greenland's annual loss.[20] Thus, significant warming has occurred beyond the Antarctic Peninsula to cover most of West Antarctica, an area comprising almost a third of the continent.[21] West Antarctica warming exceeds 0.1°C per decade over the past 50 years, and is strongest in winter and spring.

Although East Antarctica offsets this partly due to autumn cooling, the continent-wide average near-surface temperature trend is positive.

These trends are of concern for emperor penguin populations because the Terre Adelie colony has experienced population collapses when the sea ice shrinks; for example, an 11% decrease in sea ice was accompanied by a 50% abrupt decline of the penguin colony population.[22] Winters with extensive sea ice enhance krill abundance, and emperor penguins mainly feed on fish species that in turn depend on krill and other crustaceans. The median population size of emperor penguins is projected to decline from ~6,000 breeding pairs to ~400 breeding pairs going forward to 2100, with a 36% risk of quasi-extinction.

Glaciers

Glaciers in the mid-latitudes are at great risk of melting into oblivion from global warming. There has been an 81% decrease of ice on Mt. Kilimanjaro from 1912 to 2000. The decrease has been from approximately 12.5 square kilometers to 1.8 square kilometers.

NOTES FROM THE FIELD

In 1970, I hiked to the summit of Mt. Kilimanjaro and rounded the crater to Uhuru Point, which is at the very summit of 19,340 feet. I saw the several-meter face of a summit glacier. Twenty-nine years later, in 1999, my daughter Nicole hiked with a climbing party to the summit and rounded the crater to the same Uhuru Point. There was only a small snowfield remaining of the mighty glacier that once stood guard.

Other mid-latitude glaciers are at risk as well. Some of the larger concerns are Andean glaciers above Lima, Peru, because these provide the fresh water supply to 10 million inhabitants. The city lies in a desert, with the Pacific on one side and with the Andes blocking access to the Amazon basin, leaving the city at considerable risk. In mid-latitudes, the temperature has increased 0.11°C per decade, compared with global average of 0.06°C per decade in the tropical Andes, increasing melting of glaciers that supply drinking water to Quito, Ecuador, Lima, Peru, and La Paz, Bolivia. This warming has also decreased water flows to hydroelectric plants due to the shrinking ice packs. Once the glaciers have melted, there would be no water for drinking or for running the hydroelectric plants. Glaciers throughout the Alps are receding, leaving hydroelectric dams and electricity supplies at risk. Switzerland has lost 50% of its glacial surface area over the past 150 years (half of this in the past thirty years), and 100 out of 2000 of their glaciers have disappeared. What's more, landslides have become commonplace as mountainsides melt. The Himalayas and Kun Lun have 100 times as much ice as the Alps. Seven Asian Rivers from these mountain glaciers serve 40% of the world's population. The Tibetan Plateau is often referred to as the "Third Pole." Glacier National Park in northwest Montana may lose its glaciers in two decades under continued warming scenarios, and its local denizen, the bull trout, may be in trouble, since it thrives on very cold icy water from glacial melt in the late summer. W. Tad Pfeffer chronicled Alaskan glacial retreat in his 2008 book, *The Opening of a New Landscape: Columbia Glacier at Mid-Retreat,*[23] and discusses the natural landscape that melting has rendered unrecognizable. Columbia Glacier had pushed 18 miles into its fjord over the span of 1,000 years and stayed there for about 300 years before receding. Since 1994 it has receded 9 miles.

NOTES FROM THE FIELD

In April 2008 I rode a dogsled with the Thule Polar Inuit down Inglefield Fjord past Josephine Peary Island; our 2003 map showed the glacier reaching the island, but our experience showed that it had retreated approximately 8 km up the fjord toward the Greenland ice sheet.

Sea Level Rise

The gradual rise of sea level is one of the most troubling aspects of global climate change, especially because it is likely to accelerate in the future as global warming progresses. Two processes are involved: an increase in the mass of water in the oceans largely derived from melting of ice on land (**eustatic**); second, increase in the volume of ocean due to thermal expansion without change in mass (**steric**). The Fourth IPCC Report estimates the rate of sea-level rise in the twentieth century is a mean of 15 cm/century (range 10–20 cm). For the twenty-first century, 14 inches (range 7 to 23 inches) rise in sea level is expected. The Institute of Arctic and Alpine Research calculated the most likely glacial melting scenarios, which suggested a range of sea-level rise to 2100, including increased ice dynamics, to be between 0.8 and 2.0 meters.[24] More than 100 million people live within one meter of mean sea level, and sea-level rise is especially urgent and serious for the low-lying small island nations of the world. The IPCC estimates, "Sea level has risen at an average rate of 1.8 mm/year (1.3–2.3) from 1961 and at an even faster pace since 1993, at a rate of 3.1 mm/year (2.4–3.8)."

Biodiversity

The evolutionary diversity of species could be limited by global warming, leading to climate change. The world's **biodiversity** is at risk from global warming. Global warming has been linked to the loss of 67% of the 110 species of Costa Rican harlequin frog and golden toad. The pathogenic chytrid fungus shifted its growth optimum, with global warming consequently harming and endangering the harlequin frog.[25] Extinction may engulf 15–37% of species by 2050 in the mid-range climate warming scenarios.[26] Global warming will make it more difficult to achieve biodiversity in the U.S. National Parks.[27] For example, climatic change has caused wetland desiccation in Yellowstone National Park that has led to precipitous declines in populations of once-common amphibian species.[28] Computer models are highly uncertain but predict large-range shifts, high global extinction rates, and reorganized communities. Moritz and colleagues quantified nearly a century of climate change on the small mammal community of Yosemite National Park in California by resampling a broad elevational transect from 60 to 3,300 me above sea level that Joseph Grinnell and colleagues surveyed from 1914 to 1920.[29] There was a ∼500 m average increase in elevation for affected species, which was consistent with estimated warming of +3°C. High-elevation species typically experienced range contractions, whereas low-elevation species expanded their ranges upward. The pika may retrench to small, high mountain islands in order to survive.

Climate change may alter the snow conditions in the Arctic, where periods of warming can melt the snow, followed by freezing and leading to a sheet of ice over the tundra. This makes food difficult to reach for herbivores such as Peary reindeer, muskoxen, and lemmings. Lemmings thrive in a subnivean (a zone under the snow layer) space that is a gap created by warmth from the ground melting a small layer of snow above it, leaving a space where lemmings can feed on mosses without threat of predation.[30] Climate change now means that the subnivean space does not exist for as much of each year as it used to, and worse still, the space itself is less likely to form. These changing snow conditions are a major factor in the change of lemming population dynamics, leading to lack of predicted peak rodent years since 1994. Scarcity of lemmings means that predators such as foxes turn their attention to other species, including willow grouse and ptarmigan, adversely affecting their populations.

Polar bears are also likely to be affected by global warming. They face more difficult hunting of their prey, seals, with increasing open ice. Already their populations in the western Hudson Bay region have experienced a dramatic decline. More than half of the Arctic's estimated 20,000 polar bears are likely to disappear over the next two decades. King penguins in the Antarctic are seeing their population being threatened by Southern Ocean warming,[31] primarily because of declines in food supply. Population dynamic models describe a 9% decline in adult survival for a 0.26°C warming from nine years of observation on Crozet Island, where two-thirds of the King penguins breed. The IPCC Fourth Report forecasts an ~0.2°C further warming per decade for the Southern Ocean.

Henry David Thoreau initiated a dataset of Walden Pond, Massachusetts, flora that spans 150 years and provides information on changes in species abundance and flowering time.[32] Although the Concord area has many underdeveloped natural areas, climate change is thought to be responsible for 27% of species becoming locally extinct and 36% existing in such low-population abundance that their extirpation may be imminent. Species that have been lost are overly represented in particular plant families, suggesting that extinction may be phylogenetically biased. Mean annual temperature in the Concord area has risen 2.4°C over the past 100 years, and this temperature change is associated with a shift in species' flowering time, which has moved seven days earlier than in Thoreau's time.

Deforestation

Deforestation is a major threat to the climate change scenarios, with approximately 20% of GHG emissions coming from deforestation. Deforestation leads to less CO_2 uptake and results in increased wildfires, producing even more CO_2. Deforestation of the Amazon is at a pace of 5.8 million acres per year due to roads, hydroelectric plants, forest burning, and soybean farming. Most of the large virgin trees are removed by illegal loggers who cut the trees in situ and remove finished lumber on their boats. More than 11 million hectares (29 million acres) of forest are destroyed each year—in three decades, an area roughly the size of India.[33] Second-growth forest probably can keep pace with the CO_2 transpiration needs, though.

In the temperate forests in the northern hemisphere, black ash and red maple are moving north, replacing spruce, white cedar, sugar maple, and pine species. There is a forty-year trend of maple sugaring in Vermont of the sap running two weeks earlier, and most troublesome, the sugar maple is expected to be replaced by the end of the twenty-first century with oak, hickory, and pine.

Major wildfires are expected to increase with global warming, especially in the arid and drought-stricken regions. The 1997 Borneo peat fires released 40% of global CO_2, burning 5.2 million acres. Suharto started a mega-rice project that was abandoned, but the canals that were dug to drain the peat bogs dry then caught fire and burned. In 2003, forest fires in Siberia burned 48 million acres, releasing 250 million tons of CO_2.

Bleaching of Coral Reefs

Reefs are the dynamic centers of the most concentrated biodiversity on Earth.[34] They support up to 800 types of coral, 4,000 fish species, and countless invertebrates.

Their value to society has been estimated at more than \$300 billion per year. There is an increased occurrence of bleaching of coral reefs. There may be multiple causes of this crisis: ocean warming, increasing acidity of oceans from anthropogenic increases in CO_2, and increased ocean pollution. Excess heat disturbs a symbiotic partnership that coral animals normally maintain with algae termed **zooxanthellae**. Zooxanthellae supply corals with essential nutrients produced by photosynthesis, particularly carbon, in return for the shelter and access to sunlight provided by the reefs. The algae impart color to the reefs, but the dinoflagellates are sensitive to increases in temperature, causing them to die and leave the corals to starve and turn white, a process known as **coral bleaching**. There have been multiple (>six) periods of mass coral bleaching since 1979. In 1997–1998, 16% of the world's reef-building corals died due to the El Niño increase in sea surface temperatures. Bleached coral is susceptible to numerous diseases, for example, white pox, yellow band disease, and white plague.

Another negative impact on reefs is ocean acidification, with pH going from 8.16 to 8.05 from carbonic acid due to increasing CO_2. Ocean acidification affects reproduction of species that live among coral reefs and reduces fish populations, with attendant effects on coastal populations dependent on them for food. Experimentally, acidification affects bleaching more than calcification.[35] Ocean acidity dissolves outer casings of coccolithopores, tiny plankton that form the basis of food webs. Of 704 species of coral that could be assigned conservation status, 32.8% were in categories with elevated risk of extinction.[36] Twenty percent of the world's 285,000 square km of known reefs have been destroyed, and elkhorn and staghorn corals in the U.S. Virgin Islands have been labeled as threatened species. Bleaching leaves coral colorless and is widespread from Florida to Puerto Rico and through the eastern Caribbean. The IPCC Fourth Assessment Report warned that the Great Barrier Reef off the coast of Australia will become functionally extinct because of coral bleaching during the twenty-first century due to global warming. Recent data from Australia in *Porites* looking at annual coral growth rings showed a decline in calcification from 1990 to 2005 from 1.76 to 1.51 gm/cm^2 or 14.2% compared to a stable growth rate going back 400 years.[37] They surmised that increasing sea surface temperature was the key heat stressor, although the contribution or synergism with ocean acidification may also play a role.

Hurricanes and Tropical Storms

Global warming and climate change are also known to increase the intensity of hurricanes and tropical storms.[38,39] There is agreement on intensity but less on frequency.[38] Since 1957, the oceans have accumulated 22 times as much heat as the atmosphere. Data from the National Climatic Data Center indicate that, since the 1970s, extreme weather events have increased in the continental United States. The increase in water surface temperature increases evaporation, cloud formation, and consequently heavy downpours. Droughts have become longer and bursts of precipitation more intense (>2 inches over 24 hours).[40] Such events were greater in the 1980s than the 1970s, and more so in the 1990s than in the 1980s. Damage due to weather-related catastrophes has risen fifty-fold since the 1970s, and major insurers Swiss Re and AIG have taken steps to alert their customers that mitigation steps of their carbon footprint is warranted. As return periods between disasters decrease, and the rate of unusual, novel weather events rises, the costs for society and for insurers have risen stepwise twice: from $4 billion a year to $40 billion a year in the 1990s, then $123 billion in 2004 and $200 billion in 2005. The percentage of insured losses also tripled, from 10% to more than 30%, as more weather disasters hit Europe, Japan, and the United States. We are in the midst of a natural twenty- to thirty-year cycle of increased hurricane activity (driven by conditions in the Pacific Ocean), but climate change—particularly the warming of the deep ocean—is exaggerating

FIGURE 10.5   Hurricane Katrina: Climate change may increase storms

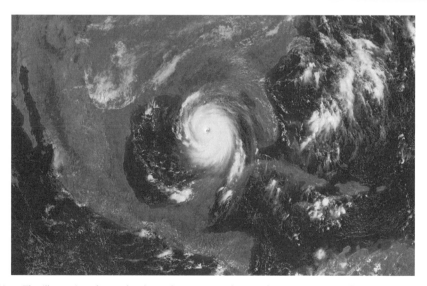

Note: The illustration shows the three-day average of sea surface temperatures from August 25, 2005, through August 27, 2005 (bottom), and Hurricane Katrina growing in strength and breadth as it passes over the unusually warm Gulf of Mexico. Light areas are at or above 82°F (27.8°C), the temperature required for hurricanes to strengthen. Since the 1970s, the number of category 4 and 5 hurricanes has increased as sea temperatures have risen.
Source: Reprinted with permission from the National Aeronautics and Space Administration.

natural variability, and insurers and reinsurers are bracing for more consecutive years with enormous losses.[41]

The U.S. Climate Change Science Program has been criticized as leaving local and regional officials unprepared for potentially catastrophic changes. The IPCC Fourth Assessment Report predicts that by the end of the twenty-first century climate change will bring water scarcity to between 1.1 and 3.2 billion people; an additional 200 to 600 million people across the world would face food shortages; and coastal flooding would hit another 7 million homes.

Extreme events such as drought or flooding can complicate public health responses. Increased rain and storms can increase risk for flooding, as seen in China, Haiti, Venezuela, and other places. Significant health issues include drowning with the rapid rise of rivers, diarrheal diseases such as cholera, typhoid fever, and cryptosporidiosis, and chemical contamination of the water by pesticides, metals, and organic chemicals. Increased intensity of storms and hurricanes will increase traumatic injuries.[39,40] The health effects of extreme weather events range from loss of life and acute trauma, to indirect effects such as loss of homes, large-scale population displacement, damage to sanitation infrastructure (drinking water and sewage systems), interruption of food production, damage to the health care infrastructure and post-traumatic stress disorder. Storm-water runoff from heavy precipitation events can also increase fecal bacterial counts in coastal waters as well as nutrient load, which, coupled with increased sea surface temperature, can lead to increases in the frequency and range of algal blooms (red tides). The western and southeastern United States may experience severe droughts as their climate changes due to regional precipitation declines.

Thermohaline Gulf Stream

On a physical scale, the Gulf Stream is part of a great ocean "conveyor belt" that helps to stabilize the climate and bring moderating temperatures to northern Europe. Due to all the warming near the North Pole[42] and more rain evaporating off warm tropical seas and falling at high latitudes, a cold, freshwater lens is forming near Greenland. Cold, salty water is heavy and sinks, and this forms an overturning pump that pulls the Gulf Stream north and drives the ocean conveyor belt. **Thermohaline circulation** (the part of the large-scale ocean circulation that is driven by global density gradients created by surface heat and freshwater fluxes) has slowed some 30–50% in the past half-century,[43,44] and it could possibly shut down. A shutdown of the Gulf Stream could place the United Kingdom and Europe at risk of far cooler temperatures. Given the current level of CO_2 buildup and the projected degree of global warming, we have truly entered uncharted seas.[44,45]

Human Health Effects

Most assessments of health and climate organize health issues categorically, as a direct effect, an indirect effect, or due to a social or economic disruption. Downstream effects include changes in food yields and water supplies that could result in malnutrition or dehydration.[46] The Centers for Disease Control and Prevention (CDC) has called for expansion of environmental public health tracking systems for health surveillance of climate sensitive pathogens and vectors.[47] There may be future changes in infectious diseases such as "year-round influenza" in the tropics. Near the equator, there is no influenza season, so as the temperature rises, the tropical areas will expand and there will be more year-round influenza. More research will be needed to investigate the interconnectedness of climate and infectious diseases. The World Health Organization estimates that the warming and precipitation trends due to anthropogenic climate change of the past thirty years already claims more than 150,000 lives annually.[48] Given the case for increases in temperature, particularly in cities, health effects attributed to global warming will be increased mortality from heat waves, increased cardiovascular and pulmonary diseases from synergy with ground-level air pollutants, and increases in vector-borne illnesses described later in this section.

Heat Stress

Heat stress is the most direct health effect of global warming. Heat stress is characterized by *heat exhaustion*, where the skin may be damp and looks flushed, and *heat stroke*, where the skin may be dry but the temperature is markedly increased and dehydration may be followed by convulsions and loss of consciousness. Extreme heat events cause an increase in mortality due to ischemic heart disease, diabetes, stroke, respiratory disease, accidents, homicide, and suicide. Hospitalized patients with chronic obstructive pulmonary disease (COPD) without appropriate climate control are at severe risk of death. In addition, heat exposure is linked to increased occurrence of heat cramps, heat syncope, heat exhaustion, and heat stroke (defined clinically as core body temperature >40.6°C accompanied by hot, dry, skin and central nervous system abnormalities). An increase in average temperature is projected to increase the number and severity of extreme heat waves in some areas.[44] Studies indicate that the probability of extreme heat events has doubled or even quadrupled with global warming.[48] This change would exacerbate an already large urban heat island effect. The heat island effect is due to the black asphalt and buildings that absorb more visible light and infrared radiation, resulting in a 2–10°C increase in temperature in the localized area. Mid-latitude cities that experience irregular heat waves appear to be most susceptible to these effects—cities such as Washington, D.C., St. Louis, Chicago, and New York. A mean rise of 2–5°C in the next fifty to one hundred years will increase the number of days with temperatures over 38°C. Washington, D.C., which now averages one to two days a year with temperatures over 38°C, may be expected to average twelve such days by the middle of the twenty-first century. This would cause an increase in illness and death, particularly among the very young, the elderly, the frail, and the chronically ill.

The deaths of 726 people that were attributed to the heat wave in Chicago in the summer of 1995 is an extreme example. Most survivors recovered near-normal renal, hematologic, and respiratory status, but disability persisted, resulting in moderate to severe functional impairment in 33% of patients at hospital discharge. At one year, no patient had improved functional status, and an additional 28% of patients had died.[49]

Another instance of heat stress occurred during the August 2003 heat wave in France, during which the mean maximal temperature exceeded the seasonal norm by 11–12°C on nine consecutive days.[50] In 2003, a summer heat wave in Europe resulted in 32,000 excess deaths, wilted crops, set forests ablaze, and melted 10% of the Alpine glacial mass. France alone experienced almost 15,000 excess heat-related deaths, with a peak of 2,000 heat-related deaths on one day. For August 2003, these deaths were a 60% increase over the normal August mortality rates.[51] There were an estimated 23,000 excess deaths due to hyperthermia, heat stroke, dehydration, and respiratory, cardiac, and nervous system causes.[52,53] Mortality was 15% higher in women than men, and increases were noted among the aged, widowed, single, divorced, and among those living in retirement institutions.[54,55] In a study from Lyon, France, there were eighty-three patients who presented with heatstroke from August 1 to 20, and twenty-eight-day and two-year mortality rates were 58% and 71% respectively.[56] Hazard ratios were increased for patients presenting on antihypertensive medication, anuria, coma, or cardiovascular failure. A positive association exists between heat waves and mortality in the elderly, specifically elderly women and those experiencing social isolation.[57]

Excess mortality was observed at hospitals (42%), homes (32%), and nursing homes (19%).[58] A crucial element in all these heat waves is the lack of letup at night. Minimum temperatures are projected to increase more rapidly than average temperatures with global warming.[59] A warmed atmosphere holds more water vapor (6% more for each 1°C); thus we are observing increased cloudiness (and nighttime and winter warming), increased humidity in heat waves, and more extreme precipitation events. Air conditioning could reduce the number of sufferers, but air conditioning expends much energy and increases the consumption of fossil fuels that create the greenhouse gases.

Higher surface temperatures, especially in urban areas, promote the formation of ground-level ozone and have been demonstrated to further increase mortality.[60] The researchers analyzed time-series trends for nine French cities with deaths regressed on temperatures and ozone levels and found that the excess risk of death was significant (1.01% 95% CI [confidence interval] 0.58–1.44) for an increase of 10 $\mu g/m^3$ in O_3 level.

The increase in mortality may be offset to some extent by a decrease in winter deaths from hypothermia and cold; nonetheless, there is a clear need to develop an adequate warning system to alert the public and government agencies when oppressive air masses are expected. High temperature in U.S. cities increases mortality for diabetes and cardiovascular causes especially among Blacks.[61] They isolated extreme temperatures from fifty U.S. cities and conducted a case-only analysis using daily mortality and hourly weather data during 1989–2000. Increased odds ratios were found for older subjects, Blacks, and those dying outside a hospital were more susceptible to extreme heat. Over a five-year period, from 1999 to 2003, a total of 3,443 heat-related deaths were reported in the United States.[62] There has been a significant upward trend of approximately 20% in the frequency of heat waves from 1949 to 1995 for the eastern and western United States.[63]

Air pollution studies show that a 10°C increase in temperature on the same summer day was associated with an increase in cardiovascular mortality by 1.17%, and there was an 8.3% difference comparing the highest level of ozone concentrations to the lowest in the National Morbidity and Mortality Study from ninety-five large U.S. communities from 1987 to 2000.[64] Schwartz and colleagues found an association between elevated temperatures and short-term increases in cardiovascular-related admissions for twelve U.S. cities.[65] In Wuhan, China, surrounded by mountains and called an "oven city" because of its hot summers, mortality from 2001–2004 showed significant associations between PM_{10} and temperature for cardiovascular and cardiopulmonary deaths.[66] The PM_{10} effects were strongest on extremely high temperature days (daily average temperature 33.1°C).

Alana Hansen and colleagues in Australia used health outcome data from Adelaide from 1993 to 2006 to estimate the effect of heat waves on hospital admissions and mortalities for mental, behavioral, and cognitive disorders.[67] Above a threshold of 26.7°C they observed an association between temperature and hospital admissions for mental and behavioral disorders of 7.3% compared to non-heat wave periods. Illnesses included symptomatic mental disorders, dementia, mood disorders, neurotic, stress-related, and somatoform disorders, disorders of psychological development, and senility. Mortalities attributed to these disorders increased during heat waves in the 65- to 74-year age group.

Allergic Diseases, Asthma, and Hay Fever with Increased Pollen and Global Warming

Allergic rhinitis (hay fever) affects approximately 40 million Americans, and asthma prevalence is estimated by the CDC to be 7.5% or 16 million.[68] The self-reported prevalence of asthma increased 75% from 1980 to 1994 in both adults and children but increased 160% in preschool-aged children.[69] Climate change has resulted in phenological changes in plants, advancing the spring allergenic pollen season. Ragweed grown at twice the ambient CO_2 from 350 to 700 ppm has greater biomass and 40–60% more pollen.[70] Laboratory experiments using an enzyme-linked immunosorbent assay for ragweed's major allergen, Amb a 1, showed that protein levels remained unchanged as CO_2 increased; however, Amb a 1 increased 1.8 times as CO_2 increased from 280 to 370, and increased 1.6 times as CO_2 increased further from 370 to 600 ppm.[71] An ubiquitous allergenic fungus, *Alternaria alternata*, produced nearly 3 times the number of spores and twice the total antigenic protein at 500–600 ppm CO_2.[72] Field experiments show an urban gradient with increased pollen in urban environs with high temperature and CO_2. The U.S. Department of Agriculture planted ragweed in and around Baltimore in 2001 during August into early September, with higher CO_2 in the urban plot and the pollen count in the urban plot much higher at 12,138 pollen grains/m^3, compared to 3,262 in the suburban plot and 2,294 in the rural plot. Longer-term plots have seen an increase in pollen-bearing trees at the expense of weeds such as ragweed. Beggs has stated, "This suggests that the future aeroallergen characteristics of our environment may change considerably as a result of climate change, with the potential for more pollen and mold spores, more allergenic pollen, an earlier start to the pollen and mold season, and changes in pollen distribution."[73]

Aeroallergen biomonitoring has been recommended as an adaptation strategy. This will allow for notification of children and adults susceptible to allergic rhinitis and asthma.

Biomass Burning and Hut Lung

Biomass burning contributes to black soot, which has recently been identified as an anthropogenic cause of global warming. Lower respiratory tract infections in children and chronic obstructive lung disease in women from indoor air pollution from biomass burning have emerged as major health risks in developing countries. Chronic exposure to biomass smoke is implicated as the leading cause of chronic bronchitis among nonsmokers in rural countries and accounts for up to 50% of the total disease burden among the rural poor.[74] Inhalation of silicates from food grinding on stones, as well as biomass burning inside houses, has been called "hut lung." Hut lung[74] individuals may present with cough, sputum production, and shortness of breath. The chest radiograph may show small rounded and irregular opacities. There may be reduced pulmonary function. Biopsies of lung tissue show alveolar macrophages engorged with black particulate material, and dark anthracotic pigment can be found in the peripheral small airways in a peribronchiolar distribution. Change to cooking with gas or more efficient stoves can reduce the burden of disease and also reduce the black carbon contribution to global warming.[75,76]

Vector-Borne Diseases

Climate change will have an impact on infectious diseases, such as vector-borne diseases including malaria and dengue fever. Temperature can affect pathogen development within vectors and interact with humidity to influence vector survival. The seasonality and amounts of precipitation in an area can strongly influence the availability of breeding sites for mosquitoes and other species that have aquatic immature stages.[77] There may be an expansion in the range of vectors that carry Lyme disease and West Nile virus.

Malaria continues to have 247 million cases per year with 881,000 deaths, primarily among African children. The theory is that global warming will move the range of mosquitoes to more temperate latitudes and higher altitudes, exposing more people to malaria risk. Increasing temperature shortens incubation time of the malaria parasite inside the mosquito. In East Africa, open treeless habitats or those near crops have warmer midday temperatures, increasing *Anopheles gambiae* mosquitoes per house in these areas and survivorship in pools of water. An increase in temperature of ~0.5°C can cause a 30%–100% increase in mosquito abundance over 1950–2002 using nonlinear singular spectral analysis.[78] Patz and Olson suggested their findings confirmed the importance of nonlinear and threshold responses of malaria to the effect of regional temperature change.[79] They said that the biological response of mosquito populations to warming can be more than an order of magnitude larger than the measured change in temperature; this suggested a nonlinear relationship—a stunning finding. The epidemic potential of malaria transmission has been projected to increase 12%–27% as a result of climate change.[80]

Recently, data spanning more than three decades of malarial surveillance from hospitals in the tea highlands of western Kenya was correlated to temperature and rainfall stored in local meteorological stations.[81] Using a computer model, predicted malaria cases exhibited a highly nonlinear response to warming. Actual cases exceeded the predicted trends, suggesting that climate change had already played an important role in the exacerbation of malaria in this region.

Dengue Fever

Dengue fever (DF) and Dengue hemorrhagic fever (DHF) are caused by the RNA Flavivirus, which has four distinct serotypes (DEN-1, DEN-2, DEN-3, and DEN-4). Infection with one of these serotypes provides immunity to only that serotype for life, so persons living in a dengue-endemic area can have more than one dengue infection during their lifetimes. From 1977 to 2004, 3,806 suspected cases of imported dengue were reported in the United States, and 864 (23%) were confirmed as dengue. Dengue fever is a severe illness with flu-like symptoms, severe headache, and muscle and joint pains (thus the name "break-bone fever"), pain behind the eye, and rash. Other symptoms include chills, dizziness, loss of appetite, and bleeding from the nose, mouth, or gums. Patients with DF are febrile for a period of about six to seven days, during which they are also infectious if bit by a mosquito vector. Often DF is misdiagnosed, especially when mild and when not accompanied by a rash. The bite of an infected mosquito is followed by an incubation period of three to fourteen days, most commonly four to seven days, before symptoms might appear. Thus many travelers unknowingly help in the transportation of this disease. Treatment for dengue consists of rest and fluids with acetoaminophen given to reduce fever and pain.

In Dengue hemorrhagic fever, the illness begins with a sudden high fever and other flu-like symptoms, accompanied by a facial rash. Convulsions may occur, and symptoms of confusion, irritability, and lethargy occur early followed by full DHF. The temperature may drop and be accompanied by increased vascular permeability, internal bleeding, circulatory failure, and shock. Treatment consists of intravenous fluids to maintain blood pressure. In 2003, the Bill & Melinda Gates Foundation pledged $55 million over six years to foster development of a vaccine for dengue fever and stop its global spread.

Dengue fever has increased nearly thirtyfold in the past 50 years and has become the most important viral mosquito-borne disease in the world. Dengue infects at least 50 million people a year in more than 100 countries, mainly across Asia, Africa, and South America. In 2007, there were more than 890,000 reported cases of dengue in the Americas, of which 26,000 cases were Dengue hemorrhagic fever. As a result, any predicted weather patterns that enlarge mosquito larval breeding grounds or allow increased transmission of dengue could have significant implications.

Dengue has infected primarily the poor in urban areas in the past, but now its distribution cuts across class. Dengue fever is transmitted by *Stegomyia aegypti* (formerly *Aedes aegypti*) and *Aedes albopictus* mosquitoes; recently, the J. Craig Venter Institute and the University of Notre Dame sequenced the Stegomyia genome, finding 1.38 billion base pairs containing the insect's estimated 15,419 protein coding sequences. Since Stegomyia transmit yellow fever as well, these mosquitoes were eradicated from the Americas during the 1950s and 1960s but the United States ended its eradication programs in 1970, with Latin American countries following suit thereafter. *S. aegypti* has adapted to urban life, preferring to live in homes and breed in household or yard containers. These mosquitoes bite during daytime, so bed nets are not as useful as household insecticide spraying. Maximum adult survival rates are in the range of 20–30°C. Higher temperatures yield faster development and smaller adult mosquitoes.

Using modeling techniques, Hales and colleagues estimated that about 5–6 billion people would be at risk of dengue transmission by 2085, but if climate change did not take place, then only 3.5 billion people (35% of the population) would be at risk.[82]

Global Warming and the International Community

The Intergovernmental Panel on Climate Change was established in 1990 at a meeting of the World Meteorological Organization and the United Nations Environment Programme (UNEP) to provide an "objective, balanced, and internationally coordinated scientific assessment of the understanding of the effects of increasing concentrations of greenhouse gases of the Earth's climate and on ways in which these changes may impact socio-economic problems."[1] The IPCC does not conduct primary research; rather it builds consensus from the collective efforts of scientists worldwide. It has three working groups: Working Group I focuses on current scientific data; Working Group II focuses on the environmental and socioeconomic impact of climate change; and Working Group III is charged with formulating response strategies to these impacts. Each Working Group has a core membership of thirteen to seventeen countries. A bureau comprised of the IPCC chair, three IPCC vice chairs, and the co-chairs and vice chairs of each of the working groups oversees all IPCC activity.

To date, the IPCC has released four assessment reports on global climate change and has chosen 831 members for the fifth report due in 2014. The IPCC 4th Assessment of 2007 numbered >1,600 pages in its main science report and was compiled by 150 scientists as main authors, another 400 scientists as contributing authors, a team of review editors, and some 600 reviewers. The IPCC reports are consensus documents that by nature are conservative, and their models can even miss events such as the disintegration of the Larsen B ice shelf collapse along the Antarctic Peninsula on January 31, 2002.[2] According to the IPCC 2007 Fourth Assessment Report, global surface temperature increased 0.74 ± 0.18°C during the twentieth century. Most of the observed increase in temperature since the middle of the twentieth century was caused by increasing concentrations of greenhouse gases, which results from human activity such as fossil fuel burning and deforestation.

Summary

Climate change poses a range of challenges to human health, but many of the linkages are complex and a range of other social, behavioral, and environmental factors also affect the health outcomes in question.[83] Because of the wide-ranging potential impacts of global warming, GHG emissions need to be decreased substantially, including emphasis on energy efficiency, renewable energy technologies, and planning to mitigate adverse health outcomes.[84] Ramanathan and Feng state that the GHGs since the preindustrial era have committed the Earth to 2.4°C warming and that any future increase would pass the tipping point of dangerous anthropogenic interference.[85]

Key Terms

Bark beetles

Biodiversity

Climate

Climate change

Coral bleaching

Eustatic

Glaciers

Global warming

Greenhouse gases (GHG)

Heat stress

Intergovernmental Panel on Climate Change (IPCC)

Radiative forcing capability

Steric

Thermohaline circulation

Weather

Zooxanthellae

Discussion Questions

1. How does the IPCC write its reports?
2. What did the IPCC conclude about humanity's role in climate change?
3. Describe the scientific explanation for global warming.
4. What are some significant environmental effects of climate change?
5. Name some of the potential negative effects to human health that could result from climate change.

CHAPTER 11

NATIONAL GREEN ENERGY PLAN

LEARNING OBJECTIVES

- To become familiar with the ways in which energy efficiency can be improved
- To understand how we use various energy sources and how they may affect the environment
- To understand the economic and political underpinnings of energy use
- To comprehend the negative health effects of obtaining, distributing, and using various energy forms

Global climate change is now recognized as an impending worldwide emergency. President Jimmy Carter stated on April 17, 1977, that we had a moral command to act on our energy crisis (and his White House rooftop solar panels have been in storage since that time). The baseline case for business as usual would increase our carbon emissions from approximately 7 billion metric tons in 2008 to 13 billion metric tons in 2050. However, if we are to stabilize the global temperature at 2°C above preindustrial levels and CO_2 concentration at 450 ppm, then we will have to reduce carbon emissions to 1.5 billion metric tons by 2050. This represents an 80% reduction from current levels.

The world's major contributors to global warming are the United States (30.3%), Europe (27.7%), Russia (13.7%), and China (which in 2008 surpassed the United States as the world's leader in carbon emissions). In developing a national green energy plan, we need to control two major sources of greenhouse gases (GHG): electricity generation and transportation. The U.S. CO_2 emissions by end-use sector are transportation, industrial, residential, and commercial. U.S. energy consumption consists almost completely of fossil fuels (petroleum 40%, natural gas 23%, coal 23%), 8% from nuclear, and only 6% from renewables (hydroelectric, biomass, wind, solar). Current electricity generation comes from the following sources: coal 52%, nuclear 20%, natural gas 16%, hydropower 7%, oil 3%, and renewables 2%. In revamping the energy utilization scenarios, most experts begin with the opportunities available in conservation.

Energy Efficiency

Energy conservation, increasing efficiency of end products, and enhancing renewable sources of energy technologies could provide a giant step toward the U.S. carbon emissions reductions that will be needed to limit the atmospheric concentration of CO_2 to between 450 and 500 ppm. Since 1970, increased **energy efficiency** helped to effectively meet approximately 50% of Americans' increased energy demands. Going forward, we could save more electricity if households used more efficient appliances or if we demanded more efficient standards. California promulgated efficiency standards and saved $700 billion since 1979. California refrigerator manufacturers opposed the efficiency standards but lost and assigned engineers the task of redesigning them. The following decade, standards were imposed on refrigerators nationwide, with the result that refrigerator size grew by more than 10% while the price in inflation-adjusted dollars was cut in half and the energy use dropped by two-thirds. In 1982 the California Public Utilities Commission decoupled utilities' sales and profits. Decoupling incentivizes utilities toward energy conservation strategies with protected profits rather than increasing profits only with increased energy sales. Chargers (cell phones, computers) and televisions draw power when they are still plugged in, and remote controls can switch them off, saving considerable power.

The Electrical Grid

In Canada and the United States the grid carries a million megawatts; more than 150,000 miles of high-voltage transmission lines carry power from 5,400 generating plants owned by more than 3,000 utilities. A major efficiency enhancement would be to improve the electrical grid. Currently, about 10% of electricity is lost in transmission. Increased electrical efficiencies would provide a substantial portion of future energy needs. Distant generation of wind and other energy sources for major population centers could be transported these long distances if there was a more efficient electrical grid. For example, thinking outside the norm, an underground superconductor of H_2 surrounded by liquid nitrogen and two layers of insulation could offer us a new way to ship electricity from the Great Plains to the East. Alternating current emerged over direct current (DC) largely because it can easily be stepped up with transformers, transmitted, then stepped down again to a safer household voltage of 110 or 220. High-voltage DC is preferred for very long distances because, although it is harder to produce than alternating current (AC), it loses even less power.

The 2007 Energy Independence and Security Act authorized $100 million to encourage utilities to implement smart grid technologies. For example, Xcel Energy Company plans a $100 million initiative called SmartGridCity in Boulder, Colorado, that will rely on a network of fiber optic cables, high-tech meters, and sensor-laden transformers to provide power stations with real-time data on demand all along the grid, allowing them to fine-tune the electrical supply, detect failing equipment, and predict overloads. Additionally, under this plan consumers will be able to utilize Web-enabled control panels in their homes, allowing them to regulate their energy consumption more closely, for example, setting their air conditioning systems to automatically reduce power use during peak hours. To accommodate green energy, the grid needs more storage, and one way to achieve this is through lithium-ion batteries in electric cars that could serve as two-way flow, providing energy in times of need and recharging when there is excess wind or sunlight.

Lighting

Lighting presents another significant opportunity to improve the end-use efficiency of electricity, since the 100-year-old incandescent light bulb is only 5%

efficient, meaning that 95% of the energy it receives is lost in generating light. Newer compact fluorescent light bulbs are 7%–9% efficient, last 9–10 times longer than incandescent bulbs, and produce equivalent brightness and a better quality of light than incandescent bulbs. They also fit into a standard light socket, although decorative lights and dimmers are still difficult to use with them. There is some concern about mercury pollution upon disposal of compact fluorescent bulbs. Currently the compact fluorescent bulb market is $2 billion per year, and the incandescent bulb market is $10 billion per year. Australia has banned use of the incandescent bulb after 2011. Wal-Mart set a goal of selling 100 million compact fluorescent light bulbs by 2007 and surpassed this goal three months early. The new LED (light-emitting diode) lighting fixtures being developed portend even greater energy efficiency.

Oil

Oil is the ultimate fossil fuel because it can be used for electricity generation, heating, and transportation. It is easy to obtain and deliver and is inexpensive, but more than half of the world's oil has already been consumed. Retrieving the remainder will come at increasing environmental risk and cost, with continuing production of greenhouse gases.

Consumption

There are an estimated 1,245 billion barrels of oil remaining (OPEC 662; other 404; Arctic 118; and deepwater 61), with 1,078 billion barrels already produced. Beyond these sources, there are other, unconventional reserves, including approximately 704 billion in oil shale extracts, 592 in enhanced recovery, 444 extra-heavy, and 758 in "exploration potential." (See Figure 11.1.) The world consumes approximately 85 million barrels of oil per day, with the United States using 25 million barrels/day. (See Figure 11.2.) This global rate of consumption reaches 29.2 billion barrels per year, and at that rate, we will consume the remaining 1,245 billion barrels in forty-one years! However, the daily rate of consumption is rising, and the exploration potential has not been accompanied by any announcements of major new discoveries in years.

Economic Costs

Seventy percent of oil consumed in the United States was imported in 2007, up from 58% in 2000. The top ten suppliers of U.S. oil imports in September 2008

FIGURE 11.1　Global oil reserves

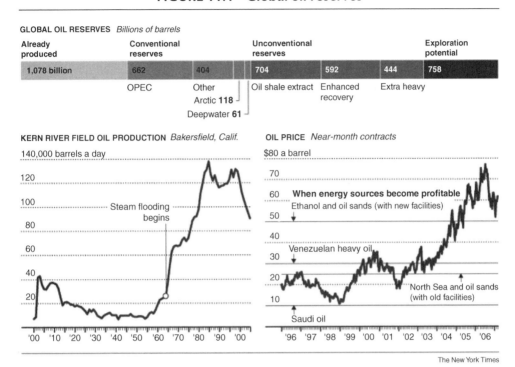

GLOBAL OIL RESERVES *Billions of barrels*

Already produced	Conventional reserves		Unconventional reserves			Exploration potential
1,078 billion	662	404	704	592	444	758

OPEC　　Other　　　Oil shale extract　Enhanced　　Extra heavy
　　　　　Arctic **118**　　　　　　　　　recovery
　　　　　Deepwater **61**

KERN RIVER FIELD OIL PRODUCTION *Bakersfield, Calif.*

140,000 barrels a day

Steam flooding begins

OIL PRICE *Near-month contracts*

$80 a barrel

When energy sources become profitable
Ethanol and oil sands (with new facilities)

Venezuelan heavy oil

North Sea and oil sands (with old facilities)

Saudi oil

The New York Times

Sources: Cambridge Energy Research Associates; Chevron; Simmons & Co.; Bloomberg Financial Markets. Reprinted with permission from the New York Times, Business Section: Jad Mouawad, "Oil innovations pump new life into old wells," March 5, 2007.

were Canada, Saudi Arabia, Venezuela, Mexico, Iraq, Nigeria, Angola, Algeria, Ecuador, and Brazil. Peak petroleum production was predicted as the Hubbert peak for the lower forty-eight states as of the early 1970s, and the global peak has been predicted for somewhere near 2010.[1] Federal oil and gas leases continued almost unabated during the George W. Bush administration, with 8.3 million acres of the Gulf of Mexico offered in 2006 and Alaska's Bristol Bay opened; under President Obama, Secretary of the Interior Ken Salazar cancelled proposed offshore lease sales in Bristol Bay and the Arctic Ocean. Of the 36 billion barrels of oil believed to lie on federal land, mainly in the Rocky Mountain West and Alaska, nearly two-thirds are accessible or nearing completion of environmental reviews. Of the 89 billion barrels of recoverable oil believed to lie offshore, four-fifths is open to industry, mostly in the Gulf of Mexico and Alaskan waters. The oil companies appear not to be using the land they have already

FIGURE 11.2 World oil consumption

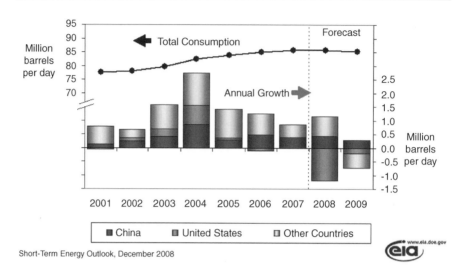

Short-Term Energy Outlook, December 2008

Source: Reprinted with permission from the Energy Information Administration: Department of Energy: Short Term Energy Outlook World Oil Consumption.

leased from the federal government; 68 million acres of the 90 million acres that the oil companies have leased are not being used to produce energy. This underlies further opening of coastal waters for drilling, when a 1981 congressional moratorium on offshore drilling was promulgated to protect coastal economies that depend on clean water and coastlines.

The primary use of oil is in transportation. In the United States there are approximately 136 million cars on the road and 105 million sport utility vehicles (SUVs) and trucks. In 2050 we will have 2 billion cars in use worldwide. According to the Environmental Protection Agency (EPA), each gallon of gasoline sends ~20 pounds of CO_2 out the tailpipe. Since 1975, U.S. vehicles have increased acceleration from 0 to 60 mph from 14.4 seconds to 9.9 seconds, and increased average weight from 3,200 pounds to 4,100 pounds. In Europe, half of all motor vehicles use diesel, which consumes 30% less fuel.

The **corporate average fuel economy (CAFÉ) standard** was 27.5 miles per gallon (mpg) in 1975, and from 1987 to 2007 it declined from 22 to 21 mpg. When Toyota introduced the Prius in 2003, the car achieved 48 mpg with average GHG emissions of 4 tons, compared to the 2003 Toyota Sequoia 4WD at 15 mpg and 12.3 tons annual GHG emissions. International comparisons of CAFÉ equivalent 2008 passenger car standards were 47 mpg in Japan, 44 mpg in the European Union, 36 in China, 32 in Australia, and 27.5 in the United States.

The National Highway Traffic Safety Administration (NHTSA) regulates CAFÉ standards; they will be issuing regulations to comply with the 2007 CAFÉ revisions that no longer grant exemptions to light trucks classified as SUVs or passenger vans. The 2007 Energy Independence and Security Act set a goal for the national fuel economy standard of 35 mpg by 2020. However, achieving 40 mpg would cut CO_2 300 million tons per year, save $45 billion at the gas pump, and save 3 million barrels of oil per day. The Obama administration mandated new CAFÉ standards of about 5% annually from today's level of 23 mpg for trucks and 27.5 mpg for cars to 30 mpg for trucks and 39 mpg for passenger cars by 2016, for an average of 35.5 mpg overall. The Obama administration states that the new measures will save 1.8 billion barrels of oil over seven years. This mandate overruled a California standard that had been adopted by fourteen other states but had been challenged by the automobile industry in court.

Transitioning off of fossil fuels will require moving to hybrid engines with battery power, when a small gasoline engine will extend mileage for long-distance driving; in addition, all-electric vehicles are being developed, and genetically engineered biofuels may extend possibilities for a liquid-fueled engine. The plug-in hybrid vehicle is rapidly being developed with batteries that have enough power to propel basic passenger vehicles >200 kilometers followed by gasoline engines to go further before a recharge. Lithium batteries have been developed for computers and cell phones as the immediate technology. Batteries have leaped ahead of expensive hydrogen fuel cells as the technology of choice for getting beyond oil. Battery technology is simple: chemical bonds trap ions in one electrode until the circuit is turned on when ions then flow through a separator to a second electrode where they release electrons generating an electric current. In a rechargeable battery, the chemical reaction has to be reversed to store energy. A battery must meet challenges of cost, safety, durability, power, and sheer capacity. The lead acid battery can only go about 150 km, and the next generation battery, nickel metal hydride, travels only 50% further on a charge. Lithium-ion batteries are compact and have a high capacity. The lithium cobalt oxide battery has potential safety problems and is being replaced by manganese oxides and iron phosphates. The electric car Chevrolet Volt for 2011 is designed to travel 40 miles on its battery with a 1.4 liter gas engine used to extend its range. This differs from the Toyota Prius, which uses braking to charge the battery to improve overall fuel efficiency. The Chevrolet Volt will have a 400-pound lithium battery that costs $10,000, although there may be a $7,500 tax break for purchasers. Better Place, a commercial venture, has decided to sell mobility shares or monthly leases through which the consumer can use an electric car that goes up to 160 km, and the driver plugs in the vehicle after the journey. The plug-in can take advantage of renewable energy (wind, solar), and several small countries—for example, Israel and Denmark—are testing the idea. Lithium will be in demand to manufacture batteries; Bolivia, home to the world's largest lithium deposits, has stated its intention to become a major producer and manufacturer of lithium batteries rather than just a raw materials supplier.

Tar Sands

Canada's Alberta tar sands cover 57,000 square miles—about the size of Florida—and consist of a heavy mixture of hydrocarbons known as bitumen. There is an extraordinary 1.7 trillion barrels of synthetic crude in this deposit, but only a fraction, perhaps 10%, is recoverable. Currently 1.2 million barrels of synthetic crude are exported, but this has been forecasted to double by 2010 and triple by 2015. For each barrel of synthetic crude, 4,500 pounds of tar sands need to be dug in open pit mines. Bitumen must be separated from the tar sands using hot water tanks that spin down the sand and siphon off the liberated bitumen. The hot water must be stored in tailings ponds that are contaminated with mercury and other toxins. Bitumen is then "cracked" or refined to less than 20 carbon-containing hydrocarbons that are viscous by heating to more than 900° F. Steam-assisted gravity drainage can be used for in situ extraction of the oil. Oil from oil sands generates 1,030% more greenhouse gases than conventional crude. Toxins from the mines and tailings ponds are descending the Athabasca River to Lake Athabasca, and lake trout and pike are beginning to show signs of toxicity in verbal reports from Cree and Athabascan natives in Fort Chipewyan. Tailings ponds have been a hazard for migrating birds. The Natural Resources Defense Council has estimated that 6 million to 166 million birds would be lost over the next thirty to fifty years because of disruption of the boreal forest and tailings ponds. U.S. policy decision makers have approved a pipeline leading to Chicago from the Canadian tar sands, enabling this technology to have a U.S. market, albeit primarily in the Midwest. The tar sands exploitation has prevented Canada from meeting its Kyoto Treaty goals, because their carbon footprint has not decreased; because the oil is exported to the United States, this has implications for U.S. fossil fuel use and policy.

Environmental Effects

Drilling for oil in sensitive environments may contaminate surface areas including marshlands, rivers, oceans, and forest. There have been numerous oil spills due to piping mishaps in the Arctic, hunters targeting the Alaska pipeline, accidents in Ecuador, and sabotage in the Niger Delta. The largest oil spills have been from oil tankers running aground. The largest of these is considered to be the *Exxon Valdez*, which ran aground on Bligh Reef in Prince William Sound of Alaska in 1989. Approximately 11 million gallons or 257,000 barrels were spilled, soiling 1,300 miles of pristine shoreline. It took four summers of cleanup efforts, and not all beaches were cleaned. At its peak, the cleanup effort included 10,000 workers, about 1,000 boats, and roughly 100 airplanes and helicopters, costing $2.1 billion. Bioremediation was used on many beaches where fertilized bacteria were used to eat hydrocarbons. Best estimates were that 250,000 seabirds, 2,800 sea otters, 300 harbor seals, 250 bald eagles, up to 22 killer whales, and billions of salmon and herring eggs were lost. Wildlife were injured by oil on their fur that destroyed their insulation value or were poisoned by eating and drinking the oil, causing toxicity to their livers, kidneys, and reproductive systems.

The Deepwater Horizon Mississippi Canyon-252 explosion in April 2010 and the ensuing 35,000–60,000 barrels per day (5 million barrels total) of oil flooding into the Gulf of Mexico has focused the nation's attention on environmental health. Eleven workers on the rig lost their lives and seventeen others were injured. The Deepwater well head is 5,000 feet below the ocean surface. The resulting oil slick covered at least 2,500 square miles, fluctuating from day to day depending on weather conditions. There were also immense underwater fumes of oil not visible at the surface. The effort to plug the leak and to clean up the environment has exposed many hundreds of oil and gas workers to oil, smoke, and particles through respiratory and skin routes of exposure. President Obama has emphasized that 5,400 skimmers have been working on boats and skiffs to break up the sheen on the surface and collect oil into booms. Twenty-seven thousand oil clean-up workers have trudged up and down the Louisiana beaches picking up tar balls and collecting oil in garbage bags. More are cleaning oil from marsh grass and soiled birds. Exposure to oil results in many toxics potentially harmful to humans: volatile organics containing aldehydes, alcohols, esters, aliphatic hydrocarbons, aromatics including benzene, and polycyclic hydrocarbons with cancer-causing attributes. Almost a million gallons of oil dispersants have been administered in the mile deep waters. The Corexit 9527 dispersant is about 4 times more toxic to aquatic species than is crude oil. Corexit contains petroleum distillates 10%–30%, organic sulfonic acid, propylene glycol, and 2-butoxyethanol. Their toxicities to humans and the environment are largely unexplored. The mixtures of crude oil, gas, and dispersants need scientific review.

Epidemiologic studies of oil spill disasters stemming from the *Exxon Valdez* (just three days worth of oil compared to the Deepwater Horizon oil flood disaster), the *Prestige* oil spill in Spain in 2002, and the *Braer* oil spill in 1993 in the United Kingdom have evaluated workers and residents affected on the beaches in the clean-up. There were significantly increased symptoms related to the eyes, upper respiratory tract, skin irritation, nausea, and fatigue. Those directly involved in the bird cleaning and physical tasks had an increased rate of injuries. But much more striking was the stress (post-traumatic stress disorder) or anxiety among the residents and workers involved. This may be from the direct exposure, or even the ecological losses or the direct and indirect financial losses. However, there have been no long-term studies of liver, kidney, or respiratory function or long-term risks for cancer, cardiovascular, reproductive, or neurological or brain disorders. The National Institute of Environmental Health Sciences will study 55,000 Gulf oil spill workers in an open-ended study rather than one focused on a specific number of end points.[2] Contaminants of concern include benzene and polycyclic aromatic hydrocarbons; exposed individuals include workers with chemical exposures, for example, the National Institute of Occupational Safety and Health tallied 52,000 workers responding to the Gulf oil spill by August 2010. Through the Superfund laws and amendments, NIEHS has experience in workers' education and training in environmental health and has trained more than 20,000 workers in the Gulf region already. NIEHS has academic centers trained in clinical epidemiology and translational medicine.

The U.S. government has named British Petroleum (BP) as the responsible party for the Deepwater Horizon spill, and officials have committed to hold the company accountable for all cleanup costs (already more than $2 billion and climbing) and other damage to local industries (a $20 billion down payment has been committed to President Obama by BP for disbursement to affected parties).

Oil and the Government

Oil Pollution Act of 1990 In response to the *Exxon Valdez* spill, the U.S. Congress passed the Oil Pollution Act of 1990 (OPA). This was a comprehensive oil spill liability, response, and compensation statute. The legislation included a clause that prohibits any vessel that, after March 22, 1989, has caused an oil spill of more than one million U.S. gallons (3,800 m^3) in any marine area from operating in Prince William Sound. As of 2002, OPA had prevented eighteen ships from entering Prince William Sound. OPA also set a schedule for the gradual phase-in of a double-hull design, providing an additional layer between the oil tanks and the ocean. While a double hull would likely not have prevented the *Valdez* disaster, a Coast Guard study estimated that it would have cut the amount of oil spilled by 60%. Liability was established for oil removal costs and damages resulting from the incident to the responsible party (this varies depending on type of vessel or facility). The Oil Spill Liability Trust Fund was established for the President for payment of oil removal costs consistent with the National Contingency Plan. Liability for responsible parties at onshore facilities and deepwater ports was up to $350 million per spill; holders of leases or permits for offshore facilities were liable for up to $75 million per spill. An Interagency Coordinating Committee on Oil Pollution Research was established to coordinate a comprehensive program of oil pollution research, technology development, and demonstration among federal agencies, in cooperation and coordination with industry, universities, and state governments.

The Deepwater Horizon disaster was a public health emergency. The charge was to immediately develop cohorts of potentially exposed and comparison groups (see Chapter 8 on the World Trade Center (WTC) disaster). There are at least three at-risk groups: high-exposed BP workers (similar to the Fire Department of New York (FDNY) workers at the WTC Dust disaster); skimmers on the water exposed to oil sheens; and beach clean-up workers. Their exposures need to be carefully assessed to crude oil, volatile organics, time of exposure, intensity of exposure, and so on. Health evaluations and questionnaires assessing symptoms need to be planned early to capitalize on WTC Dust experience. Blood, respiratory function, exposure assessments, and general health evaluations need to be planned in advance. Data entry and databases, central laboratories, and blood repositories need to be established.

It will be important to have a central coordinating health research-oriented agency. The WTC Dust disaster led to a mélange of overlapping jurisdictions of federal, state, local, academic, and other agencies with different expertise and missions. The experience of the WTC Dust disaster required congressional earmarks for funding to perform clinical health examinations of FDNY workers, funding to a central coordinating center and five clinics for clean-up worker health evaluations, and a New York City Health and Hospitals Clinics for residents' health. A critical gap was the restriction for health evaluations without the important research component to answer compelling scientific questions or inquiries of epidemiology and study design to elicit disease patterns and studies on the mechanisms of diseases.

The Department of the Interior's Minerals Management Service had responsibility for encouraging industrial development on federal lands and the outer continental shelf, collecting the royalties due the federal government, and regulating the same industry to determine that it had complied with relevant federal laws. This made for numerous conflicts of interest and was sharply criticized by the Interior's inspector general for being beholden to the industry that it regulated. The new Bureau of Ocean Energy Management under the Assistant

Secretary for Land and Minerals Management will be responsible for the sustainable development of the outer continental shelf's conventional and renewable energy resources, including resource evaluation, planning, and leasing. The new Bureau of Safety and Environmental Enforcement, also under the same assistant secretary, will be responsible for ensuring comprehensive oversight, safety, and environmental protection in all offshore energy activities. The new Office of Natural Resources Revenue under the Assistant Secretary for Policy, Management, and Budget will be responsible for the royalty and revenue management function including the collection and distribution of revenue, auditing and compliance, and asset management. The Minerals Management Service has been reconstituted as the new Bureau of Ocean Energy Management, Regulation and Enforcement (Bureau of Ocean Energy or BOE) created on June 18, 2010. President Obama chartered a BP Commission chaired by former Florida senator Bob Graham and former EPA administrator William K. Reilly to investigate the cause of the BP accident and recommend solutions and regulatory reform to prevent such accidents in the future. Their final report stated, "Minerals Management Service became an agency systematically lacking the resources, technical training or experience in petroleum engineering that is absolutely critical to ensuring that offshore drilling is being conducted in a safe and responsible manner. For a regulatory agency to fall so short of its essential safety mission is inexcusable."

Natural Gas

Natural gas is 90% methane but includes significant quantities of ethane, propane, butane, and pentane. Before natural gas can be used as a fuel, it must undergo extensive processing to remove almost all materials other than methane. The by-products of that processing include ethane, propane, butanes, pentanes, higher molecular weight hydrocarbons, elemental sulfur, and sometimes helium and nitrogen. The major difficulty in the use of natural gas is transportation and storage because of natural gas's low density. Pipelines carry it across North America, and liquefied natural gas carriers can be used to transport liquefied natural gas across oceans; tank trucks can carry liquefied or compressed natural gas over shorter distances. Significant amounts of methane (1.4%) leak from gas pipelines. A minute amount of odorant, t-butyl mercaptan, with a rotting cabbage-like smell, is added to the otherwise colorless and odorless gas so that leaks can be detected. Electricity is generated by combining gas turbines with a steam turbine in combined cycle mode. Natural gas is a major feedstock for the production of ammonia, via the Haber process, for use in fertilizer production. It can be used to power cars, buses, and trucks, burning more cleanly than gasoline, and can be used to produce hydrogen.

Natural gas releases 45% the CO_2 of coal and 30% less CO_2 than burning petroleum. According to the Intergovernmental Panel on Climate Change (IPCC) Fourth Assessment Report, in 2004 natural gas produced about 5,300 million tons per year of CO_2 emissions, while coal and oil were double this. However, this will double by 2030, and since natural gas is mostly methane, it has 22 times the climate forcing compared to CO_2 as a GHG in increasing surface temperature. The global production is approximately 2,600 billion m^3/year, and 550 billion m^3/year is produced in the United States. Supplies in the United States could last several hundred years by tapping shale formations like the Barnett in Texas, the Marcellus in Appalachia, and the Haynesville in Louisiana. Estimated reserves are more than 2,037 trillion cubic feet currently, with proven reserves at 284 trillion cubic feet from the Energy Department. The Potential Gas Committee estimated gas reserves at 1,800 trillion cubic feet, including 616 trillion cubic feet from shale gas (Marcellus Shale estimates are 500 trillion cubic feet). Natural gas is being promoted as a natural back-up for alternative sources of energy, since it could fire up power plants rapidly when the wind is not blowing and during cloudy periods. Natural gas could serve as an interim solution for climate change since it could replace coal in power plants in the eastern United States and still be relatively inexpensive and plentiful. Hydro-fracking to extract natural gas from shale deposits in Appalachia may contaminate ground water, with various chemicals requiring close monitoring by state and federal environmental agencies.

A major concern about natural gas is the inadvertent methane leaks from oil and gas wells, pipelines, and storage tanks. Estimates are that 3 trillion cubic feet of methane are leaked each year, with Russia leading at 427 billion cubic feet, the United States second at 346 billion cubic feet, and Ukraine third at 225 billion cubic feet. The EPA has estimated that natural gas leaks have the warming power of more than half the coal plants in the United States. With Energy Department projections showing a 50% increase in gas production over the next twenty years, there will be more developments and pipelines to monitor. The original EPA greenhouse gas reporting rule would exempt the >700,000 oil and gas wells in the United States, but EPA officials will be issuing rules explicitly for this industry.

The expansion of natural gas drilling in the United States, especially in the shales in New York and Pennsylvania, has raised environmental concerns over hydraulic fracking, which uses proprietary chemicals in pressurized water to increase flows of natural gas. Up to 8 million gallons of water may be used to frack a well, and a well may be fracked multiple times. These chemicals include benzene, toluene, xylene, and ethylbenzene. Natural gas wells are typically 8,000 feet deep, and the water table usually is 1,000 feet deep. The natural gas may enter the water supply if the cement casing leaks around the natural gas well. The larger problem is that the injected water is contaminated with the fracking chemicals and must be properly disposed of in buried disposal pits. Moreover, there are many volatile organic compounds that are vaporized from the contaminated water, and these chemicals can contribute to ground-level ozone or smog production. The New York Marcellus shale covers much of the New York City watershed, and these lands have been declared off-limits for gas drilling by New York State's Departmental of Environmental Conservation.

Hydrogen Gas

Although futuristic, a hydrogen-based energy economy appears to be the most challenging. Hydrogen is difficult to compress since it is a gas at room temperature and it is an energy carrier rather than an energy source. This means that hydrogen is not readily available and must be made from splitting water into hydrogen and oxygen, which requires energy. Most of that energy is recovered when hydrogen is combusted. Splitting water can be accomplished using renewable energy sources, and storage and distribution systems could be developed. Currently, hydrogen can yield thermal energy in a combustion engine or electrical energy in a fuel cell. Fuel cells are two orders of magnitude more expensive than internal combustion engines due to precious metal catalysts to produce power. Developing a hydrogen power train for a fuel cell and/or electric motor remains technically difficult. Focusing the hydrogen program on basic research will give this important alternative appropriate long-term consideration.

Coal

The United States has 275 billion tons of recoverable coal out of reserves of 496 billion tons. Approximately one billion tons are produced per year with 1.16 billion tons mined in 2006.

Coal mining itself has several attendant hazards. First, coal dust can produce coal worker's pneumoconiosis (CWP), though it has declined dramatically over recent years due to improved ventilation and dust controls. CWP occurs mainly among underground miners (one-third of U.S. coal comes from underground mines) and is due to coal mine dust in the lung with tissue reaction including focal emphysema and peribronchiolar fibrosis. Second, progressive massive fibrosis (PMF) can occur in heavily dust-exposed miners. It is characterized by fibrosis in the mid–upper lung zones and reduced pulmonary function. Coal can activate macrophages to release monocyte chemotactic factor to attract macrophages that release reactive oxidant species, fibronectin, and fibrotic growth factors that stimulate collagen accumulation. Neutrophil elastase contributes to the focal emphysema. Twelve thousand miners died from black lung disease (CWP and PMF) between 1992 and 2002.

The deadliest year in U.S. coal mining history was 1907, when 3,242 deaths occurred. That year, America's worst mine explosion killed 358 people near Monongahela, West Virginia. There was an all-time low of twenty-three coal mining fatalities in 2005, compared to thirty-four coal mining fatalities in 2007. The fatality rate for coal mining in 2006 was 49.5 fatalities per 100,000 workers, up from a rate of 26.8 recorded in 2005, compared to that of total private industry workers, which was four. Of the forty-seven coal mining fatalities recorded in 2006, 43% were due to fires and explosions, 34% resulted from contact with objects and equipment, and 19% were transportation incidents. Since 1900, nearly 100,000 coal miners have been killed in mine accidents and explosions, including twenty-five miners who died in an explosion in early April 2010. Coal mine explosions come from methane seepage that can mobilize large amounts of coal dust, which has even greater explosive characteristics. Methane is also released to the environment during coal mining, and the EPA estimates that 26% of all energy-related methane emissions in the United States come from coal mining.

Federal and state laws were promulgated to better advise and regulate the mining industry, to extend coverage to all types of miners, to require or encourage use of successful safety procedures and technology, to provide effective miner training, and to focus on reducing or eliminating the most serious hazards. The most far-reaching laws were the Federal Coal Mine Health and Safety Act of 1969, which provided a worker's compensation program for black lung, and the more comprehensive Federal Mine Safety and Health Act of 1977. This law created the Mine Safety and Health Administration (MSHA), which was moved to the Department of Labor. MSHA reporting rules listed 4,881 injuries and thirty-four fatalities in 2007, a 4.21 and 0.03 incidence rate per 200,000 employee hours respectively. Coal mining has to use underground techniques for deep coal seams, but surface mining is much cheaper, safer, and productive. Surface mining in Wyoming has propelled that state into the lead in quantity of coal mined. Additionally, that coal is low in sulfur, helping to solve the SO_2 and acid rain problems.

Mountaintop Removal

Mountaintop removal in West Virginia and Kentucky has led to a resurgence in coal mining in both states, but the blasting off of mountain tops dumps tons of material into adjacent ravines and destroys streams and rivers. Between 1985 and 2001, mountaintop removal coal mining in Appalachia cut down more than 7% of the region's forests and buried more than 1,200 miles of streams. The Interior Department, in concurrence with the EPA, has a written rule that allows the coal companies to dump mountaintop waste into rivers and streams of adjacent valleys. The EPA said the rule had been revised to protect fish, wildlife, and streams as well as federal and state water quality standards. The Council of Environmental Quality in the White House coordinates such rules and announced that the White House Office of Management and Budget had approved the rule—the last hurdle before publication in the Federal Register. The National Mining Association, a trade group, welcomed the rule, but environmental organizations, including the Sierra Club, the Environmental Defense Fund, Earthjustice, and the Natural Resources Defense Council decried it. They claimed that it would accelerate "the destruction of mountains, forests, and streams throughout Appalachia." The governors of Kentucky and Tennessee, both Democrats, wrote to the Bush administration not to approve the rule. Under President Obama, the EPA issued a guidance for protection of water quality under the Clean Water Act for mine companies to meet when mountaintop fill was used in river valleys. A final guidance that was expected in April 2011 was delayed while the Office of Information and Regulatory Affairs in the Office of Management and Budget reviewed this major rule that had an effect of $100 million or more on the economy according to Executive Order 12866.

Coal mining released more than 13 million pounds of toxic chemicals to landfills or directly to streams in 2004. Every year, coal-fired power plants in the United States generate 130 million tons of ash and sludge containing toxic substances, including chromium, arsenic, and nickel. About half of these plants dump their waste in surface ponds, only 26% of which are lined to prevent pollution from escaping. On December 22, 2008, 1.1 billion gallons of coal fly ash slurry spilled at the Kingston Fossil Tennessee Valley Authority (TVA) plant. It traveled downhill, covering the surrounding land with up to 6 feet of sludge, damaging homes, and flowing into nearby waterways.

Coal-Fired Power Plants

There are more than 500 major coal-fired power plants in the United States, and 154 are planned by 2030, with only twenty-four using advanced coal-burning technologies. This would add 37.7 gigawatts of capacity and produce 247.8 million tons of CO_2 per year. A 500 megawatt (MW) coal plant powers 500,000 homes and produces as much CO_2 emissions as 750,000 cars. CO_2 makes up 14% of flue gases; this must be scrubbed before capture. Amine solutions take up CO_2 and release it when heated. The United Kingdom, Germany, and Poland produce more than half of their power from coal. Global plans are stunning: by 2012 the world faces the prospect of having 7,474 coal-fired power plants in seventy-nine countries pumping out 9 billion tons of CO_2 emissions annually, out of 31 billion tons from all sources in 2012.

Coal liquefaction can produce coal-based diesel using a technology known as Fischer-Tropsch, named for German chemists of the 1920s. The Natural Resources Defense Council has labeled this as a brown path, not a green path, in using synthetic fuels (synfuels). The gas is produced by high temperatures and pressure and is channeled to a reactor where catalysts re-unite carbon and hydrogen to form hydrogen chains of varying lengths, including diesel and petrol. Mercury and sulfur can inhibit the reaction and are removed from the gas before liquefying it. Consequently, coal-liquefied diesel has less mercury, sulfur, particulates, and volatile organic compounds than diesel from oil. However, it takes one ton of bituminous coal to produce two barrels of coal-based oil. This process is very energy intensive, such that even with carbon capture and storage (CCS), coal-derived fuels will release 80% more CO_2 than petroleum-derived fuels.

Carbon Capture and Storage

In order to prevent further accumulation of anthropogenic CO_2 in the atmosphere, carbon capture and storage will be important for clean coal technologies. CO_2 is heavier than air and would tend to remain in deep wells. Germany has an experimental CCS site near Berlin at Ketzin, where 60,000 tons of CO_2 will be injected into an aquifer of salt water 700 meters below the surface. This CCS was singled out at G8 summit meetings. There will be scientific monitoring at the site for undesired chemical interactions between CO_2 and minerals and acidification of brine that could in principle eat away at cap-rock or contaminate drinkable ground water. CO_2 transport, storage, injection, and pumping facilities will cost at least $80 billion by 2030, which will be a small amount in comparison to the energy investments needed by then. Norway has injected 10 million tons of CO_2 1,000 meters below the North Sea into the Utsira Sand formation. Sleipner West pumps natural gas—12 billion cubic feet annually—and 9% is CO_2 that is stripped onsite to be injected below. Since 1996 they have been injecting about one million tons of CO_2 per year.

In Southern California, the BP Carson Oil Refinery is building a $1 billion plant to burn petroleum coke to H_2 and CO_2. H_2 would drive turbines and produce electricity. CO_2 would be injected into an oil well to squeeze hard-to-reach petroleum toward the surface. Once empty, the well would be sealed forever, trapping the CO_2.

Three CCS methods are storage in deep saline brine pools below ground water, deep coal seams or porous rock such as sandstone, or depleted oil and gas fields. Saline aquifers with their large storage capacity (10,000 gigatons of CO_2) and global distribution are the most attractive. The amount of CO_2 produced by coal-fired power plants in the United States is daunting, with almost 2 billion tons of CO_2 per year to inject.

Much research is ongoing in regard to terra preta (char), which is Amazonian soil that has more carbon than surrounding soils from Indo-farmers 7,000 years ago. For example, 250 tons of carbon may be in a 2-acre plot, compared to 100 tons in unimproved soils; how to reproduce this carbon sequestration is of interest. Such char could be used for large-scale farming and carbon sequestration.

Integrated gasification combined cycle (IGCC) has 20% higher costs but CO_2 can be captured more easily. Germany is planning a $1.3 billion investment in a 450 MW IGCC plant. The U.S. Department of Energy has planned an IGCC called FutureGen since 2003 representing a $600 million investment by the Department of Energy plus >$250 million from several U.S. businesses, Australia, China, and India. This is a technology forcing demonstration plant to go online in 2012. It would use coal to produce H_2 and electricity with **carbon sequestration**. Coal gasification is to produce H_2 and CO that will react with steam to produce additional H_2 and concentrated CO_2. H_2 will be used to drive turbines for electricity and fuel cells. IGCC plants use two thermodynamic cycles; the H_2 from the gasifier and the shift reaction drives a gas turbine, while the heat from that turbine and the gasifier drives a separate steam turbine. Having more than one cycle means that efficiencies of IGCC should go higher than the 40% of most advanced conventional coal plants. IGCC power plants in the Netherlands and Japan have routinely operated between 50% and 100% load, increasing and decreasing output in under an hour. H_2 produced at a single plant can be used to cogenerate stream and produce chemicals and liquid fuels as well as generate electric power. In 2007 site selection had been completed, with the state of Illinois chosen. By generating 275 MW of electricity, Future-Gen will be capable of powering 150,000 average U.S. homes. Costs ballooned to $6.5 million per MW, compared to less than $2 million per MW for wind turbines resulting in cancellation of the project only to be revived by stimulus funds by Secretary of Energy Stephen Chu in 2009. Early in 2010 Futurgen 2.0

was announced as a retooling of a shuttered coal-fired power plant using new oxy-combustion technology with CO_2 sequestration. The 18-month Environmental Impact Statement is scheduled to begin in the spring of 2011.

Biofuels

Biofuels have the potential to solve the transportation problem of diminishing supplies of oil, but they do produce greenhouse gases. Furthermore, the production of corn, soybeans, and other crops would compete for fertilizer and arable land, resulting in little if any greenhouse gas reduction. Algae may consume CO_2 and could be bioengineered to produce a liquid fuel. The transportation sector will be facing technology choices such as liquid fuel versus development of rechargeable batteries.

Biodiesel in the United States is primarily produced from soybean oil and in Europe from rapeseed oil. In Europe, one-third to one-half of all vehicles are powered by diesel. Diesel engines compress air in a cylinder, making it so hot that when fuel hits the air, it explodes. They are more efficient than spark plug designs and get better fuel economy. Soybean oil is 20% efficient (50 gallons biodiesel per acre), while canola achieves 40% and algae 50% (8,000 gallons biodiesel per acre). The growth of diesel in the United States charted by the National Biodiesel Board is from 25 million gallons in 2004 to 75 million gallons in 2005, 250 million in 2006, and 450 million gallons in 2007. In 2008 capacity had reached double this level, with another one billion gallons under construction.

Biodiesel is made through transesterification, whereby glycerin is separated from fat and vegetable oil. The process leaves behind two products: methyl esters and glycerin. Transesterification makes vegetable oil less viscous by adding methanol and sodium hydroxide as a catalyst, producing biodiesel and glycerin. Biodiesel is defined as mono-alkyl esters of long chain fatty acids derived from vegetable oils or animal fats. A 1998 biodiesel lifecycle study, jointly sponsored by U.S. Departments of Energy and Agriculture, concluded that biodiesel reduces net CO_2 emissions by 78% compared to petroleum diesel. Biodiesel generates 3.2 times more energy than is required to produce it. Biodiesel contains no sulfur and emits 47% less particulate but may emit 10% more NOx. Cold weather can gel biodiesel, requiring precautions or fuel heaters in very cold weather.

Starch and cellulose are more challenging biofuels, but the most efficient breakdown strategies use enzymes to break down starch and cellulose to glucose. The glucose can then be fermented by the yeast *Saccharomyces cerevisiae*, which helps to convert glucose into two equivalents of ethanol, but this process is slow. There is considerable chemical research on this process, for example, enzymes can convert glucose into fructose that can be made into a low-oxygen fuel called dimethyl furan. Genomes of higher termites have been sequenced and many carbohydrate-active enzymes identified that could be utilized in these industrial processes.[3] Whereas the conversion of starch-based feedstock results primarily in hexoses, the products from degradation of lignocellulose biomass, composed of hemicellulose, include large amounts of the pentose sugars D-xylose and L-arabinose. In contrast to the hexose sugars, the pentose sugars cannot be fermented by wild-type *S. cerevisiae*. Most fermenting organisms such as *S. cerevisiae* cannot tolerate ethanol concentrations exceeding 25%, resulting in a product that must be concentrated by distillation. *Escherichia coli*, the common intestinal bacterium, can be engineered genetically to convert algae into a commercial biodiesel and jet fuel. *E. coli* can also be genetically engineered to produce butanol and isobutanol that is superior to ethanol as a fuel because it is less hygroscopic and more closely resembles petroleum.[4]

Algae

Cyanobacteria, a blue-green algae capable of photosynthesis, and yeast have been engineered to produce isobutanol. Algae don't compete with food crops for land or even fresh water since many species can grow in brackish or briny water. They reproduce in hours and are far more productive than terrestrial plants. Algae naturally produce oils that have a 50% higher energy content than ethanol. Numerous start-up companies are researching the production of hydrocarbons from algae, for example, ExxonMobil has invested $600 million, half in Synthetic Genomics, Inc, to reengineer some strains of algae to secrete hydrocarbons from their cells. The challenge will be to scale up production in closed reactors or possibly open traditional farming methods using shallow ponds. Algae require waste CO_2 to be bubbled through to increase photosynthesis, providing a commercial opportunity for the millions of tons of waste CO_2.

Jatropha

Jatropha, grown in marginal lands in Asia, especially India, can be converted to biodiesel. It is a member of the euphorbia family, originated in Central America, and its seeds have long been used to make lamp oil and soap. Jatropha bushes live up to fifty years, fruit annually for more than thirty years, and weather droughts with aplomb. It takes about 4 kilograms of seeds to make a liter of oil, and the cost of biodiesel is the same as petrodiesel. The nutrient-rich seed cake after pressing can be returned to farmers as a fertilizer. Jatropha seed biodiesel exceeds quality measures for soya bean, rapeseed, and sunflower oils. Demonstration transesterification plants are being developed, but little is known about the agronomics of growing jatropha commercially.

Palm Oil

Southeast Asia contains 11% of the world's remaining tropical forests, and recently there has been an explosion in the planting and harvest of palm oil. Palm oil is a biofuel, but it also can be used as a cooking oil, a food additive, and in cosmetics and industrial lubricants. Currently there are 21 million tons produced per year, and this will grow to >30 million by 2010. Indonesia and Malaysia are the two major producers, and India and China are the major consumers, primarily using it for cooking.

Logging of virgin forest in Indonesia, especially Borneo, with replacement with palm oil plantations has decimated many wild areas and endangered the orangutan. To correct this imbalance, revenues could be diverted from palm oil agriculture to reserving private nature reserves and protecting forest habitats and endangered species. Approximately 25% of Indonesia and 11% of Malaysia are virgin primary forests, with 20% of Indonesia's and about 10% of Malaysia's total forest under protective covenants. One approach to increasing land protection is for nongovernmental organizations to purchase palm oil plantations, and after paying off acquisition costs in about six years, steering subsequent profits into purchasing forest for private reserves. These private reserves could protect endemic species and provide employment for local communities in ecotourism or select resource harvest. The Roundtable for Sustainable Palm Oil will certify plantations that use degraded land and promulgate good practices for sustainable harvests.

Converting rainforests, peatlands, savannas, or grasslands to produce food-based biofuels in Brazil, Southeast Asia, and the United States creates a biofuel carbon debt by releasing 17 to 420 times more CO_2 than the annual GHG reductions these biofuels provide by displacing fossil fuels.[5] In contrast, biofuels made from waste biomass or from biomass grown on abandoned agricultural lands planted with perennials incur little or no carbon debt and offer immediate and sustained GHG advantages, for example, jatropha.

Ethanol

Ethanol is the biofuel du jure in the United States, where we produced 5.4 billion gallons in 2008. The primary feedstock for U.S. ethanol is corn, and the ethanol plants are concentrated in the Midwest. Sugar cane produces ethanol 10 times more efficiently than corn because of a higher sugar content. Brazilian gasohol is 23% ethanol, and Brazil produces 4 billion gallons per year. This potentially reduces 26 million tons of atmospheric CO_2. Ethanol reduces CO_2 only 12%, compared to 41% for biodiesel.[6] The 2007 U.S. Energy Act prescribes a goal of 36 billion gallons of ethanol by 2022, with 15 billion of that to come from corn ethanol by 2015. There are 16 billion gallons to be derived from cellulosic (plant-derived) biofuels and 5 billion gallons per year of other renewable fuels such as biodiesel. There is a strong Midwest lobby for utilizing corn as the ethanol feedstock, and high tariffs blocking importation of Brazilian sugar cane as a feedstock to protect the smaller U.S. sugar industry. The U.S. sugar beet and sugar cane industries are located in Louisiana, Florida, northwestern Minnesota, and California, where there are no or few ethanol refineries.

Fertilizing, harvesting, and refining corn into fuel takes a lot of energy, and the sugar conversion process wastes most of the plant's biomass, primarily cellulose. Switching all U.S. corn and soybean to ethanol and biodiesel would offset only 12% of U.S. gasoline and 6% of diesel; the most appropriate use of ethanol would be as an oxygenate at 10%–20%.[6] Oxygenates prevent engine "knocking" ever since lead has been removed from gasoline, and methyl tert-butyl ether, the original oxygenate, was found to contaminate ground water following leaking from underground gasoline storage tanks. Replacing 10% of U.S. motor fuel with biofuels would require about a third of the total cropland now devoted to cereals, oilseeds, and sugar crops. Cellulosic ethanol from switch grass or agricultural waste is the most efficient. This could supply up to half of the 135 billion gallons of gasoline consumed per year in the United States.

The debt repayment (energy consumed to energy produced) of biofuels varies dramatically when one calculates the clearing of land, farming, and so on: Brazilian sugarcane is best at 17 years, palm oil grown in tropical peatland at 420 years, corn grown on fallow land at 48 years, and corn grown on U.S. grasslands at 93 years. Most of these calculations suggest that carbon mitigation is best achieved by saving and restoring forests rather than conversion to biofuels.[7] A 10% substitution of petrol and diesel fuel is estimated to require 43% and 38% of current cropland area in the United States and Europe, respectively. Searchinger and colleagues used a worldwide agricultural model to estimate emissions from land use change, finding that corn-based ethanol, instead of producing a 20% savings, nearly doubles GHG emissions over thirty years and increases GHG for 167 years.[8] Biofuels from switchgrass, if grown on U.S. corn lands, increases emissions by 50%. The sterile hybrid grass *Miscanthus x giganteus* can convert 1% of solar energy into biomass that could be harvested to make cellulosic ethanol. That's 10 times the standard 0.1% efficiency cited for plants, and compared to switchgrass, 3 times as much harvestable biomass can be produced on the same amount of land. Such dramatic increases in biomass have also been observed with mixtures of up to fifteen prairie grasses rather than just switchgrass monocultures. The 2007 Energy Act requires refiners to produce an estimated 61 billion liters of cellulosic biofuels by 2022 as a stimulus to this industry.

In the United States there is a 51 cents per gallon tax allowance given to blenders who mix ethanol with petrol, and a 54 cents per gallon tariff on imported ethanol, which primarily serves to largely keep low-cost Brazilian ethanol from sugar cane out of the country. The commercial product that promotes ethanol biofuel is E85, which is 85% ethanol and 15% gasoline. E85 is available at 850 service stations out of 169,000 service stations nationwide. The reason that it has not caught on includes capital costs of $200,000 for an E85 storage tank, and that E85 delivers only three-fourths the energy of gasoline.

Nuclear

Nuclear energy provides 20% of U.S. electricity. There are 104 operable nuclear energy plants and 27 new ones under consideration. There are 439 nuclear reactors worldwide with a capacity of 370 gigawatts, and 20%–30% of today's reactors will be decommissioned between 2011 and 2030. The U.S. nuclear industry is aging, with more than 80% built before 1990 and 25% in the 1960s and 1970s. Of the thirty nuclear plants under construction, nineteen are in Asia, six are in Russia, five are in Europe, and none are in the United States. There are several technologies involved, but most are pressurized water reactors that generate steam to drive turbines. These are light water reactors (LWR) using ordinary water to slow neutrons and cool the reactor. Uranium is the fuel, but 99% of this is unburned, and long-lived nuclear wastes such as plutonium, americium, and curium are produced that require geologic isolation. New technologies could spur nuclear development.

Integrated fast reactors (IFR) have been designed and tested at U.S. national laboratories; they keep neutrons "fast" by using liquid sodium metal as a coolant instead of water and can burn existing nuclear waste and surplus weapons-grade uranium and plutonium, making electrical power in the process. *Integral* means that all fuel reprocessing is done within the reactor facility. Another concept is the **Liquid-Fluoride Thorium Reactor (LFTR)** that uses a chemically stable fluoride salt for the medium in which nuclear reactions take place. Both IFR and LFTR are lower pressure reactors than LWR and are 100–300 times more fuel efficient. The pebble bed reactor (PBR) is a graphite-moderated, gas-cooled nuclear reactor that is also known as a high-temperature gas reactor. In the PBR, tennis ball–sized pebbles are made of pyrolytic graphite containing thousands of fuel particles consisting of fissile 235U surrounded by a coated ceramic layer of SiC for structural integrity. In the PBR, 360,000 pebbles are placed together to create a reactor, and it is cooled by an inert gas such as helium, nitrogen, or CO_2. Breeder reactors (none are yet commercial) make plutonium from uranium isotopes that are not themselves useful for power production and can effectively create more fuel than they use. Breeder reactors might get 60 times more energy out for every input kilogram of natural uranium.

The risks of nuclear power are real including accidents, nuclear waste, terrorist attacks, and financial. Federal insurance is available to reduce this risk. The **Price-Anderson Nuclear Industries Indemnity Act** (renewed in 2005 for a twenty-year period) partially indemnifies the nuclear industry against liability claims arising from nuclear incidents while still ensuring compensation for the general public. The Nuclear Regulatory Commission provides nuclear power plant operators an operating license. Also, the 2005 Energy Policy Act offers loan guarantees of as much as 80% for energy companies willing to build nuclear power plants, cellulosic ethanol plants, coal sequestration facilities, or other low-polluting technologies.

In 1979, the Three Mile Island nuclear accident occurred in Pennsylvania. A core meltdown at one of its reactors, with resulting political backlash, has prevented any construction of new plants. Seventy million dollars were paid out under Price-Anderson for this accident. It took years to dismantle the partially melted core and place radioactive debris into containment vessels and ship to Idaho storage sites.

The much worse disaster at the Chernobyl reactor in the Ukraine in 1986, in which more than fifty people died, led to an abandonment of the badly contaminated cities of Pripyat and Chernobyl. A failed safety test and explosion in reactor 4 spewed 6.7 tons of radioactive isotopes over 200,000 kilometers of Europe. A sarcophagus was constructed over the stricken reactor and 3,500 workers labor to prevent further releases. Engineers want to construct a containment arch to allow them to dismantle the reactor; the arch will be the world's largest mobile structure and will take until 2065 to completely dismantle the sarcophagus and parts of the reactor. More than 5,000 cases of thyroid cancer have been seen in people who were children at the time of the accident and lived in contaminated areas of the former Soviet Union. This is more than tenfold more than expected, and most were caused by drinking milk contaminated with radioiodine. A public health program of distributing potassium iodide following nuclear accidents, staying inside, and banning the sale of food and milk around the plant is necessary.

On March 11, 2011, an earthquake registering 9.1 on the Richter scale and a tsunami struck northeastern Japan, devastating 200 miles of coastal cities, including Sendai. More than 20,000 people were lost or missing. The Fukushima Daiichi nuclear power plant, with six reactors, suffered considerable damage including cracks of the containment vessels of several reactors. In addition, the diesel engine back-up for the pumps that circulate the cooling water were damaged by flooding on the lower floor. The subsequent loss of cooling water allowed the nuclear rods to overheat and create accumulations of hydrogen gas that exploded in several reactors. Sea water was dumped and routed into the reactors to keep them cool. All of the citizens within 15 miles were evacuated, and many more were told to stay inside their homes. Both iodine-131 and cesium-137, which has a half-life of thirty years, have been detected indicating a partial meltdown. The United States is developing new technologies, like sealed pumps that are maintenance free for sixty years, and using passive gravity or convection to bypass valves and increase safety of water cooling.

The Yucca Mountain nuclear waste storage site in a remote Nevada desert is predicted to come online in 2017. Fifty-six thousand tons of highly radioactive waste have already piled up at power plants across the nation. In 1987, Congress, via an amendment to the Nuclear Waste Policy Act of 1982, selected Yucca Mountain from a group of three previously identified potential repository sites. The 1982 act had mandated detailed study of all three sites before selection of a finalist. The courts have also been involved: the U.S. Court of Appeals for the D.C. Circuit in 2004 ruled that the EPA should revise its Yucca Mountain standard for permissible releases of radioactivity to the environment to encompass a time frame from 10,000 years (EPA preference) to one going from hundreds of thousands to a million years. To demonstrate compliance, computer models have been constructed to simulate the interaction of all the geochemical, hydrogeologic, and other geologic processes that are currently believed to control the release of radionuclides to the environment over the next several hundred thousand years. The Yucca Mountain site is to be constructed 300 meters above the water table within consolidated volcanic strata, a physical setting that facilitates retrieval and monitoring high-level wastes. The Obama administration is proposing to find a new site, since current storage at nuclear facilities is adequate for a full century. In contrast, France (as well as Russia, Japan, and the United Kingdom) have taken the route of reprocessing nuclear waste, since spent fuel rods are still 95% uranium and 1% plutonium, both of which can be reprocessed and enriched to be used as fuel. The danger of reprocessing plutonium is its potential for nuclear bomb fuel. An alternative to the Yucca Mountain Repository is to use the funds collected from nuclear utilities to accelerate development of fast and thorium reactors.

Uranium mining health hazards include accidents from transport of heavy moving equipment, underground roof collapses, and dust-induced lung diseases and cancer. Dust-induced lung diseases include silicosis, a pneumoconiosis, from silica-containing dusts that are inhaled. Silica is phagocytosed by alveolar macrohages that become activated to release injurious reactive oxidant species, fibrotic growth factors, cytokines, and chemokines. A rapidly progressive form of silicosis called "acute silicosis" has been described from very high exposures to dust containing many fine particles. Advanced silicosis is caused by heavy dust exposures, usually over many decades, and is called "complicated pneumoconiosis" or "progressive massive fibrosis." Uranium miners inhaled radon gas containing alpha particles that released high energy for the bronchial epithelium, resulting in an increased risk of lung cancer. Early in the development of underground uranium mining with inadequate ventilation, there was a synergistic interaction with smoking and radon daughters with predominantly small cell lung cancer occurring.

Nuclear fusion is experimental; the first International Thermonuclear Fusion Project in Cadarche, France, with subcontracts to Japan and other producing countries, is planned to come online in 2015. This will be the first fusion experiment that will generate more energy than it uses. It will be a $\sim$500 MW plant costing $\sim$\$9 billion. Fusion is a hot plasma confined in a floating doughnut shape by superconducting magnets (a tokomak reactor).

Wind

Wind has a very promising future to provide green, renewable energy. Advanced windmills can produce 3 MW while turning. A 1.5 MW wind turbine generates enough electricity to power about 500 homes. One hundred and ten thousand MW of wind turbines on the Great Plains could cost 5.4 cents/kWh (kilowatt hour) or about the same as coal. The American Wind Energy Association says the potential for wind electrical energy is 10 trillion kWh or twice the amount of electricity currently generated in the United States (see Figure 11.3). There is currently 40,181 MW available in the United States, with 5,116 MW added in 2010. Wind energy constituted 35% of energy installed in the United States over the past four years, second only to natural gas. The U.S. wind power capacity represents more than 20% of the world's installed wind power.

An impediment to expanding the use of wind energy is the difficulty of shipping power to the east coast from the Great Plains since there is no direct current transmission. To achieve a goal of 5% of U.S. electricity from wind by 2020

FIGURE 11.3   Annual direct normal solar radiation
(two-axis tracking concentrator)

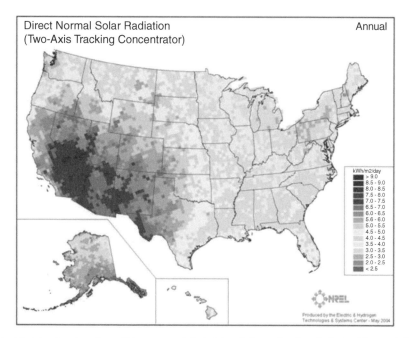

Direct Normal Solar Radiation
(Two-Axis Tracking Concentrator)

Annual

kWh/m2/day
> 9.0
8.5 - 9.0
8.0 - 8.5
7.5 - 8.0
7.0 - 7.5
6.5 - 7.0
6.0 - 6.5
5.6 - 6.0
5.0 - 5.5
4.5 - 5.0
4.0 - 4.5
3.5 - 4.0
3.0 - 3.5
2.5 - 3.0
2.0 - 2.5
< 2.5

Produced by the Electric & Hydrogen
Technologies & Systems Center · May 2004

Note: Model estimates of monthly average daily total radiation using inputs derived from satellite and/or surface observations of cloud cover, albedo, and so on sampled to a 40 km resolution.
Source: Courtesy of Department of Energy/National Renewable Energy Laboratory.

will require $60 billion in investment with $1.2 billion for farmers' leases, but the wind energy industry will create ~80,000 jobs. The average price to lease land for a wind turbine is approximately $2,000 per year. Currently there are 300,000 MW of proposed wind projects, but they cannot move forward due to the lack of transmission capacity for this electricity; this amount of wind energy would meet 20% of our nation's electricity needs. Wind electricity is intermittent, which complicates the full utilization of transmission grids. There is also the problem of a "Not in My Backyard" syndrome for coastal projects such as the 140 MW wind farm off of Jones Beach, New York, that was canceled. The Cape Wind in Nantucket Sound would have 130 wind turbines to produce 420 MW of renewable energy and reduce greenhouse gas emissions by 734,000 tons per year. The $2 billion Cape Wind project was approved by Interior Secretary Ken Salazar, who took in local citizens' complaints about loss of their view and also the Aquinnah Wampanoag Tribe on Martha's Vineyard, who said the project would interfere with sacred rituals. Resolving wind power siting issues would go a long way in wind power development and solving the nation's energy crisis.

China is the world's leader in the development of wind power, with 41,800 MW by the end of 2010. Germany and Spain lead the European Union. Ireland and Denmark had led Europe in installing wind power, but their power grid could not respond to the power surges that were put on the network; currently Denmark sells its wind power to Norway and Sweden. Norway and Sweden use this extra wind power to pump underground water into upstream reservoirs to produce more hydropower.

Another important consideration for wind is the need for back-up sources of power, since wind turbines historically generate just 20% of their capacity. Wind turbines are also responsible for approximately 40,000 American bird deaths per year, far less than the millions that succumb to domestic cats. Migratory bats have also been killed by windmills, leading to increasing amounts of research to learn more about migratory bats.

The federal renewable energy production tax credit is the primary stimulus to the industry since its inception in 1992, but the tax credit has been extended in one or two-year intervals. A renewable electricity standard or a renewable portfolio standard is a policy that sets hard targets for renewable energy in the near and long term to diversify electricity supply, reduce pollution and promote the wind and solar industries. In 2011 twenty-nine states have renewable electricity standards and seven states have renewable energy goals, but the renewable portfolio standard does not exist at the federal level.

Geothermal Energy and Hydropower

Geothermal Energy

Geothermal energy produces 2,800 MW with forty-six power plants at seven sites in California, including the Geysers at 1,000 MW. This provides 0.3% of the electricity in the United States but 17% of its renewable energy. The current plants prevent 22 million tons of CO_2 from being emitted. Geothermal energy can be tapped by drilling 3 or more miles deep underground in areas where 300°F rock exists, followed by applying high water pressures to open fractures in the rock. Injection wells are then drilled to circulate water in the human-made reservoir and extract steam to the surface to run electric turbines. Approximately 2% of the U.S. geothermal resource base could yield nearly 2,000 times the power that the nation now consumes each year, for example, 100,000 MW of electricity could be envisioned by fifty years. The U.S. Geologic Survey estimates that geothermal regions spread across thirteen states could continually produce a total of 9,000 MW of electricity. Hydro-fracking for tapping geothermal energy of magnitudes envisioned would need to be tested so that it doesn't touch off earth tremors nearby. Venture capital and government partnering would be necessary to demonstrate the economic feasibility of geothermal plants—certainly this would reduce CO_2 emissions.

Geothermal power can now be harnessed at lower temperatures than is required for boiling water by using closed circuits and liquid compounds with lower boiling temperatures. For example, Chena Hot Springs in Alaska, located about 65 miles from the electricity grid, uses a geothermal closed circuit to generate 500 kilowatts of geothermal electricity per day to heat the resort's forty-four buildings, run a greenhouse, and a café made of carved ice. In October 2008, the DOE awarded $43 million in cost-sharing grants to twenty-one geothermal research projects. At the same time, the Department of the Interior took initial steps to open 200 million acres of federal lands to geothermal development. Several of these projects have been halted due to earth tremors and actual earthquakes that may have been triggered by the deep drilling near tectonic plates. More research needs to be done on this potential drawback.

Hydropower

The World Energy Council estimates that the world has 45,000 large dams that have a generating capacity of 800 gigawatts, and they currently supply one-fifth of the electricity consumed worldwide. China's Three Gorges Dam has a claimed full capacity of 18 gigawatts that can generate twice as much power as all the world's solar cells. The Hoover Dam on the Colorado River in the United States can produce about 1.8 gigawatts of electricity. One hundred and sixty countries use **hydropower** to some extent. Brazil, Canada, China, Russia, and the United States currently produce more than half of the world's hydropower. Europe has exploited 75% of its feasible hydropower, but Africa and Asia have large unharnessed capacities.

There are adverse environmental effects, though; in the past few decades, millions of people have been relocated in India and China because of flooding upstream of dams. Dams have ecological effects on the ecosystem upstream and downstream and present a barrier to migrating fish. Sediment build-up can shorten dams' operating lives, and sediment trapped by the dam is denied to those downstream. Biomass that decomposes in reservoirs releases methane and carbon dioxide. Climate change could itself limit the capacity of dams in some areas by altering the amount and pattern of annual runoff from sources such as the glaciers of Tibet. Hydropower in the United States is maximally harnessed, and there is current planning for decommissioning dams on the Klamath and Columbia rivers to allow salmon to spawn and protect these critically endangered species.

Adverse effects of hydropower are loss of wild rivers, inundation of scenic areas such as Lake Powell in southern Utah Red Rock Country, or cities and cultural heritage such as the Three Gorges on the Yangtze River, China, and effects on migratory spawning fish. Hydropower is dependent on adequate water levels. Northern Canada has lost exceptional wilderness in this regard. Manitoba Hydro dammed the Nelson River to provide power to Winnipeg. However, to provide for future growth, they then dammed the Churchill River at Southern Indian Lake, flooding the lake into a reservoir, draining the lake in a southerly direction to the Nelson River to provide more water to the Nelson River Hydroelectric scheme. The lower 500 miles of the Churchill River became essentially dry, obliterating the wildest rapids on the North American continent.

NOTES FROM THE FIELD

I was one of the next-to-last people to run the rapids of the Churchill River by canoe in 1967 when we paddled from the Rockies across 1,517 miles of Canadian voyageur waterways. It took ten days to paddle the last 500 miles from Pukatawagan to Churchill on Hudson Bay. We paddled down 17 miles of rapids in Portage Chute. There were cliffs on one side of the river and high snowbanks on the other. We traveled more than 81 miles in just one day down the mighty Churchill current. Another American group after mine took three weeks for the same route.

Quebec Hydro did the same on the other side of Hudson Bay by damming the East Main and Great Whale rivers, which were once wild canoe routes from interior Quebec to the bay. The Cree in Quebec and at Southern Indian Lake had to be moved, with loss of their native hunting grounds and much of their local culture. Chile repeated the same mistake by building a dam on the Bio Bio River, with wild river rafting losing another section of wild river.

Biomass and Hut Lung

Biomass is used by 3 billion people to cook their meals and represents 10% of the energy consumed globally. Biomass consists of tree and bush branches, wood, dung that is usually dried against the outside walls of houses, and charcoal. Branches, wood, and dung burn very inefficiently. Charcoal and coal are more efficient; however, all forms of biomass emit tremendous amounts of smoke when used in primitive stoves in millions of homes. This is the major cause of indoor air pollution in Asia, Africa, and Latin America. Biomass constitutes 80% of domestic energy consumption in India. The World Health Organization (WHO) estimates 1.6 million premature deaths per year from indoor pollution (twice that from outdoor pollution) from burning biomass. It ranks fourth in developing countries' burden of disease. The predominant victims are women, who may spend 6–8 hours per day cooking indoors with biomass, and their preschool-aged children, who are on their backs in papoose-style carry-alls as infants or playing in the house as toddlers. Women develop "hut lung" from inhaling particles: they develop small rounded and irregular opacities noted on their chest X-rays and increased chronic bronchitis with cough, phlegm, and dyspnea, all characterized as chronic obstructive pulmonary disease (COPD).[9] Their children have increased lower respiratory tract infections, with increased mortality. Additionally, chronic exposure to biomass smoke can cause genetic damage, cardiovascular disease, and stroke. The prevalence of chronic bronchitis in populations that use biomass as the principal source of energy ranges from 22% in Bolivia to 8% in Guatemala to 18% in Nepal. Particulate counts have been measured as high as 30,000 $\mu g/m^3$ per hour in Bolivia and South Africa. By 2030, WHO estimates mortality from biomass burning to be 9.8 million. Lung cancer is also increased in these women.

Using efficient cookstoves that cost less than $25 or switching to propane or kerosene ameliorates this problem. A public–private partnership sponsored by the UN Foundation called the Global Alliance for Clean Cookstoves will target 100 million households with clean cookstoves by 2020. "Today we can finally envision a future in which open fires and dirty stoves are replaced by clean, efficient and affordable stoves and fuels all over the world—stoves that still cost as little as $25," said Secretary of State Hillary Rodham Clinton in September 2010 at the UN Foundation. "By upgrading these dirty stoves, millions of lives could be saved and improved. Clean stoves could be as transformative as bed nets or vaccines." The U.S. Department of State, U.S. Department of Health and Human Services–National Institutes of Health and Centers for Disease Control, U.S. Department of Energy, U.S. Environmental Protection Agency, and the U.S. Agency for International Development will mobilize top experts, key financial resources, and research and development tools to help the alliance with a financial commitment of $50.82 million over the next five years.

Biomass, diesel, and open burning are sources of black carbon that absorbs all wavelengths of sunlight contributing almost a million times the effect of CO_2

on global warming. However sulfate and organic carbon reflect light negating much of the warming effect of black carbon. Developing countries emit 77% of the black carbon while North America and Europe emit diesel that accumulates on Greenland and Arctic ice, respectively. Black carbon emissions have dropped 50% from 1989–2008 recorded by the twenty-two California black carbon monitoring stations. This probably reflects controls on diesel emissions. California is retrofitting their pre–2007 diesel heavy-duty trucks and buses over 2012–2025 for a cost of $2.2 billion.

Solar

Solar energy produces 8,775 MW as of 2007 and is expected to grow substantially in the near term. Solar energy installment responds dramatically to government programs such as rebates and research. California will have solar panels as a standard option for new home buyers in 2012. Federal tax credits give homebuyers a $2,000 solar tax credit for solar panels, and further credits may be obtained at the state level; however, these are for primary residences. The solar industry has benefited recently from spectacular policy-driven growth in the form of financial rebates, for example, shipment of photovoltaic modules increased twelvefold from 1999 to 2006. Further stimulus to include second homes or vacation homes would be a huge benefit to the industry.

One of the supply bottlenecks for solar is high-purity polycrystalline-grade silicon, the basic feedstock required to make photovoltaic solar cells; refining capacity at existing plants is limited, and marked growth may be accompanied by painful downturns resulting in cautious business plans. The polysilicon supply shortage is generating interest in other technologies for converting solar energy into electricity—most notably, thin films made of amorphous (noncrystalline) silicon and/or of compounds such as gallium arsenide, cadmium telluride, copper indium diselenide, and copper indium gallium diselenide.

The Solar Energy Research Institute (SERI) was established by President Carter, who considered the U.S. Energy Crisis the "moral equivalent of war." He gave SERI a $100 million budget, and 1,000 scientists were hired. This was slashed to $30 million and 435 scientists under President Ronald Reagan and was reorganized as the National Renewable Energy Laboratory. The federal budget was $7.7 billion in 1979 and declined to $3 billion for all energy research and development in 2008.

Silicon Valley entrepreneurs have entered the photovoltaic panel market to design new approaches to harnessing solar power. Google built a 1.6 MW solar project atop its headquarters in Mountain View, California. Google is trying to provide a market for solar and wind power that operates on windy and sunny days by investing in advanced batteries in plug-in hybrid automobiles that would take advantage of this green power surge. Google calls this initiative "RE<C," denoting "renewable energy cheaper than coal."

Concentrated solar power, for example, the parabolic trough, could be cost competitive with other sources of energy, especially in southern California deserts. Solar thermal plants are being envisioned for the Sahara Desert that can ship power to Europe. Solar thermal power uses solar energy stored in special heat-retaining fluid to drive a turbine and create power.

Summary: The Future U.S. Energy Plan

Although it is difficult to predict the future, abating climate change provides opportunities and consequences; this will be evaluated from the perspective of the private sector, for example, the investment firm Alliance Bernstein with more than \$800 billion in institutional assets analyzed strategic change in relation to climate by 2030. There were 8,000 sources that emitted 45% of all CO_2, with 150 stationary sources emitting as much CO_2 as all of the cars in the world in 2010. These sources were geographically concentrated in the United States, Europe, China, South Africa, and Japan. Alliance Bernstein estimated that approximately \$5 trillion would be spent by 2030 by owners of power plants and factories to reduce CO_2. Billions more will be spent on improving motor efficiencies of automobiles, industrial motor systems, and large consumer appliances such as refrigerators and washing machines. They estimated a decline to 26 million metric tons of CO_2 emissions and calculated an increasing demand for electricity at conservative growth of 2.2% per year from 18 trillion kilowatt-hours to 30 trillion. Global demand for electricity has grown 3.6% a year on average since 1971, more than double the 1.7% demand growth for all energy uses combined. They predict a doubling of power from renewables, almost a tripling of nuclear's contribution, a 40% increase in coal, and a small increase in natural gas.

Capturing and storing CO_2 from fossil fuel generation, principally coal power, will be absolutely critical if atmospheric CO_2 levels were to rise no higher than 450 ppm. Capturing, compressing, and transporting CO_2 from coal and natural gas power plants as well as some factories will create new industries. This will create value for depleted oil and gas fields that are geologically suitable for CO_2 storage. The global daily volume of CO_2 captured and sequestered will exceed 7 billion cubic feet (bcf) per day by 2012, approach 70 bcf by 2020, and reach 500 bcf a day before 2030—roughly double the amount of natural gas currently flowing through pipelines worldwide on a daily basis. Wind and solar will increase from 80 gigawatts today to nearly 900 gigawatts by 2030; however, the overall increase in electricity production from these sources will be significantly less than the increase in capacity because of their low utilization rates, since power is generated only when the wind is blowing and the sun is shining.

By 2030 there will be nearly one billion hybrid and plug-in hybrid vehicles on the road, dwarfing the 365 million conventional vehicles at the present. These vehicles will increase electricity demand by 7%, but oil demand by these vehicles will be reduced by over 50%. The product category that may benefit most is lithium-based batteries that should grow from the $9 billion lead acid battery market to one more than $150 billion for automotive batteries. Adoption of plug-in vehicles will reduce demand for gasoline and oil producers and refiners will be challenged by the market changes.

The International Energy Agency asserted that nearly a quarter of global electricity could be generated from nuclear power by 2050. This would require the construction of about thirty 1-gigawatt nuclear plants each year during 2010–2050, as well as significant infrastructure capacity and development of adequate nuclear safety and environmental regulations.

The United States will undoubtedly develop a national energy plan that has greater regulation, as the BP Commission will be recommending how we move forward with our more than 3,600 offshore oil rigs and more than thirty-three deep water platforms.

Many of these energy goals have been articulated by President Obama in 2011:

- Reduce our oil imports that are currently 11 million barrels of oil per day by a third.
- Improve safety for offshore drilling with approval of permits (thirty-nine shallow-water and seven deep-water permits).
- Incentivize natural gas by converting U.S. government vehicles to use compressed natural gas rather than oil.
- Convert half of the Air Force jets to biofuels by 2016.
- Build biorefineries with advanced technologies and reform biofuels incentives.
- Establish the first-ever fuel economy standards for heavy-duty trucks.
- Purchase all government vehicles using alternate fuels or electric by 2015.
- Install more energy-efficient technologies in residences and businesses.
- Review nuclear safety strategies.
- Adopt a clean energy standard (80% of electricity in the United States would be generated by clean sources by 2035), which would promote private investment in innovation, particularly in solar and wind.

Key Terms

Biodiesel

Biomass

Carbon sequestration

Corporate average fuel economy (CAFÉ)
  standard

Energy efficiency

Geothermal energy

Global climate change

Hydropower

Integrated fast reactors (IFR)

Integrated gasification combined cycle
  (IGCC)

Jatropha

Liquid-Fluoride Thorium Reactor (LFTR)

Natural gas

Nuclear fusion

Price-Anderson Nuclear Industries
  Indemnity Act

Discussion Questions

1. What are some of the ways in which energy efficiency can be improved?
2. What are some of the environmental effects of oil extraction, distribution, and use?
3. In what ways is natural gas a more efficient energy source than other sources?
4. What are some of the health hazards associated with coal mining?
5. What is a major complaint about using wind energy?
6. What are the causes of hut lung?
7. What are some economic problems with expanding the use of solar energy?

CHAPTER 12

CLIMATE CHANGE POLICY OPTIONS

LEARNING OBJECTIVES

- Become familiar with international efforts to combat global warming
- Understand the role of state and local governments in addressing climate change
- Comprehend the interactions among the different branches of the federal government in addressing climate change
- Understand what needs to be done to escape the harmful effects of global warming
- Become familiar with the current efforts to establish climate change legislation

To achieve a "cap and trade" national program to control CO_2 emissions we will need a consensus of public opinion.[1] A **cap and trade** program is government driven, with a maximal limit on greenhouse gas (GHG) emissions that progressively decline over time. In order to meet these limits, sources of pollution that are regulated need to have permits authorizing limits on their GHG pollution. Since these permit amounts decline over time, the polluter needs to plan to meet reduced GHG emissions, for example, closing an older plant, building in pollution controls, and so on. The mandate allows the polluter to choose the controls and technologies harnessing the private market system.

Public opinion in favor of carbon controls is helpful for congressional action, although executive regulatory action can take place according to an administration's goals. In this regard, the administration of President Barack Obama has signaled that it prefers congressional action to control GHG and pursue renewable energy strategies but in absence of congressional action will permit the Environmental Protection Agency (EPA) to move forward with regulatory actions to control CO_2.

In 2007, the *National Journal* released its Congressional Insider's Poll that asked the following question:

> Do you think it's been proven beyond a reasonable doubt that the Earth is warming because of man-made problems?
>
> - 95% of Democrats responded Yes or scientific consensus; Republicans said Yes 13% with 84% No.
> - 88% of Democrats supported mandatory limits on CO_2 emissions; Republicans were at 19%.
> - 83% of Democrats supported cap and trade; 42% Republicans did.
> - Democrats 83% to Republicans 45% on higher fuel efficiency standards for automobiles.
> - Democrats 95% to Republicans 71% increased spending on alternative fuels.

Since this poll in 2007, the two parties have diverged further on environmental regulation.

A Gallop Poll in 2007 of 1,009 adults asked the following questions:

> [Are] the "Greenhouse effect" or global warming among your concerns?
>
> - Great deal 41%,
> - Fair amount 24%

○ Only a little 18%
○ Not at all 16%

Thinking about what is said in the news, in your view, what is the seriousness of global warming?

○ Generally exaggerated 33%
○ Generally correct 29%
○ Generally underestimated 35%

From what you have heard or read, do you believe increases in the Earth's temperature over the last century are due more to the effects of pollution from human activities or natural changes in the environment that are not due to human activities?

○ Human activities 61%
○ Natural causes 35%,
○ No opinion 5%

Vice President Al Gore contributed to public awareness by turning his book *An Inconvenient Truth* into a movie that won Oscars in 2007 for Best Documentary and Best Song for his theme, "I Need to Wake Up." In addition, he gave testimony to a combined House Energy and Commerce Committee and Senate Environment and Public Works Committee stating that we needed to freeze CO_2 emissions, use the tax code to help renewables and tax polluters, provide help to low-income groups on energy, be part of a strong global treaty on climate change; he also called for a moratorium on new coal power plants that do not have CO_2 sequestration.

American public opinion expresses substantial doubt about the anthropogenic cause and the level of scientific agreement underpinning anthropogenic climate change. In June 2010, Anderegg and colleagues published in the *Proceedings of the National Academy of Sciences* an extensive dataset of 1,372 climate researchers and their publications and citation data showing that 97%–98% of the climate researchers most active in publishing in climate science support the tenets of anthropogenic climate change outlined by the Intergovernmental Panel on Climate Change, and the relative scientific prominence and expertise of climate deniers were substantially below that of the convinced researchers.[2] Polls suggest that about 70% of the American public generally trust scientists' opinion on the environment. The disinformation campaign experienced by the public is multifactorial, financed by some in the fossil fuels industry through "think tanks," political action committees, and support of media who provide equal time as "balanced" for those scientists unconvinced by the scientific evidence as those who are convinced.

International Efforts to Prevent Climate Change

Kyoto Climate Treaty

At the 1992 Earth Summit in Rio de Janeiro, the United States and 170 nations agreed on reducing greenhouse gases to 1990 levels by 2000. This was one of the first efforts at international consensus to consider the global effects of greenhouse gases. President George H. W. Bush attended the meeting.

The Kyoto Protocol was negotiated in 1997 with U.S. Vice President Al Gore in attendance; he was able to move negotiators and achieve a consensus treaty. Three disagreements were the binding amount of greenhouse gas reductions and the gases involved, whether developing countries should be included in the requirements for GHG reductions, and whether to include emissions trading and joint implementation (which allows credit to be given for emissions reductions to a country that provides funding or investments in countries that bring about the actual reductions). The Kyoto Protocol to the United Nations Framework Convention on Climate Change was signed on December 11, 1997. The goal for the United States was to lower CO_2 by 7% below 1990 levels by the period 2008–2012. Canada, Japan, and Poland agreed to 6%, and the European Union had an 8% reduction. Thirty-eight nations had reductions (average 5.2%), and developing nations only had to set voluntary limits.[3]

The goal of the Kyoto Protocol was to enhance energy efficiency, protect GHG sinks and afforestation, promote sustainable forms of agriculture, promote research on renewable forms of energy and CO_2 sequestration, phase out subsidies for GHG-emitting sectors, encourage reforms to reduce emissions of GHG, and limit CH_4 emissions in waste management. Databanks were to be established to determine carbon stocks in 1990 and data to include forestry and agriculture to establish sinks (sinks absorb CO_2). Annual reports of progress were required, with total CO_2 emissions calculated.

Eighty-two countries signed the protocol, including the United States; 142 countries' legislatures ratified it by February 16, 2005, the date that the **Kyoto Climate Treaty** went into effect. As of 2009, 187 parties have ratified the protocol (exception: the United States). The countries committing to targets in 2005 accounted for 64% of 1990 emissions.[4] The Byrd-Hagel Resolution in the U.S. Senate, approved by ninety-five senators, mandated that developing countries had to be included before the United States would sign the treaty. The Kyoto Protocol has not been submitted to the Senate for ratification because it would not muster the two-thirds majority in order to pass.

China, India, Brazil, and other developing countries already emit half of the GHG emissions and are not subject to Kyoto reductions since they are considered developing countries. A multi-gas strategy could greatly reduce the costs of fulfilling the Kyoto Protocol compared to a CO_2–only strategy, making it more palatable to conservative U.S. senators.[5] Including sinks and abatement opportunities for gases other than CO_2 could reduce the cost of meeting Kyoto requirements by 60%. The only other Western country to not sign the treaty was Australia, but that country had a change of government and immediately signed it, leaving the United States alone. The United States would have to reduce carbon emissions by 550 million tons below the reference value with allowance for reforestation accounting for only 9% of this.[4,5]

The European Union and Climate Change

The European Union (EU) started a mandatory emissions trading system in 2005. Carbon-hungry companies could buy credits from companies that had emissions to spare. The clean development mechanism (CDM) gave credits to developed countries to help poor countries by funding alternative energy or reforestation. There were 4,000 CDM projects in place or planned that could save 2.2 billion tons of CO_2 by 2012; this could amount to 7 times the total CO_2 that the EU needs to save by 2012. In addition to CDM, there is the joint implementation mechanism that covers green projects in industrialized countries in Central and Eastern Europe. Developing-country cities will have considerable lack of equity in environmental health as they face large in-migrations from poor rural areas that suffer from drought and severe weather events, coastal location with exposure to rising sea levels, exposure to the urban heat island effect, high levels of indoor and outdoor pollution, high population density, and poor sanitation.[6] Laggards were Japan (CO_2 grew 8% and needs to cut 14% by 2012) and Canada (CO_2 grew 25% with a conservative pro-oil government and needs to cut 40%). Canada is the first to admit that it will fail to meet the 2012 target. Ukraine and Russia had carbon credits to sell. Countries missing their targets would be suspended from carbon trading and must make up the shortfall plus a 30% penalty in the second commitment period after 2012. Negotiations to build a post–Kyoto Treaty began in earnest in Copenhagen in 2009. Kyoto's structural elements like carbon markets and compliance mechanisms, as well as the CDM Adaptation Fund, have no expiry date.

Copenhagen COP15

Copenhagen was the fifteenth Conference of Parties to the UN Framework Convention on Climate Change in 2009. One hundred and ninety-five parties met to negotiate a new climate treaty. Kyoto enters its second phase in 2013, with two-thirds of the major emissions sources—United States, China, India, and Brazil—not covered, providing a need to act with dispatch. Key issues became more acute as the world entered into a deep recession in 2008. Major industrialized nations were pressed to reduce emissions; China, India, and Brazil were to rein in their emissions; and the group of seventy-seven developing nations bargained for funding to alleviate their climate crisis. The Group of 77 requested a 40% cut in emissions by major industrialized nations, using 1990 as a baseline, to limit global warming to a 1.5°C rise, but the European Union pledged only 20% with a possibility of 30%, and the United States offered only 3%–4%. The United States was constrained by legislative language committing a 17% reduction by 2020 from a 2005 baseline and 80% by 2050 from the Waxman-Markey bill (see later in chapter). The commitment to the poorer nations was only $10 billion a year for three years; this was increased by Secretary of State Hillary Clinton to $100 billion per year for adjustments to the impact of global warming and to develop green energy, coming from both private and public sources, beginning in 2020, given that meaningful reductions in emissions committed to could be measured, reported, and verified (MRV) in a transparent manner.

Developing countries insisted they must deal with immediate poverty reductions and social issues and should be assisted with mitigation actions, as they did not cause climate change and have fewer resources to deal with it. A program in Reducing Emissions from Deforestation and Degradation (REDD) could gain carbon credits for reduced deforestation. The Least Developed Countries and Association of Small Island Developing States wanted urgent action and boycotted the discussions for several days, losing critical time, whereas oil-producing states preferred to stall negotiations and seek less ambitious actions. The issues surrounding measurements and verification of cuts and the legal binding framework proved the most difficult, especially to China.

President Barack Obama and Secretaries Clinton, Steven Chu, Alphonso Jackson, Tom Vilsak, Ken Salazar, and many other U.S. dignitaries as well as other countries' leaders attended the final days of the meeting. President Obama in his opening remarks emphasized mitigation, transparency, and financing as the clear formula for agreement. Secretary Chu described Climate REDI, a $350 million fund that will quick-start technology to reduce emissions by accelerating solar home systems, assisting with high-efficiency appliances and LED (light-emitting diode) lanterns in low-income countries. Individual commitments came from China to reduce carbon intensity 45% going forward; Brazil pledged an 80% cut in its emissions from deforestation; India offered to cut its carbon intensity emissions 25%. By 2020 China's emissions will have grown to be 40% larger than America's. In the final moments of Copenhagen, President Obama negotiated a political agreement with China, Brazil, India, and South Africa to pursue their individual goals to abet climate change. This was not a binding international agreement with specific near-term and long-term targets that the delegates had envisioned. It did provide for a system for monitoring and reporting progress toward national pollution reduction goals, and it called for hundreds of billions of dollars to flow from wealthy nations to those most vulnerable to a changing climate. It set a goal of limiting the global temperature rise to 2°C by 2050. President Obama called this only a tentative start down a long road; many of the delegates were terribly disappointed in such a meager outcome. Since the accord does not go into effect until 2015, this first step would be further negotiated in Cancun in November 2010. In Cancun, the parties mostly agreed on targets for protecting forests and to continue pursuing renewable and clean energy paths.

State, City, and Private Actions on Global Warming

State and Regional Actions

Since the George W. Bush administration recommended a voluntary program to reduce CO_2 emissions by 18% by 2012, there was an opportunity for state and local governments to act on reducing GHG emissions. This vacuum of leadership at the federal level was filled by the states, cities, and regional governmental approaches.

Eleven states (including New York, New Jersey, and Connecticut) enacted regulations on CO_2 from cars. These states represent 30% of the auto market. In 2002 California passed AB 1493, mandating a 30% reduction in CO_2 emissions by new automobiles sold after 2009 to be achieved by 2016. Auto industry executives state that this was a back-door CAFÉ standard and sued California, since CAFÉ is part of the National Energy and Conservation Act under which California has no special status. EPA ruled against California on December 20, 1997, refusing to allow California the right to regulate CO_2 and stating that this required a national solution; this was overruled by the Obama administration.

Eighteen states have adopted requirements that 10%–20% of electricity come from renewables. They defined renewables as wind, solar, biomass, hydroelectric, and geothermal. California and Minnesota required 25% by 2020. The California Global Warming Solutions Act (AB 32) caps CO_2 for all major industries, requires achievement of a 25% reduction in GHG emissions by 2020, and has penalties for noncompliance. Governor Bill Richardson signed a New Mexico executive order to reduce CO_2 10% below 2000 levels by 2020 and 75% by 2050. California's governor Arnold Schwarzenegger signed executive orders pledging to reach 2000 GHG levels by 2010, 1990 levels by 2020, and 80% below 1990 by 2050. California's 35 million people produce 13% of the U.S. gross domestic product. California policies and regulations tend to lead the nation, since manufacturers prefer to make one product for the national market rather than target one state.

States have not only worked individually to combat global warming, but there have also been regional initiatives from groups of states to promote GHG ideas. The northeastern states have a Regional Greenhouse Gas Initiative (RGGI) pledging to reach 10% below 1990 levels by 2020. These states release 10.7% of U.S. emissions and include Connecticut, Maine, Massachusetts, New Hampshire, Delaware, Rhode Island, Vermont, New Jersey (left RGGI in 2011), Maryland, and New York. This Regional Greenhouse Gas Initiative allows the purchase of offset credits from projects certified by the Kyoto clean development mechanism. The Western Regional Climate Action Initiative includes governors from California, Arizona, Washington, New Mexico, and Oregon who have agreed on their own cap and trade program. Each state will set its own caps. They release 11.2% of CO_2 emissions. Governor Schwarzenegger remarked that this agreement showed the power of states to lead our nation in addressing climate change. The problem of regional initiatives on climate change is a lack of mechanisms for enforcing such small-scale programs.

City Actions

The U.S. mayors have developed their own climate protection agreements. In 2005 the U.S. Conference of Mayors voted unanimously in favor of the Climate Protection Agreement that matches the Kyoto Protocol's goal of reducing global warming pollution by 7% below 1990 levels by 2020. The conference represents 1,183 cities from all fifty states. As of July 2011, 1,049 cities have signed the agreement. Prior to the 2008 primary in New Hampshire, 140 towns had passed global warming resolutions, sending a clear message to Congress and the White House that immediate action was needed to curb global warming pollution. Most U.S. cities have initiatives to encourage alternative fuels in their fleets and policies to make buildings more energy efficient. On October 29, 2007, it was reported that Seattle met its target reduction in CO_2 in 2005, reducing its greenhouse gas emissions by 8% since 1990. Cities are energy gluttons; they account for three-fourths of greenhouse gas emissions the world over, and buildings are responsible for 40% of emissions. At the 2007 G-8 Summit, fifteen cities signed on to a $5 billion program to make older buildings more energy efficient. Other programs include congestion charging in London and distributing rooftop rain barrels in Chicago that pipe 55 million gallons of rainwater into Lake Michigan every year.

Private Actions

Businesses have also taken the lead in green initiatives. The U.S. Green Building Council is a coalition of industry officials that rates new buildings based on site development, water savings, energy efficiency, construction materials, and design and indoor environmental quality. The **Leadership in Energy and Environmental Design (LEED)** Green Building Rating System encourages and accelerates global adoption of sustainable green building development practices through the creation and implementation of universally understood and accepted tools and performance criteria. LEED is a third-party certification program and the nationally accepted benchmark for the design, construction, and operation of high-performance green buildings. LEED projects are in progress in forty-one countries, including Canada, Brazil, Mexico, and India.

Private partnerships with nonprofit entities can influence power company decisions. TXU Energy in Texas planned eleven pulverized coal power plants but was purchased by a New York investment firm and Pacific Group, with a former EPA administrator (William K. Reilly) on the board, who contacted the Natural Resources Defense Council (NRDC) and Environmental Defense to negotiate a $400 million renewable energy investment and build only three coal-fired power plants with advanced technology. Several banks, including Citigroup and Bank of America, have pledged to tie GHG emissions to its loan review process for power plants and other GHG polluters.

The Pew Center for Climate Change formed the U.S. Climate Action Partnership with several U.S. and global industrial giants and nonprofits: Alcoa, BP, Caterpillar, Duke Energy, DuPont, FPL Group, General Electric, PG&E Corporation, PNM Resources, Environmental Defense, Natural Resources Defense Council, and World Resources Institute. Forty-two companies have joined Pew's Business Environmental Leadership Council. The U.S. Climate Action Partnership recommends enactment of national legislation in the United States to slow, stop, and reverse the growth of GHG emissions over the shortest period of time reasonably achievable. These corporations believe that climate change will create economic opportunities that will require innovation and efficiency and create new markets. Their environmental goals were an economy-wide, market-driven approach that includes a cap and trade program that places specified limits on GHG emissions. They urged that the U.S. climate protection program should create:

- A domestic market that will establish a uniform price for GHG emissions for all sectors and promote the creation of a global market
- A national emissions baseline

- A federal technology research and development program with demonstration and development projects with joint public/private cost sharing and oversight
- A roadmap to guide research and development with stable, long-term financing
- An international engagement and linkage post–2012 for a global framework for international GHG markets
- Assistance for vulnerable populations and support for climate-friendly technology in developing countries

U.S. Judiciary Branch and Climate Change

The EPA, Greenhouse Gases, and the Supreme Court

Since the EPA refused to regulate CO_2 as a primary pollutant under the Clean Air Act (CAA) under the Bush administration, aggrieved parties became involved in legal action. Aggrieved parties need to have legal standing in order to sue; for example, a private citizen probably cannot say he or she represents the public interest, but an individual may join a nonprofit environmental organization that then may have standing in order to sue, or a state's attorney general may sue on the behalf of a state that is an aggrieved party for a U.S. governmental decision regarding federal legislation and its enforcement. In 1998 the EPA's general counsel ruled that CO_2 and other GHGs were air pollutants under the CAA, and in 2003, under the Bush administration, EPA reversed itself and has since steadfastly denied it has such authority. The State of Massachusetts sued the EPA, stating that it had misinterpreted the CAA and that CO_2 indeed was a primary pollutant and that EPA had authority to regulate CO_2. Massachusetts stated that it had "standing" to bring the lawsuit because it was at risk from rising ocean levels in Boston Harbor and Cape Cod and increasing storm damage and flooding along its northern coast (*Massachusetts et al. v. Environmental Protection Agency*).

Amicae curiae (friend of the court) briefs were joined by the states of California, Connecticut, District of Columbia, Illinois, Maine, New Jersey, New Mexico, New York, Oregon, Rhode Island, Vermont, and Washington, and Samoa. Cities include New York and Baltimore. Others groups were the Center for Biological Diversity, Center for Food Safety, Conservation Law Foundation, Natural Resources Defense Council, International Center for Technological Assessment; four previous EPA administrators; Aspen Skiing Company, Environmental Defense, Friends of the Earth, Greenpeace, National Environmental Trust, National Wildlife Federation, Sierra Club, USPIRG (U.S. Public Interest

Research Groups), Union of Concerned Scientists; and scientists James Hansen and Sherwood Rowland.

Madeleine Albright, former U.S. Secretary of State, argued against the EPA statement that if United States reduces CO_2 it has no bargaining chip of reducing emissions of foreign countries. The CAA defines a pollutant as "any air pollution agent . . . including any physical, chemical, biological, radioactive substance or matter which is emitted into or otherwise enters into the ambient air." The U.S. Supreme Court agreed with the plaintiffs in a 5–4 decision April 2, 2007; Justice John Paul Stevens, in writing for the majority (Anthony Kennedy, David Souter, Ruth Bader Ginsburg, and Stephen Breyer), stated that the petitioners had standing because Massachusetts owned a great deal of the territory alleged to be affected, that EPA's failure to dispute the existence of a causal connection between human-made GHG emissions and global warming and its refusal to regulate such emissions contributed to Massachusetts's injuries, and because EPA's argument that it would be unwise to regulate GHG at this time rested on reasoning divorced from the statutory text. While the statute conditions EPA action on its formation of a "judgment," that judgment must relate to whether an air pollutant causes or contributes to air pollution that may reasonably be anticipated to endanger public health or welfare. Under the act's clear terms, EPA can avoid promulgating regulations only if it determines that GHG do not contribute to climate change.

California's Automobile Regulation

California's Air Resources Board proposed a regulation for CO_2 emissions from cars and trucks by cutting CO_2 emissions 30% by 2016. This regulation was submitted to the EPA for a waiver under the Clean Air Act. Carmakers stated that only EPA had authority to regulate CO_2 and California had been granted no exception. California traditionally receives waivers to apply more stringent regulations to achieve compliance of the CAA and requested so in 2005, but this was denied for GHG emissions by the EPA in 2008. This was reversed by President Obama's EPA in June 2009, with Governor Schwarzenegger stating this would spur his state's emerging green economy, create new jobs, and bring Californians the cars they want while reducing GHG emissions. EPA determined that there were unique air pollution problems in California and that the waiver opponents did not adequately demonstrate that California no longer needed its motor vehicle emission program, or that the impacts from global climate change in California were not compelling or extraordinary. EPA also found that California had a rational basis for its GHG emission standards considering the absence of applicable federal standards. Thus, California's standards were not arbitrary and capricious. California and thirteen other states agreed with carmakers that meeting President Obama's CAFÉ standard for 2012–2016 of 35.5 miles per gallon announced in 2009 would meet their GHG regulation.

Global Warming and the Endangered Species Act

Another case is the *Center for Biological Diversity, the National Defense Resources Council, and Others v. Dirk Kempthorne,* former Secretary of Interior, in which the plaintiffs are suing under the Endangered Species Act, alleging that the government must limit threats from CO_2 emissions to species such as polar bears and corals. This case was settled in the summer of 2006 when the United States agreed to evaluate the status of polar bears. The U.S. Fish and Wildlife Service after nine months and a ninety-day comment period agreed to list polar bears as "threatened." However, the U.S. Interior Department then issued a rule that the Endangered Species Act could not be used to regulate CO_2 through the back door as in this lawsuit.

Private Companies and CO_2 Emissions

In September 2009, the New York Second Circuit Court of Appeals ruled that power companies could be sued by states and land trusts for emitting CO_2 (*American Electric Power et al. v. Connecticut et al.*). In 2004 six states (Connecticut, New York, California, Iowa, Rhode Island, and Vermont) and three land trusts (Open Space Institute, Open Space Conservancy, and Audubon Society of New Hampshire) had sued American Electric Power, Southern Corporation, TVA, Xcel, and Cinergy Corporation for creating a "public nuisance" by emitting CO_2 and damaging their environments and properties. They emit 650 million tons of CO_2 per year, about 10% of the U.S. total. The U.S. district court ruled that this was a political case for the executive or legislative branch and dismissed the case; the Second U.S. Circuit Court reinstated the case, stating that the plaintiffs had standing and that a public nuisance could be regulated under the Clean Air Act under the interstate commerce clause of the constitution. The U.S. Superme Court ruled on June 20, 2011, by a vote of 8-0, that the Clean Air Act and the EPA's implemention of the act displace any federal common-law right to seek abatement of carbon dioxide emissions from fossil fuel–fired power plants.

U.S. Executive Branch and Climate Change

The Climate Change Science Program

The United States **Climate Change Science Program (CCSP)** coordinates climate change research among thirteen federal agencies. The 2002 reorganization was to tackle a wider array of research activities than the prior decade under the U.S. Global Change Research Program. The CCSP's explicit goal was to connect research on climate change and the development of technologies to address it. However, the budget had a significant shortfall in supporting all of the activities in the strategic plan. The effects of climate change on ecosystems and humans was particularly underfunded. The CCSP had a plan to provide synthesis and assessment reports that needed to provide information for state and regional decision makers about rising coastal sea levels, droughts, and decisions about policies to reduce GHGs. The CCSP needed independent oversight so that political influence would not discredit the program. Moreover, stakeholders needed input on scientific reports.

The CCSP operates in ten-year time frames and integrates well with the National Research Council of the National Academy of Sciences. CCSP coordinates an extensive Earth monitoring program, including thirty orbiting satellites with more than 120 major instruments, ocean buoys, and land stations, and NASA aircraft. To establish a more permanent system, the U.S. government is building the National Polar-Orbiting Operational Environmental Satellite System, which will include weather, climate, and space weather sensors on four bus-sized satellites.

Changes under the Obama Administration

President Obama named Carol Browner, EPA administrator under President Bill Clinton, as a climate change czar to coordinate climate change approaches in the White House with his economic team, congressional legislation, EPA approaches, international negotiations, and climate change science. Additionally, the Obama EPA has announced that it will promulgate rules (**GHG Reporting Rule**) for reporting greenhouse gases for entities that release >25,000 tons per year, which are responsible for nearly 70% of greenhouse gas emissions in the United States. The EPA found CO_2 pollution to endanger public health and welfare (so-called endangerment finding under the NAAQS). Also starting in 2011 the EPA has announced that it intends to regulate CO_2 emissions under the Clean Air Act. Different political parties use the executive agencies to promulgate policy in diametrically opposed directions. The leaders of the executive agencies are political appointees who carry out policies of elected officials, and the staffs of civil servants carry them out under either political party. Following the Republican victories in the 2010 midterm elections and capture of the majority in the House, several bills were introduced abrogating EPA regulation of GHG. The 2011 budget eliminated the climate change czar position, but President Obama, in signing language accompanying his signature to the bill, stated that he was committed to executive leadership in coordinating policy among federal agencies with jurisdiction over climate change, that is, he would continue with a czar position as necessary.

Congress: The Climate Stewardship Act of 2003 Through the Climate Security Acts of 2008 and 2009

Climate Stewardship Act

Affected industries and environmentalists preferred congressional action on a climate and energy bill. This would provide legislative and regulatory certainty to electrical utilities and industries planning long-term investments. However, there are constraints and local political considerations that constrict the ability to move forward; for example, coal-mining states and states that contain many coal-fired power plants do not want to harm those industries; Republicans do not wish to add costs to business or taxes; oil- and gas-producing states do not wish to harm their fossil fuel industries; subsidies to industries are frowned upon in a period of deficit spending; Midwestern interests wish to promote ethanol from corn; Republicans prefer nuclear technologies, whereas Democrats prefer renewables; oil exploration is opposed in wilderness study areas and the Arctic National Wildlife Refuge by Democrats, whereas oil exploration in these areas and off the continental shelf is generally encouraged by Republicans ("Drill, Baby, Drill").

The first bill to be debated on the Senate floor was the 108th Congress's S. 139 **Climate Stewardship Act of 2003**, better known as the McCain-Lieberman bill. Cosponsors were Senators Dick Durbin (D-IL), Daniel Akaka (D-HI), Dianne Feinstein (D-CA), Olympia Snowe (R-ME), Patty Murray (D-WA), Frank Lautenberg (D-NJ), and Bill Nelson (D-FL).

Title I covered Federal Climate Change Research. This title would provide National Science Foundation scholarships to study climate change under mentorship. The secretary of commerce would direct technology transfer from federal laboratories to private entrepreneurs. There was to be a report on the impact of signing the Kyoto Protocol on U.S. industry. There would be support for international cooperation on scientific research and environmental climate change mitigation. The National Science Foundation would have a research program on climate change, especially abrupt change. The National Institute of Standards would provide GHG measurements.

Title II provided for a National GHG Database and Registry. Secretaries of commerce, energy, and agriculture would be charged to set up the database. The EPA administrator would collect GHG emissions for covered utilities. Title III would provide for market-driven GHG reductions. The EPA was designated the lead agency.

By 2010 each entity in electrical, industrial, commercial, and petroleum would submit one tradable allowance for every ton of GHG to the EPA. Transport was separate but could sell credits if average miles per gallon exceeded CAFÉ standards by 20%. A Climate Change Credit Corporation would be established as a nonprofit corporation without stock. EPA would establish tradable allowances for 5,896 million tons of CO_2 reduced by the amount of GHG in 2000 for the years 2009–2016. The reductions would be implemented in two phases, with an emissions cap in the year 2010 based on affected facilities' 2000 emissions (for any entity that emits more than 10,000 metric tons of GHG) and a further reduction cap imposed in the year 2016, based on affected facilities' 1990 emissions.

By year 2010, S. 139 would reduce GHG by 5% relative to business as usual but still 27.7% above 1990 levels, although Phase 2 would involve a reduction down to 1990 levels. In 2015 there would be 5,123 million tons minus the 1990 amount. This was the only climate bill to reach the floor of the U.S. Senate and to be debated in the autumn of 2003; forty-four senators voted for it. This was an encouraging beginning, and most observers thought that the momentum had swung in the direction of passage in the next year's Congress. Most bills take several years and several dozen drafts before consensus is reached and a bill passes both houses of Congress and a conference committee reconciling differences between the two houses.

The Sanders-Boxer Bill, the New McCain-Lieberman Bill, and the Kerry-Snowe-Kennedy Bills, 2009

In the 109th Congress there were a host of cap and trade bills introduced into Congress. They followed the format design of the original McCain-Lieberman bill in that there were titles for federal research, a GHG database, and a cap-and-trade mechanism for CO_2 usually using the EPA as the lead agency. The Sanders-Boxer bill, the New McCain-Lieberman bill, and the Bingaman bill focused on 2020 as a goal to reduce CO_2 emissions to 1990 levels or, in the case of Bingaman, to limit growth. By 2050 only Sanders-Boxer reduced emissions ~80% below 1990 levels in order to achieve stabilization of GHG at 450 ppm. The Sanders-Boxer bill required EPA to establish a competitive grant program for CO_2 sequestration and carry out a global climate change standards and processes research program. The bill stated that the sense of the Senate would encourage funds to be appropriated for clean, low-carbon energy research and deployment and that this should be doubled each year for ten years.

The Sanders-Boxer Bill, S. 309 Global Warming Pollution Reduction Act, directed the EPA to promulgate requirements concerning electric efficiency and to establish a renewable energy credit program; the secretary of agriculture to establish standards for accrediting certified reductions in CO_2 through biological sequestration activities; EPA to receive reports on GHG emissions from major stationary sources; EPA to establish market-based programs to achieve GHG milestones reduction; require each fleet of automobiles sold by a manufacturer beginning in 2016 to meet emission standards; require that electric generation units meet an emission standard that is not higher than the emission rate of a new combined cycle natural gas generating unit; establish a low-carbon generation trading program; and require covered generators to provide a minimum percent of electricity produced for sale from low-carbon generation.

The S. 280 Lieberman-McCain Climate Stewardship and Innovation Act differed in its establishment of a climate change credit corporation through which EPA would determine the allocation of the number of tradable allowances for each sector. A climate technology financing board would develop joint venture partnerships in reducing GHG, with loans for up to three integrated gasification combined cycle (IGCCs) with sequestration, three advanced nuclear reactors, three biofuels plants using cellulosic biomass, and three concentrated solar facilities.

The S. 485 Kerry-Snowe-Kennedy Global Warming Reduction Act of 2007 would amend the Clean Air Act to establish an economy-wide global warming pollution emission cap and trade program to assist the economy in transitioning to new clean energy technologies and to protect companies and consumers from significant increases in energy costs. The EPA administrator was to promulgate regulations to achieve 1990 CO_2 levels by 2020, by 2030 another 25%, and between 2030 and 2050 3.5% CO_2 reductions per year. There would be market-based caps that would then allow trading.

Compromising on Policy Related to Climate Change

As chair of the Environment and Public Works Committee, Sen. Barbara Boxer (D-CA) decided on a compromise bill that would have the greatest chance of bipartisan support from the whole Senate. To achieve this support, she engaged Sen. John Warner (R-VA), a widely respected conservative senator, to join with Sen. Joe Lieberman (I-CT) on a compromise bill to obtain Republican support but not lose any Democrats. What emerged was the Lieberman-Warner **Climate Security Act** of 2007 S. 2191. It was cosponsored by Senators Tom Harkin D-IA, Norm Coleman R-MN, Elizabeth Dole (R-NC), Susan Collins (R-ME), Ben Cardin (D-MD), Amy Klobuchar (D-MN), Charles Schumer

(D-NY), Ron Wyden (D-OR), and Robert Casey (D-PA). It defined GHG as six gases: CO_2, CH_4, N_2O, SF_6, HFC, and perfluorocarbon. It directed the EPA administrator to develop a GHG Registry with quarterly reports by facilities (10,000 CO_2 equivalents) and develop an electronic format and consistent policies for calculating carbon content and GHG emissions. An emission allowance account was specified for CO_2: 2012, 5,200 million tons; 2015, 4,912; 2020, 4,432; 2025, 3,952; 2050, 1,560 million tons. The electric utility, transportation, and manufacturing sectors would reduce 15% of CO_2 below 2005 levels by 2020 and 70% by 2050. These are 80% of U.S. GHG emissions. Each facility would submit to EPA an emission allowance. They would have to reduce emissions as a condition of obtaining an operating permit. There would be deductions of allowances in the future if there are excess emissions and assessments for new projects. There would be a Carbon Market Efficiency Board with seven members with oversight functions. There would be a bonus allowance of 5% for CO_2 sequestration projects, forestry projects, GHG sequestration in agriculture, and a 3% allowance for foreign forest projects. There would be an emissions allowance set aside each year for new-entrant covered electric power sector facilities and new-entrant covered industrial sector facilities.

Furthermore, there would be a climate change credit corporation that would auction the carbon credits and auction up to the emission allowance. There would be an energy assistance fund for low-income persons (20% of auction proceeds) and a climate change worker-training fund (5% of auction proceeds). The Department of Interior's Fish and Wildlife Service would get an adaptation fund (20% of auction proceeds). Most of the proceeds (55%) would go to energy technology deployment: 45% for low carbon technologies, 28% for advanced coal and sequestration technologies, 7% for cellulose biomass ethanol, and 20% for advanced technology vehicles.

Additionally, there would be an Interagency Climate Change and National Security Council made up of Departments of State and Defense, EPA and National Intelligence that would report on how other countries are reducing GHG and potentials for conflicts. Energy efficiency would be addressed with residential boilers, regional standards for space heating and air conditioning products, and building energy codes. There would be a global effort to reduce GHG where State and EPA would carry out a U.S./UN Framework Convention on Climate Change to establish binding agreements committing all major GHG emitting nations to contribute equitably to the reduction of GHG emissions. It would amend the Safe Drinking Water Act to require the administrator to permit commercial-scale underground injection of CO_2 for purposes of geological sequestration. There would be a National Academy of Sciences review every three years that would report on the extent emission reductions are being achieved, the contributions from other countries, the predicted amount of warming, the predicted changes in ocean's rise, the status of science to avoid GHG emissions, the auction's effectiveness, and the impact on low- and moderate-income individuals. The EPA would report on transportation-related programs. The secretary of energy would study CO_2 sequestration facilities and pipelines for CO_2 transport. It directed the EPA administrator to establish a task force to study the cost implications of potential federal assumption of liability with respect to closed geological storage sites. It authorized the president to waive the act's requirements in a national security emergency. Last, it required the Securities and Exchange Commission to direct securities issuers to inform investors of material risks related to climate change.

S. 2191 would achieve substantial reductions in U.S. GHG reductions over a nearly forty-year period beginning in 2012 and culminating in 2050, with reductions in total U.S. GHG emissions below 2005 levels of as much as 66%. (See Figure 12.1.) Considerable funding streams were added to help states and industries to adjust to a low-carbon future; an $800 billion tax relief fund through 2050 would help consumers in need of assistance related to energy costs. The Natural Resources Defense Council and World Resources Institute estimated that the bill would reduce emission levels by up to 13% below 1990 levels by 2020 and up to 60% below 1990 levels by 2050. In addition, S. 2191 would raise substantial resources from the industries responsible for GHG emissions, including electric

FIGURE 12.1 Lieberman-Warner Climate Security Act allows dangerously high levels of greenhouse gas emission

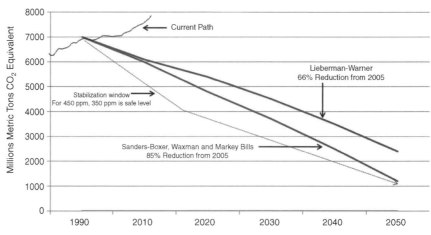

Source: Center for Biological Diversity.

utilities and other businesses, and recycle those resources, largely to the private sector in order to (1) spur the rapid development and commercialization of clean energy, energy conserving, and other GHG emission-reducing technologies that will trigger substantial growth in domestic green collar jobs; (2) assist communities, individuals, and companies that could be affected by the costs of transitioning to lower GHG-emitting energy sources; and, (3) support efforts to protect people and ecosystems from the effects of rapid climate change.

A key feature of the GHG reduction program is its cap and trade architecture. Through cap and trade, S. 2191 would assure that the intended reductions in GHG emissions were actually achieved. At the same time, the program would enable GHG sources to engage in emissions trading; this would afford full flexibility for businesses operating under the program and create a dynamic market for GHG emissions reductions. Coupled with the Climate Security Act's comprehensive GHG emissions reduction program is a similarly comprehensive program for fostering the development and commercialization of new, clean technologies, with a particular focus on the electricity and transportation sectors. The act establishes an Energy Technology Deployment Program as well as an Energy Transformation Acceleration Fund, which would be administered by the Advanced Research Projects Agency of the Department of Energy. These funds would operate through financial incentives to speed the development and commercialization of sustainable energy technologies, low-carbon electricity technologies, advanced biofuels, like cellulosic ethanol, CO_2 capture and storage systems, electric and plug-in hybrid electric vehicles and high-efficiency consumer products.

Despite such bipartisanship in writing this bill, there still was opposition, and the bill passed the committee by an 11–9 vote with Sen. Warner the only Republican supporting it. The EPA stated that global CO_2 concentration in 2095 would be lower than 491 ppm, and S. 2191 would achieve significant global warming pollution reductions at an affordable price. The EPA analysis did not estimate the tens of thousands of clean energy jobs from the 61 gigawatts of renewable energy—equal to 120 new 500 MW power plants spurred by this bill. S. 2191 required carbon capture and sequestration; this would reduce the average annual GDP 2010–2050 by only 0.04%. EPA estimated no increase in electricity rates until 2020 and then a one-fifth increase until 2040. The cost of the CAA Acid Rain program effect on electricity rates was 8.1 cents/kwh in 1990, which declined to 7.5 cents/kwh in 1995 and to 7.6 cents/kwh in 2000, all in 2000 dollars. Industry calculated that CO_2 would cost $55 per ton in 2020 for allowances, and EPA projected the cost at $26/ton. The Congressional Budget Office estimated the costs of the act to be $90 billion each year during the 2012–2016 period. The intergovernmental mandate costs under Unfunded Mandates Reform Act estimated costs of $136 million for 2008.

The Warner-Lieberman bill was forwarded to the Senate Majority Leader Harry Reid but it couldn't muster the sixty required votes to overcome a Republican filibuster (forty-eight voted to end the filibuster) for debate and a vote on the floor. The business interests—aligned against the costs of dealing with global climate change, particularly cap and trade, asserting this was a tax—had won the day.

S. 2191 framed the full complement of executive agencies to deal with climate change in a novel legislative manner. But legislative solutions require political compromise and public support. The complexity of climate change stems from the many diverse groups from environmentalists to dozens of affected industries, each with their own agenda. Critical aspects of achieving compromise are the economics of climate change, whether a tax could achieve necessary GHG reductions, and would the indirect costs from GHG pollution rise to the point that legislative compromise could be achieved.

Economic Factors Surrounding Global Warming and Potential Solutions

The Stern Report

At about the same time Nicholas Stern, a former vice president of the World Bank, estimated the economic costs of dealing with global warming (Stern Review on the Economics of Climate Change, Oct 30, 2006). He estimated it would cost 1% of global economic activity in 2050 to cut CO_2 60%–80% below 1990 levels. The costs would be 5 to 20 times higher if we didn't act now. The worst effects of climate change could be avoided by 4% of gross domestic product (GDP), with an upper bound of 20%. Most people valued future benefits less than current costs and would invest only if the projected payoff was large enough. The **Stern Report** treated current and future generations equally. He estimated $7 trillion in costs if we didn't blunt global warming within a decade. "Our actions over the coming few decades could create risks of major disruption to economic and social activity, later in this century and in the next, on a scale similar to those associated with the great wars and the economic depression of the first half of the 20th century," he stated.

Economics of Cap and Trade

The European Union has a system of CO_2 caps on 12,000 industrial facilities.[7] The EU committed to 20% of its power to come from renewable sources by 2020 and running 10% of its cars and trucks on biofuels. The global carbon market was worth $11 billion in 2005 and climbed to $30 billion in 2006. Carbon is destined to become one of the world's biggest commodities markets, with the EU mandating power plants to purchase permits to emit CO_2 beginning in 2013. Under a plan proposed in Australia's eight states and territories, electricity companies would have to hold tradable permits to emit GHGs starting in 2010. The Edison Electric Institute, American Gas Association (AGA), and AFL-CIO back mandatory curbs on CO_2 and other GHGs. The AGA represents 200 utilities, and the Edison Electric Institute members generate 60% of electricity in the United States; their board has fifty members who are chief executive officers. The IPCC Fourth Report estimates a 60% increase in energy demand by 2030, with the energy sector responsible for two-thirds of emissions.

Economics of Global Warming Solutions

Pacala and Socolow have written about the scientific, technical, and industrial know-how to solve the carbon and climate problem for the next half-century.[8] A portfolio exists to prevent the doubling of CO_2; this portfolio was divided into seven equal wedges. Seven of the following fifteen options must be accomplished by 2050. The first category, efficiency and conservation, included four possible options for wedges:

1. Increase the fuel economy of two billion cars (four times as many as today) from 30 mpg to 60 mpg.
2. Reduce the average annual distance driven of 2 billion cars from 10,000 miles to 5,000 miles.
3. Reduce mid-century CO_2 emissions from buildings by about one-fourth
4. Increase efficiency of coal-fired power plants from 40% to 60% and still allow for a doubling of the quantity of coal-based electricity.

The second category is to decarbonize electricity and fuels:

5. Increase natural gas for power by fourfold and displace 1,400 GW of baseload coal.
6. Install carbon capture and storage (CCS) at 800 GW baseload coal plants or equivalent to 3500 Norwegian Sleipner projects.
7. Institute CO_2 capture and storage with a sixfold increase in hydrogen from coal and natural gas plants for off-site use.
8. Institute CO_2 capture and storage with synfuels equivalent to 200 South African Sasol projects.

9. Build more nuclear fission power plants at the pace of 1975–1990 for 700 GW baseload coal capacity.
10. Increase wind turbines about 50 times today's deployment, covering 3% of the area of the United States.
11. Increase photovoltaics by 700 times today's deployment.
12. Produce hydrogen for automobile fuel cells from wind turbines at about 100 times today's wind turbine deployment. Or
13. Produce 34 billion barrels of ethanol, which would be 50 times larger than today's output of Brazilian sugar cane and U.S. corn ethanol.

The third category is natural sinks:

14. Reduce tropical forest clear-cutting to zero over 50 years and reforest approximately 500–1,000 million acres of land.
15. Apply conservation tillage to all of the world's 4,000 million acres of cropland.

Each of these represents a considerable challenge, but seven need to be accomplished completely to stabilize CO_2 levels by 2050. Presidential leadership will be required to make this happen.

Prospects for Climate Change Legislation Going Forward

Waxman-Markey

On Friday June 26, 2009, the U.S. House of Representatives passed the first climate change bill, H.R. 2454, by a vote of 219–212. It was authored by Representatives Henry Waxman (D-CA), chair of the Energy and Commerce Committee, and Edward Markey (D-MA), chair of the Select Committee on Global Warming. Earlier, Henry Waxman had succeeded in defeating the former chair of the committee, John Dingell (D-MI) who lacked enthusiasm for going forward with climate change legislation, in the Democratic Caucus, and Speaker Nancy Pelosi (D-CA) had appointed Edward Markey as chair of a Select Committee on Global Warming to develop a climate change bill. Only eight Republicans voted for the bill, and forty-four Democrats voted against it. The split was so one-sided primarily because regulating GHG was seen as a tax on the fossil fuel industries.

The American Clean Energy and Security Act of 2009 (ACES) bill grew from more than 600 pages to more than 1,400 to accommodate numerous last-minute compromises. The final bill was based on cap and trade, with a goal of reducing GHG 17% below 2005 levels by 2020, and 83% by 2050 (see Figure 12.2).

FIGURE 12.2 Emission reductions under the Waxman-Markey discussion draft, 2005–2050

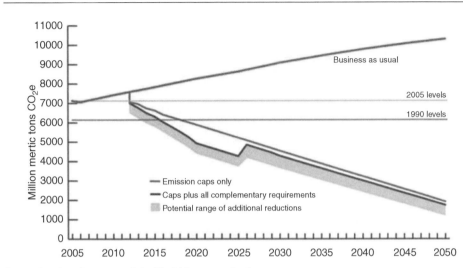

Source: Reprinted courtesy of the World Resources Institute.

The cap and trade program was scheduled to begin in 2012 with the estimated price of a permit to emit a ton of CO_2 at about $13; the price was projected to rise steadily as emission limits declined. The bill would grant a majority of the permits free in the early years of the program to keep costs low. This provision also accommodated regional differences: some states were further along on solar and wind and did not need permits, whereas others had more dependence on coal and coal-fired power plants. President Obama praised the bill but opposed a last minute provision inserted by Rust Belt State lawmakers that required the president to impose a tariff on certain goods imported from countries that did not act to limit their global warming emissions by 2020 and prohibited the EPA to regulate GHG under the Clean Air Act.

The Senate also has several committees with jurisdiction over parts of climate change legislation. First, the Energy and Natural Resources Committee approved a bill that included a nationwide renewable electricity standard, and committees covering finance, commerce, agriculture, and foreign relations plan to be involved. On September 30, 2009, Senators Boxer and John Kerry (D-MA) of the Environment and Public Works Committee introduced their 800-page bill S. 1733. It would parallel the House version but have a more ambitious 2020 target of 20% reduction in CO_2 compared to 2005. Titled the "Clean Energy Jobs and American Power Act," it proposed a pollution reduction and investment system that targeted carbon emitting businesses. These 7,500 facilities account for nearly three-fourths of U.S. carbon pollution. The sponsors of the bill hoped to change the debate from cap and trade to pollution reduction. The bill passed the EPW Committee 11–1 with all of the Republicans boycotting the final mark-up and committee vote. Thus, the future of cap and trade in the U.S. Senate was cast in doubt; however, the EPA is ready and willing to regulate the major emitters of greenhouse gases.

Summary

The 2009 Copenhagen meeting to write a new international treaty to reduce GHG emissions resulted in a disappointing failure. Yet there was agreement to limit the rise in global temperature to 2°C. How to get there with a world economy built on fossil fuel sources driving modern life will take a sea change of adaptation, lifestyle change, technology, and global cooperation.

Clearing the legislative hurdle in the U.S. Senate has proved to be a considerable challenge for climate change in the United States. Disagreements among senators persist on cap and trade or a carbon tax and their effects on industry in an economic recession. A simple carbon tax proposal by House Democrats has gained no traction. The Gulf oil spill of 2010 has further challenged lawmakers on safety considerations, the Department of Interior's regulatory role, environmental permits, design of fail-safe mechanisms on deep water drilling, clean-up authority, liability, and so on. Whether this should be included in an energy bill and whether climate change should be addressed all in one bill has not been agreed to. Further arguments can be made about executive leadership in creating a solution. President Obama has called for a green energy revolution and jobs creation in response to the oil spill. Despite this, the Energy Department is proceeding on research and demonstration on renewable energy and encouraging nuclear plant construction; the Interior Department is proceeding with regulatory reform; Senators Kerry and Lieberman continue to attempt to forge agreement among the few Republican senators willing to find a creative legislative solution; and EPA is proceeding with a regulatory framework for GHG.

Senators Maria Cantwell (D-WA) and Susan Collins (R-ME) proposed a bipartisan "cap and dividend" thirty-nine-page bill called the Carbon Limits and Energy for America's Renewal Act, or CLEAR Act. The legislation would set up a mechanism for selling "carbon shares" to the few thousand fossil fuel producers and importers through monthly auctions; 75% of the revenue would be returned to every U.S. citizen as dividend checks, averaging $1,100 for a family of four each year. The remaining 25% would finance energy research and development, help reduce emissions in agriculture, forestry, and manufacturing, and provide transition assistance for workers and communities in carbon-intensive regions. The legislation aims to reduce GHG emissions 20% by 2020 and 83% by 2050. The predictable carbon price could spur investment in efficiency and clean energy solutions.

Key Terms

Cap and trade

Climate Change Science Program (CCSP)

Climate Security Act

Climate Stewardship Act of 2003

GHG Reporting Rule

Kyoto Climate Treaty

Leadership in Energy and Environmental Design (LEED)

Stern Report

Discussion Questions

1. What were the major goals of the Kyoto Climate Treaty?
2. What are some major problems facing regional climate change agreements?
3. Describe some of the efforts by the private sector to address global warming.
4. What role has the judiciary branch played in addressing climate change?
5. How has the party affiliation of the president played a role in the EPA's decisions on climate change?
6. Describe some of the initial efforts by Congress to address climate change.
7. Describe a few of the major changes that need to be undertaken in order to stave off the effects of global warming.
8. What are two major approaches to addressing climate change that are currently being put forward in Congress?

CHAPTER 13

ENVIRONMENTAL POLICY AND THE LAND

Wilderness Preservation

William N. Rom
with Kim Elliman

LEARNING OBJECTIVES

- To understand the link between wilderness preservation and environmental health
- To become familiar with the history of wilderness protection
- To understand the numerous debates over wilderness protection
- To comprehend some of the problems associated with continuing wilderness protection
- To become familiar with current legislation regarding wilderness protection
- To become familiar with the Land and Water Conservation Fund and the Endangered Species Act

Wilderness is important for humans as places to regain our peace of mind after the stresses of society. Wilderness protects lakes, rivers and streams, forests and soils that are important for water purification, allowing us to have safe drinking water. Wilderness preserves biodiversity and the variation among genetic species. Wilderness affects human health by giving us opportunities to seek adventure, provide intellectual sustenance in studying nature, and obtain mental solace in discovering natural beauty. Adventure travel through wilderness areas involves hiking trails, climbing distant peaks, rock climbing, rafting, and canoeing—all with the goal of a destination. It is rewarding enough to reach the goal. Many prefer to observe wildlife or birds, name plants, search for new species, study fauna and flora, or engage in scientific study. Mental rejuvenation comes after a week's escape from computers, work stress, social interaction, multi-tasking, but more important capturing a view of purple tree buds with spruce understory across an ice-clad lake, a morning mist, and a changing sunset with a wilderness lake still as glass in the foreground. Those memories can last a long time.

The legislative creation of wilderness, executive agencies' role in managing and protecting wilderness values, and judicial proceedings to protect land are quintessential examples of environmental policy. Protecting land will affect public health in indirect and direct ways—including the very oxygen we breathe, as we learned from the carbon sinks related to climate change. Richard Fuller, an ecologist at the University of Queensland, demonstrated that the psychological benefits of green space are closely linked to the diversity of its plant life.[1] When a city park has a larger variety of trees, study subjects who spend time in the park score higher on various measures of psychological well-being, at least when compared with less biodiverse parks. "We worry a lot about the effects of urbanization on other species," Fuller says. "But we're also affected by it. That's why it's so important to invest in the spaces that provide us with some relief."

Several arguments are to be made on behalf of what we know as wilderness: it protects ecosystems and landscapes if at scale; it provides public ownership and use of natural resources—hunting, fishing, and recreation; it resolves and provides certainty in fundamental land use disputes, for example, protection versus exploitation, and there is no ambiguity; it preserves a natural and cultural heritage. But wilderness designation is not without flaws and issues: what constitutes public access, what sort of public access is or should be permitted, and what user groups are favored.

The History of Wilderness Protection

The United States has been an innovator in preserving wilderness by capturing the wilderness spirit with the creation of national parks as a novel idea for Yellowstone and Yosemite in 1872. In 1924 Aldo Leopold established the first wilderness area in New Mexico's Gila Mountains as part of the **U.S. Forest Service (USFS)**; the USFS was custodian to millions of acres of roadless land. Wilderness, Leopold said, "is the very stuff America is made of."[2] The first protection of USFS wilderness was by administrative fiat, and it could be changed by a subsequent Forest Service chief. In 1929, U.S. Forest Service Chief William Greeley promulgated a "primitive area" policy to protect wild areas and discourage roads as much as possible. What was needed was a law that could protect wilderness lands for future generations without the threats of logging, roads, development, mechanized vehicles, airplanes, snowmobiles, and a host of other intrusions. Aldo Leopold felt that wilderness was a fundamental basis of American culture: "There is little question that many of the attributes most distinctive of America and Americans are the impress of wilderness and the life that accompanied it. If we have any such thing as an American culture (and I think we have) its distinguishing marks are a certain vigorous individualism. . . . A certain intellectual curiosity bent to practical ends, a lack of subservience to old social forms, and an intolerance of drones, all of which are the distinctive characteristics of successful pioneers."[3] Leopold captured the essence of wilderness values to public health practice: a healthy lifestyle and a healthy mind.

The Wilderness Act

President Theodore Roosevelt established the National Forest System in 1907. He named Gifford Pinchot his first chief. Instrumental to this effort was The Wilderness Society, founded in 1935 by Bob Marshall, Aldo Leopold, Harvey Broome, Ernest Oberholtzer, Benton Mackaye, Harold Anderson, Bernard Frank, and Robert Sterling Yard.

Robert Marshall, a native New Yorker, and Aldo Leopold were founders of the Wilderness Movement in the United States and were its effective leaders from World War I to World War II. Marshall was the icon of American wilderness: he explored the Brooks Range in Alaska, writing *Arctic Wilderness* about his travels; he was a founder of The Wilderness Society and explored wilderness throughout America, including a canoe trip through the Superior Wilderness along the Boundary Waters with Sigurd F. Olson, who wrote *The Singing Wilderness* in 1956.

FIGURE 13.1   Robert Marshall

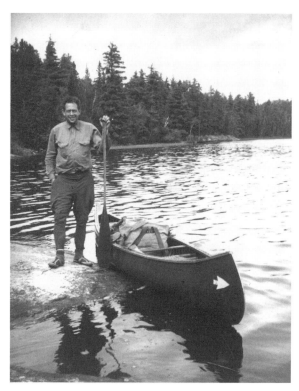

Source: Courtesy of The Wilderness Society.

Marshall, the leader of the roadless lands and wilderness policy in the USFS, advocated a Wilderness Planning Board in the 1930s to select areas of wilderness value and to assure maximum protection (see Figure 13.1). These selected areas would be designated by act of Congress. In his 1930 *Scientific Monthly* article, Marshall argued for a study to determine the wilderness needs of the country, stating that it ought to be a radical calculation: "the population which covets wilderness recreation is rapidly enlarging and because the higher standard of living may be anticipated should give millions the economic power to gratify what is today merely a pathetic yearning. Once the estimate is formulated, immediate steps should be taken to establish enough tracts to insure everyone who hungers for it a generous opportunity of enjoying wilderness isolation."[4,5]

Bob Marshall became famous for his prodigious hikes, climbing fourteen Adirondack peaks within nineteen hours—a feat that required a total ascent of

13,600 feet; his unflagging commitment to wilderness (identifying all roadless areas in the United States—an inventory that prompted President Bill Clinton's 58 million acres "roadless" designation in 2000), and his indefatigable advocacy and writing on behalf of wilderness.

Aldo Leopold discovered the wilderness ethic while exploring the woodlands of Wisconsin and contributed to the establishment of the Gila Wilderness in the 1920s. He wrote the classic *A Sand County Almanac* as a wilderness primer in 1949. Leopold explained, "The land ethic simply enlarges the boundaries of the community to include soils, waters, plants, and animals, or collectively: the land."[3]

Harvey Broome hiked in the Great Smokies. Ernest Oberholtzer envisaged the Quetico-Superior Wilderness as a great international park along the Minnesota–Ontario border. He lived on Rainy Lake and fought a hydroelectric and logging scheme that would have destroyed this great wilderness canoe country. Benton Mackaye founded the Appalachian Trail, and Bernard Frank created and protected the Rock Creek Park in Washington, D.C. Robert Sterling Yard worked with Stephen Mather to found the National Parks Service in 1916, was the creator of the National Parks Conservation Association, and helped the USFS develop the concept of "primitive areas"; he fervently believed in protecting wilderness in its wildest state and abhorred the roads and plush lodges that Mather was building in the national parks.

The Political Background to the Wilderness Bill During the 1930s, there was considerable tension between the Department of Agriculture's U.S. Forest Service and the National Park Service in the Department of Interior under Harold Ickes. Ickes wanted to transfer the U.S. Forest Service to the Department of the Interior, especially to protect the 11 million acres of Primitive Areas. By contrast, the U.S. Forest Service resisted, stating that the National Park Service would install roads and lodges that would trespass against their "primitive" wilderness idea. The National Park Service did capture Olympic National Park and Kings Canyon National Park from U.S. Forest Service primitive areas in 1938 and 1940, but Robert Marshall died suddenly in 1939. The U.S. Forest Service had only 14.2 million acres of wilderness at this time, and this number persisted up until the Wilderness Act in 1964.

Howard Zahniser had spent several years in the early 1950s building consensus among conservation groups that a practical and politically viable bill to establish a wilderness preservation program with a congressional mandate should be their priority. Rep. Wayne Aspinall (D-CO) opposed Zahniser's plan of affirmative action, whereby leaders of conservation organizations would consult with agencies about wilderness and an executive order would designate wilderness subject to the veto of Congress; rather, Aspinall insisted that each wilderness area be created through an act of Congress.

The conservation community mobilized to defeat the Echo Park Dam on the Yampa River in Dinosaur National Monument in 1956. The Bureau of Reclamation proposed a dam there on the Colorado plateau that was championed by Rep. Aspinall. Against all odds, the conservationists lobbied Congress and informed the public over a span of five years.

To lose this battle would create a damaging precedent that industrial development could proceed within a unit of the National Park System. During this conservation battle, the conservation community recognized that a law was necessary to protect wilderness on a permanent basis rather than fighting each threat alone. Zahniser had to overcome agency opposition to draft a wilderness bill; the agencies coveted the responsibility of selecting, managing, and providing wilderness stewardship. Congressional stalwarts came to his rescue by stating that wilderness selected by an act of Congress would prevent politicization of the agencies and protect them from undue influence in redrawing boundaries or altering management decisions to suit a single powerful group. Last, Zahniser had to accommodate Rep. Aspinall, who represented mining interests, grazing, water projects, and negotiated hard on the final House version of the bill.

Zahniser drafted the bill in 1955; in 1956 Sen. Hubert Humphrey (D-MN) and Rep. John Saylor (R-PA) introduced the Wilderness Bill. The bill included fifty-four areas within national forests designated as wilderness, primitive, or canoe, totaling 9.1 million acres.

The Wilderness Society mobilized public opinion and finally prevailed after many dozens of drafts by Howard Zahniser; David Brower of the Sierra Club celebrated this victory alone since Howard Zahniser did not live to see the signing ceremony. Historian Howard Nash claimed that the American wilderness movement had its finest hour.[7]

Eight years, eighteen hearings, and sixteen versions later, the **Wilderness Act** was passed in 1964 and set the course for protecting federal lands in the United States as a model for the world. The House vote was 374–1 and the Senate voted 73–12 on July 30, 1964. President Lyndon B. Johnson signed the bill into law on September 3, 1964. An act of Congress was now required for a presidential recommendation or for a bill to create a wilderness area. This was the highest level of protection, excluding commercial development, logging, roads, mining, and administrative fiat of removing areas from protection.

Defined in the act was the term *wilderness*. In contrast with those areas where humans and their works dominated the landscape, wilderness is recognized as an area where the Earth and its community of life are untrammeled by humans, where humans themselves are visitors who do not remain. An area of wilderness is an area of undeveloped federal land retaining its primeval character and influence without permanent improvements or human habitation. The Wilderness Act required that proposed land:

- Has outstanding opportunities for solitude or primitive type of recreation
- Has 5,000 acres or "sufficient size of unimpaired conditions"
- Has ecological, geological, or other features of scientific, scenic, or historical value

Secretary of the Interior Stewart Udall told senators that the wilderness bill ranked with the Homestead Act of 1862 and the National Parks of 1916 as a "great landmark conservation decision."[6] The Wilderness Act required an act of Congress to designate wilderness, providing both agencies an opportunity to propose wilderness areas and their boundaries and citizens acting alone or in groups to initiate and lobby for wilderness designation. Local community groups from chambers of commerce to environmental organizations could all contribute to supporting a proposal, and when there was a previous human disturbance within a boundary, or a nonconforming use, such as grazing, or a neighboring contrasting use, such as a ski area, controversy would need to be resolved among competing parties beforehand.

The Wilderness Act proclaimed a national policy to preserve "an enduring resource of wilderness" in perpetuity. It designated 9.1 million acres of statutory wilderness areas in the National Wilderness Preservation System. It mandated a ten-year review process with the federal agencies to study and report to Congress on hundreds of potential wilderness areas. It shifted the power to decide which areas to protect and to determine the boundaries from the agencies to Congress, requiring an act for new wilderness designations or boundary alterations. It proclaimed a common mandate for wilderness stewardship applying to all designated wilderness areas on federal lands to preserve "the wilderness character" of each area.

The National Wilderness Preservation System President Ronald Reagan signed more ($n = 43$) wilderness protection laws than any other president (10.6 million acres in thirty-one states). President Jimmy Carter designated the most wilderness acres of any other president, totaling 66.3 million acres, mostly in Alaska. The Campaign for America's Wilderness has canvassed the remaining USFS and Bureau of Land Management (BLM) lands, identifying 319 million acres that were without roads and still wild and located in parcels >1,000 acres in size that were suitable for wilderness designation.

As of 2010, the National Wilderness Preservation System contained 109.5 million acres in wilderness areas or 5% of all land in the United States (total wilderness area is about the size of California, and 2.5% is in the lower continental United States). There are approximately 44 million acres in national parks, out of 84.4 million acres in 58 national parks; 34.7 million acres in national forests, out of 192 million acres in 155 national forests; 20.7 million acres in national wildlife refuges, out of 100 million acres in 547 national wildlife refuges; and 6.5 million acres in the Bureau of Land Management, out of 260 million acres. More than half or 57 million acres are in Alaska, and more than one-third are in the eleven westernmost contiguous states. Less than 5% are in the East, and half of this is in the Everglades National Park and Boundary Waters Canoe Area Wilderness in Minnesota.

The nation's largest wilderness complex is the contiguous 12.7 million acres in Noatak and Gates of the Arctic Wilderness National Park in Alaska. The largest wilderness is the Wrangell-Saint Elias Wilderness in Alaska (9,078,675 acres). There are 756 wilderness areas. The National Park Service lags behind designating its lands as wilderness because the national parks already are protected from development. Each park must develop a proposal for public review and submit this to Congress for enactment. The Wilderness Society has urged the National Parks Service to be more aggressive in seeking wilderness status for its parks. Congress has fulfilled this role; for example, the Omnibus Wilderness Act protects Rocky Mountain National Park in 2009.

Local citizen groups became essential to the protection of wilderness, resulting in many local conservation organizations, for example, the Friends of the Boundary Waters Canoe Area Wilderness. National organizations such as The Wilderness Society opened regional offices, and the Sierra Club opened state chapters. Local groups were best able to determine boundaries of wilderness in their domains and had access to local politicians and hearings to state their views and findings. For example, the Friends of the Boundary Waters Wilderness could advocate for the Boundary Waters Canoe Area Wilderness much better than could the Sierra Club or The Wilderness Society, since their members were canoe guides and local denizens who canoed the lakes, knew where boundaries could be drawn, and also knew the opposition (Conservationists for Common Sense supported increased motorization).

U.S. government polls have asked the public about protecting more wilderness areas in their own states; 69.8% were in favor and only 12.4% opposed. Zogby Polls (2003) found that 54% of Republicans, 66% of Independents, and 75% of Democrats supported additional wilderness in their own states. Wilderness is truly bipartisan; members of both parties have supported wilderness, although those supporting limited government or development have oftentimes been opponents.

NOTES FROM THE FIELD

There is tremendous diversity among our wilderness areas, from desert landscapes to mountains, to lake country, to rugged forests; these range in size, degree of wildness, and ecosystems. I have often thought of the importance of a buffer zone around wilderness, but more important, wilderness boundaries must be sufficient, and if not, vigilance must be maintained to expand them. I remember a hike with my daughter around Agassa Lake in the winter; we snowshoed into this pristine lake with the sun glistening off the radiant snow. I reminded her that this beautiful wild lake in the Superior National Forest was entirely outside of the Boundary Waters Canoe Area Wilderness—it was our duty to attempt to protect this by enlarging the boundary or possibly risk losing this priceless lake to a circumnavigating road and cabins at every prominent rocky point. The work of protecting wilderness is never finished, and the task must be passed on to future generations.

Once wilderness is protected, regulations from the lead land agency become very important, requiring continual vigil by national or local environmental groups. Wilderness management needs to consider wilderness stewardship as priority one, preventing access roads or lenient regulations that may lead to loss of the true wilderness experience. Congress may repeatedly expand wilderness areas, as they did California's Ventana Wilderness, which started as a 55,000 acre primitive area but after four expansions is now a quarter-million acres.

The History of Wilderness Protection Evolving from New York State's Leadership (Kim Elliman)

In the eastern United States most land is privately or state-owned, limiting the role of the federal government in protecting wilderness. However, there are large state wildernesses in New York and Maine. In addition, the Northern Forest has largely recovered from the devastating effects of logging 200–300 years ago. Protecting this forest is an even greater challenge as large private tracts are now coming onto the commercial market. States and private foundations have an unprecedented opportunity to purchase and protect these lands. Their importance to public health cannot be overstated; the Catskill Preserve provides safe, clean drinking water to more than 10 million inhabitants of New York City and Westchester County. The largest population centers along the east coast have easy access to some of America's greatest wildernesses in the Adirondacks, Catskills, and Appalachian Mountains.

Sedentary lifestyle contributes to increased obesity and chronic diseases, including high blood pressure, diabetes, congestive heart failure, cancer, and stroke. The Centers for Disease Control and Prevention has called for more parks and playgrounds as one solution.

Regardless of whether New York was wilderness prior to European colonization—*wilderness* defined as the state of nature that exists absent the hand of man—or simply wild, the state was heavily forested, about 90%, by mixed hardwoods at lower elevations and conifers and hemlock in higher elevations. Suffice to say that the human footprint was evident long before the seventeenth century, but it was relatively light and was certainly sustainable and not extractive. We know, however, that Native Americans regularly burned, or permitted burning the forests for ease of travel, hunting, and agriculture.

With peace after two wars (French and Indian War, 1754–1763, and the American Revolution, 1775–1783) came more land development, settlement, and serious incursion into what had remained relatively intact forest. Veterans of the Continental Army were given land in lieu of pay, often the lands of Tories who had fled, but also "virgin land" in unsettled lands. The white pines, which were previously protected by the Crown for the British Navy for masts and spars, were felled. Lumbering was particularly extensive in the Hudson Valley, the Mohawk Valley, and into the foothills of the Catskills and Adirondacks. From the opening of the Erie Canal in 1825 (easy transport and improved access to forests) through the Civil War and its immediate aftermath (about fifty years), New York was the lumber basket of the country, producing more timber and timber products than any other region. What was left behind was a despoiled landscape, full of scraps of trees that had been trimmed, litter that became tinder boxes for the subsequent wildfires, and an impoverishment of soils, ecosystems, and wildlife.

George Perkins Marsh, in "Man and Nature," identified the importance of forests and forest preservation in the 1860s, particularly as they related to the health and maintenance of watersheds and riparian systems. Over the next decades, as New York moved fully into an industrial economy (albeit with a strong agricultural base), there were conflicting factions debating the use and protection of natural resources: forests and water. From the 1860s on, New York tried to define the role of government in protecting natural resources by assaying the natural capital and the ecosystem services of its public—and private—estate. There is a debate about which had roots in forest protection, clean drinking water, water as a power source and as a means of transport, or—as in the romantics and naturalists schools of virginal nature—the contemplative and transformative power of nature and wilderness. The leading philosophers, scientists, and writers of the day began to equate nature and unaltered lands with a state of grace.

In the 1840s and 1850s, Ralph Waldo Emerson and Henry David Thoreau, among others, increasingly denounced commerce and held up nature as a preferred state of being. Their Metaphysical School, started in Boston, visited the Adirondacks in 1858–1860 because it was the most complete expression of wilderness remaining in the eastern United States. They were joined physically and intellectually with such other cultural and scientific leaders such as Louis Aggassiz, Oliver Wendell Holmes, Thomas Cole, Robert Lowell, and William Lloyd Garrison. This same era—the second quarter of the nineteenth century—gave rise to the paintings of the Hudson River School, the novels of James Fennimore Cooper featuring the Mohawk Valley, and the writings of the metaphysical philosophers. The Hudson Valley, the Mohawk Valley, the Catskills, and the Adirondacks were epicenters of New York's natural world and best described in superlatives for their wild state of beauty and virtues.

It was not until the Adirondacks, not formally named until 1837 (an English map from 1761 labels it simply "Deer Hunting Country"), saw three events occur that dictated both its loss and recouping of its wilderness state:

1. Railroads and a country desperate for timber (another by-product of the Civil War). Until the end of Reconstruction, Congress prohibited logging of southern forests as a way of punishing southerners and rewarding northern landowners—and vast expansion and clear-cutting of the Northern Forests from Maine to Wisconsin occurred from the 1860s to the early 1900s as America industrialized.

2. Land was surveyed by New York State—by intrepid surveyor Verplanck Van Colvin. In the years he spent preparing the survey, he saw how the land had been raped and ravaged and became an advocate for public and private protection.

3. A minister from Boston, William Henry Harrison Murray (who came to be known as "Adirondack" Murray) wrote a travelogue about the joys of virgin wilderness and its natural bounties: trout jumping into his canoe; deer strolling toward his blind; colorful and amusing guides; nature in all its glory. Murray popularized what Emerson and the Metaphysical Club had earlier described in more philosophical parsing. Adirondack Murray began the outdoor movement and launched the first hunting magazine, and crowds followed his lead. Within a few years of his writings, hundreds of hunting and fishing camps were established in the Adirondacks. Logging suggested that paradise was being cut and burned. An urban polity, growing geometrically in the last quarter of the nineteenth century, was also concerned about its future drinking water needs (perhaps from the Hudson, the source of which was the Adirondacks). They were

worried that if the Adirondacks watershed faltered, Hudson River commerce would suffer, as would New York City public health. The interplay of land, natural resources, and expanding geography gave rise to a political discourse, perhaps for the first time in America, about how government should address limits to growth.

The Catskills, considered the Adirondack's (red-headed) stepsister, were afflicted and pressured by similar issues. However, deforestation in the Catskills was not as drastic or sudden as the Adirondacks for three primary reasons: (1) they were closer to urban centers, so transportation was much easier; (2) as it was less rugged and steep, agriculture was more viable in and around the Catskills; and (3) it was much smaller (about 700,000 acres versus 6.1 million acres), so getting to the interior of the Catskills was much less difficult. Because of these reasons, the Catskills were already exploited and inhabited over time as early as the Declaration of Independence, and the natural capital had been impaired by the time of the Industrial Revolution. Eventually, virtually every acre of land had been exploited in one way or another—only 5%–10% was first growth or virgin timber—the rest affected by tanning, bluestone mining, furniture manufacture, charcoal mining, and hardscrabble farming.

In the early years of the twentieth century, the Catskills became a popular destination for naturalists, and its featured natural philosopher was John Burroughs. Burroughs, unlike the earlier naturalist schools or the Adirondack wilderness advocates, preferred a mixed-use landscape. He preferred the closed views and subsistence life of a Catskills farm to the forested wilderness of the Adirondacks or the daunting power and the impersonal nature of the Hudson River.

Forever Wild

In 1892, the legislature established the Adirondack (ADK) Park and, in 1904, Catskill State Park, the first wilderness parks in the nation (the ADK Park was not wilderness until the Forever Wild 1894 amendment). Yellowstone, created by President Ulysses Grant as a preserve, was neither wilderness nor a park until President Theodore Roosevelt further protected it. In 1894, the New York state legislature called for a state convention to consider amending the state constitution, an extremely rare event. Led by New York City legislators and delegates, the convention passed an amendment (Article XIV) that called for the establishment of a forest preserve in the Catskills and Adirondacks, where the public forests would be "forever wild," not to be harvested or exploited commercially in any way.

The park's boundaries were defined by the blue line that roughly approximates the topographic footprint of the ADK and Catskill uplift. The best agricultural land lay outside the defined park boundaries. As did parks across the nation, the Catskill and Adirondack Park encompassed "rocks and ice" and little arable land. New York had created the first wilderness park, but what did it consist of?

The ADK and Catskills Forest Preserve and Park only protected the lands the state already owned, and that was not all that much. In fact, prior to Article XIV, the state had been selling land it had acquired or reacquired from tax liens to timber companies and entrepreneurs. Eventually, it selectively, then generally, retained those tax lien lands, swapped to acquire more lands, and finally began to acquire land and interest in lands. The Catskills Park started at 34,000 acres, and is now 300,000 acres (43% state owned). ADK was 550,000 and is now about 3 million (roughly 50% state owned). Within the parks—much like in the American West—it is the mountains and upland acreage (cheaper lands) that came into state ownership. The private lands tend to lie along river corridors, valleys, and more accessible low-lying lands.

In 1902, President Roosevelt, who had summered as a child in the high peaks of the Adirondacks, created a bi-state park commission—the first in the nation—the Palisades Interstate Park Commission, or PIPC. The move to protect and preserve the Palisades came, as does most protection, after the fact, from its despoliation. As New York City grew and developed affordable housing for immigrants from Europe and the American South, business interests blasted and excavated the rock face of the Palisades on the west bank and in the Hudson Highlands. The Palisades became the source of quaint village brownstones, excavated from the iconic cliffs that demark the Hudson River. However, the neighbors complained that their viewsheds were being destroyed; these neighbors were the robber barons who typically inhabited great estates across the river. They bought up the Palisades and donated (which was novel) it to a park—a bi-state park—first in the nation and the world. The purchase and preservation came too late to save some prominent and historic sites, but it led to a movement that over the first half of the twentieth century altered how parks and wilderness were aggregated, created, and perceived. PIPC also created the first linear or greenbelt park in the United States. It runs from George Washington Bridge beyond the Tappan Zee Bridge past the Bear Mountain Bridge, north of West Point, and almost to the mid-Hudson Bridge. It created a remarkable legacy and a wilderness park available and accessible to tens of millions of metropolitan residents.

The Progressive movement in American politics included land and natural resource protection as one of its key platforms. That is nowhere more apparent than in the acts of a succession of New York governors, politicians, and U.S. presidents as the twentieth century dawned. This movement was lead by many figures, including Theodore Roosevelt and continuing to Al Smith, Franklin Delano Roosevelt, Herbert Lehman, Averell Harriman, Nelson Rockefeller, and George Pataki. All greatly expanded both the physical and the political foundations of New York's parks, wilderness, and environmental conservation.

Another dam fight in New York inaugurated the birth of the modern environmental movement. Storm King Mountain lies at the north gate of the Hudson Highlands, the northernmost part of the PIPC greenway. In the early 1960s, Con Edison proposed a pump storage plant and hydroelectric facility. The top of Storm King would be chopped off, a lake created, water pumped up the side of the mountain in large penstocks, and flushed back down at times of high or peak energy demand. The opposition to Storm King, like the Palisades sixty years before, initially was led and financed by wealthy neighbors who created a citizen group that sued for standing. Out of this struggle the courts affirmed that citizens had standing to sue on behalf of nature—a sort of green class action litigation. Storm King was preserved, and the fight birthed the modern environmental movement: Earth Day, the Natural Resources Defense Council, the Scenic Hudson, and ultimately the Open Space Institute.

In the late 1960s, under the ever-sensitive political sensibilities—and of the genuine beliefs—of then-Gov. Nelson Rockefeller, New York passed a spate of landmark environmental legislation, often predicting or mirroring similar federal bills. New York has its own version of the Federal Wilderness Act (in Article XIV) and the Wild and Scenic Rivers Act, National Environmental Policy Act (NEPA) or State Environmental Quality Review, clean air, and clean water legislation. Rockefeller passed several environmental bond acts to purchase and create parks and wilderness areas. He established an environmental agency. He catalyzed and surfed a popular movement for environmental protection and an environmental agenda that expanded beyond just parks—or land—and waters. The 1960s was, in retrospect, a very progressive decade, and the legislation passed then—fifty years ago—still defines the legal underpinnings of environmental and wilderness protection. Together, President Lyndon Johnson on a national level and Gov. Nelson Rockefeller on a state stage waged an arms war over who could conceive and create a more beneficial government and progressive state using the environment as his platform.

Rockefeller appointed the Temporary Study Commission on the Future of the Adirondacks; its premise was that through designation and restrictions of both public and private lands in the park, one could achieve all of the advantages of a natural wilderness park with none of the drawbacks. Arguably, this land protection controversy created a countermovement—one that militated for more local control and more private property rights. The so-called Wise Use movement became ascendant in the mid-1990s, but it was not strong enough to

FIGURE 13.2   The signing of the historic Private Land Zoning Act

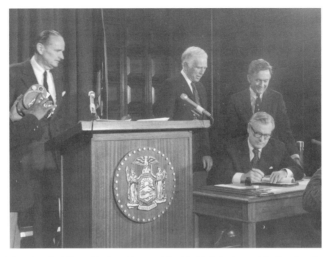

Note: Gov. Nelson Rockefeller with Sen. Bernard Smith (right), Assembly Speaker Perry Duryea (center), and Richard Lawrence Jr., chairman of the Adirondack Park Agency (left), May 22, 1973.
Source: In Defending the Wilderness: The Adirondack Writings of Paul Schaefer by Paul Schaefer. Reprinted with permission from the Adirondack Research Library.

block the most sweeping regional zoning and land use regulation in the county: the **Adirondack Park Act** of 1971 (Figure 13.2). The Act designated all lands in the park into five categories of public land use—the highest being wilderness. There were multiple categories of private land use, the highest of which, resource management, mirrored wilderness by creating large lots and limited development options. The Wise Use movement consisted of local interests, especially those favoring development of resources on public lands, that gave rise to the Sage Brush Rebellion in the West. This Rebellion, in the 1980s and 1990s, opposed further wilderness designation on federal lands, and wilderness studies were undertaken.

The Adirondacks were next protected by **conservation easements**. In a conservation easement, a landowner voluntarily agrees to sell or donate certain rights associated with his or her property—often the right to subdivide or develop—and a private organization or public agency agrees to hold the right to enforce the landowner's promise not to exercise those rights. A conservation easement is legally binding whether the property is sold or passed on to heirs and may qualify for significant tax benefits. Land is comprised of a bundle of rights or ownerships: buildings including homes and structures, timber, water, mineral, recreational use, and so on, and these rights can be segregated. The entire bundle is called fee simple. If you own the physical land it is known as "owning in fee." But the fee can be owned and held separately from other rights, most prominently development rights, but also timber, agricultural, recreational, and public access rights. As noted, Diamond International sold its assets—really auctioned themselves off—including its timberlands, mills, and outlets. The sum of those parts exceeded its public market value. This model was worrisome since northeastern forests are relatively unproductive, have a high real estate value, and are located near a global market.

One of the largest conservation organizations in the United States, the Nature Conservancy, protects 15.4 million acres, and more than 2 million acres have been protected through conservation easements granted to the conservancy. The conservancy has also assisted other U.S. land trusts and public agencies with conservation easements on an additional 1.3 million acres.

On a broader scale, 6 million acres of land have been protected in the Northern Forest that runs from Maine to New York. More than 90% of the protected land is under some form of conservation easement. Little more than a decade ago, the largest landowners in the United States were industrial timber companies, led by International Paper at roughly 13 million acres, 5% of which were in the Adirondacks. International Paper has, for all practical purposes, sold all its land in the United States, most to timber investment management organizations (TIMOs), a creature of Wall Street. This broad sell-off was prompted by tax considerations, global markets, disaggregation of mills from forests, and more efficient use of capital/balance sheet manipulations. Our forest lands, like our homes, were collateralized, commoditized, and sold off. While there has been some good news as properties changed hands, about 50% of the lands sold in the Northern Forest were not protected, and virtually every transaction resulted in parcelization of ownership and management. If the point of wilderness protection is to protect at scale, parcelization is particularly bad.

In addition to parcelization, protection of riparian areas and corridors is key. For human as well as other animal and vegetative life, waterways, watercourses, and riparian corridors are essential to collect, store, recharge, and transport water. The Adirondacks cool the humid air off the Great Lakes, which then causes rain and forms the headwaters of major rivers—the St. Lawrence and the Hudson—and many of their main tributaries—the Mohawk, Racquette, Black, Moose, Saranac, and Sacandaga. We need to protect the riparian corridors first and their critical watersheds second. For many reasons, these are the most expensive lands, since people want to build homes on lands that abut water.

In addition to riparian corridors, terrestrial corridors for migratory species are key for long-term viability and sustainability of intact ecosystems. While there is obviously much overlap with riparian corridors, discrete land corridors usually lie along valleys or bottomlands. Again, these lands generally confront more conflicting land use pressures and are higher value and more politically charged. This is where people want to live, farm, build stores, and recreate; these utility corridors are all bad for wilderness and wildlife. We do not now have a good mechanism to resolve land use disputes outside of zoning, which is parochial, or purchase, which is expensive.

The flip side to parcelization, corridor protection, or even easements, is scale. Scale is the protection of large ecosystems, for example, the Northern Forest of New England. The premise is that scale solves all other issues ultimately. It is an expensive solution, and it begs all the other land use conflicts mentioned since the only way we currently get to scale is through partial protection through easements. If zoning were an option in the northeastern United States, again we might get to scale, though again at the pain of conflicting economic and lifestyle choices that have to be addressed and reconciled. As more than one naturalist has noted, the animals and trees don't get to vote.

Debates over Wilderness

The Purity Theory

There is considerable debate on what may constitute eligible wilderness for protections, since practically all of the United States had been previously logged; roads may enter small parts of pristine areas; mines may have been extant years ago; homesteads might be found, and so on, leading to delicate compromises on boundaries of wilderness areas. One problem with both the NPS and USFS was their **"purity theory"** of what lands were wilderness, since roads had been placed in many national parks, and many now-pristine forest areas had been previously logged. There was considerable debate over buffers near roads, and exclusion of logged areas. Aldo Leopold in *A Sand County Almanac* declared that bringing wilderness areas into being may require diversity in size and degree of wildness.[2] The purity theory would exclude many wild lands in the eastern United States that were being championed by many citizen advocates of wilderness. The Eastern Wilderness Bill, introduced by Rep. Diane Saynor (R-PA) and Sen. Henry "Scoop" Jackson (D-WA) in 1973 brought this debate to the floor of Congress. Sen. James Buckley (D-NY) stated, "If we are to have a national system of wilderness areas, as the drafters of the Wilderness Act obviously intended, less than pristine standards would be necessary for practical application. As a basis for public policy I believe it would be a mistake to assume that the Wilderness Act can have no application to once-disturbed area" (*Congressional Record*, January 11, 1973, 757).

Sen. Frank Church (D-ID) told the chief of the USFS to submit the proposals to the subcommittee of the Senate. In turn, the senator would determine what belongs in a wilderness and what does not! President Gerald Ford signed the **Eastern Wilderness Act** in 1975, bringing statutory protection to fifteen eastern wilderness areas in national forests and requiring studies of seventeen additional de facto areas. Because these areas had logging and logging roads up to a century or more earlier, this ended the debate on the purity theory.

Multiple Land Use Example: The Boundary Waters Canoe Area Wilderness
(William N. Rom)

The next debate occurred over **multiple land use**. This was a forestry doctrine allowing multiple management practices in the national forests, including logging, mechanized vehicles, road access, and watershed and wilderness protection. Conservationists argued against multiple use. Their slogan was "Not every use on every acre." This argument boiled over in the debate over Minnesota's Boundary Waters. The original protection of the canoe country was as a million-acre roadless area in 1926. However, there were deletions to accommodate locals' desire for roads to service the burgeoning resort trade: the Echo Trail cut off the Little Sioux River portion of the Boundary Waters Canoe Area (BWCA), and the Fernberg Road and Gunflint Trail penetrated from the west and from the east. It took considerable energy to prevent the road builders from connecting the Fernberg Road and Gunflint Trail, which could have destroyed the heart of the roadless area.

E. W. Backus, the regional industrialist who had built the paper and pulp mill at International Falls, proposed damming all of the border lakes for a grand hydroelectric scheme and logging enterprise. Ernest Oberholtzer, a founder of The Wilderness Society who was an early canoeist in the Boundary Waters from his cabin on Rainy Lake, rallied the Quetico-Superior Council to oppose Backus's scheme through conservation organization activism. He was able to shepherd the Shipstead-Newton-Nolan Act through Congress; the act prohibited logging within 400 feet of the shoreline and preserved the shorelines intact. Following World War II, more than 400 seaplanes were operating out of Ely, Minnesota, flying into the more than 1,000 lakes of the Boundary Waters to service fishermen and the many resorts that had been built on private land inholdings in the Superior National Forest. After seeing floatplanes land in wilderness lakes after several days of portaging into the interior lakes, Sigurd Olson and colleagues requested President Harry S Truman to declare an airban on seaplanes from landing in the Superior Roadless Area.[7] Truman did so in 1949 and required private planes to fly at an altitude of 4,000 feet over the Superior Roadless Area. The pilots appealed all the way to the U.S. Supreme Court, but the Court refused to hear the case.

NOTES FROM THE FIELD

I guided Dr. Clayton Rudd, editor of the journal *Naturalist*, deep into the Kawishiwi River canoe country and hiked to a nearby small lake to witness logging direct to the shoreline. He published photographs of the logging violations of the Shipstead-Newton-Nolan Law leading to a federal USFS commission led by Minnesota's noted conservationist, George Selke, appointed by Secretary of Agriculture Orville Freeman, to consider the issues and recommend restrictions on logging. In 1964 I was able to testify before the Selke Commission as a local canoe guide to urge wilderness protection and an end to the logging. I was followed by Sigurd Olson, who said, "Wilderness holds within itself all the mystery of the universe, the story of evolution, of growth and change and beauty from the beginnings of time. Wilderness is more than lakes, rivers, and timber along the shores, more than fishing or just camping. It is the sense of the primeval, of space, solitude, silence, and the eternal mystery. It is a fragile quality and is destroyed by man and his machines."[8] I was shocked as Ely Mayor Dr. J. P. Grahek came up to Sigurd after his presentation exclaiming, "How dare you raise your children in the community of Ely." The mayor had always been in cahoots with the development interests. The Selke Commission recommended a 600,000 acre no-cut zone but left a 400,000 acre zone that would allow logging, and there were no restrictions on motors. The USFS renamed the Superior Roadless Area the Boundary Waters Canoe Area after they built logging roads into the wilderness as part of their multiple use policy. With the passage of the Wilderness Act in 1964, Sen. Hubert Humphrey kept these intrusions in the Boundary Waters Canoe Area. He did not want the acrimony over the Boundary Waters to disrupt his chances of winning passage of The Wilderness Bill.

Logging and Protection in Wilderness: The BWCA Again

During the 1950s and 1960s, the inland resorts needed to be purchased; the Thye-Blatynik Act provided funds for this purpose. By then the next battle emerged as the USFS determined that the second-growth forests in the margins of the Superior Roadless Area were ripe for timber harvesting for the emerging paper and pulp mills. They built a town on the edge of Lake Isabella named Forest Center and a railroad to deliver the logs to market. Roads were constructed miles into the roadless area to harvest timber on many tens of thousands of acres.

Mechanized Vehicles: BWCA Becomes BWCA Wilderness

The next threat came from mechanized vehicles, including motorboats and snowmobiles. Large motorboats cruised on lakes at the end of the roads and trucks on portage roads hauled these motorboats into the border lakes deep into the BWCA. At the beginning of the winter season, snowmobiles cruised to remote lakes in 1–2 hours at high speeds for lake trout fishing. After all the preservation work, wilderness in the BWCA was rapidly losing ground. The only hope was for a federal wilderness bill that would protect the Boundary Waters Canoe Area as a wilderness. Two competing bills were introduced in the U.S. House of Representatives. The first was local Rep. James Oberstar's proposal to create a national recreational area of the border lakes, allowing motorboats and protecting only the interior lakes as a wilderness. The second was Twin Cities Rep. Bruce Vento's proposal to protect the entire wilderness and restrict motorboats. There was an intense lobbying effort with Bud Heinselman, former USFS researcher who retired to lobby full time, leading the way.

NOTES FROM THE FIELD

Because I was on the faculty of the University of Utah Medical School and had worked as a guide for eight years in the BWCA and Quetico, I was assigned by the Friends of The Boundary Waters Wilderness to lobby the western representatives. I spent several days on Capitol Hill making the rounds of twenty western-state congressional offices asking to meet with the congressional legislative aides who handled environmental policy and wilderness bills. I would bring out the map of Quetico-Superior and would describe wilderness attributes and discuss all of the lakes and portages that I knew well. I pointed out the necessity of supporting the Vento version of the BWCA Wilderness bill.

Toward the midnight hour in the 1978 Congress, Representatives Vento and Oberstar came together to designate a negotiating team to blend both bills at the request of California's leader in wilderness protection, Rep. Phillip Burton. Chuck Dayton, a lawyer who had spent many years canoeing out of Ely, represented Rep. Vento with the able back-up of Miron "Bud" Heinselman. The entire BWCA would be protected as a wilderness; more than 60,000 acres would be added to protect valuable Native sites such as the Indian pictographs on Hegman Lake; the borders on Murphy and Big Moose Lakes would be moved to prevent seaplane landings and access; outboard motors would be banned, except motorboats up to 25 horsepower would be allowed on access lakes and motorboats allowed on select border lakes, including Basswood, Lac La Croix, Saganaga, Fowl Lakes, and Loon Lake; and snowmobile traffic would be banned. This bill was agreed upon, passed both houses of Congress, and was signed by President Carter in 1978. This was one of the most significant victories under The Wilderness Act!

Ontario's Quetico Provincial Park, covering 1,000 more lakes and another million acres, followed suit with a similar wilderness management plan. They did have one major difference, since they had to accommodate their Ojibway band on Lac La Croix, who had been given motorized access to several western Quetico lakes as part of their guide service. Also, Quetico employed Lac La Croix band members as park rangers. Voyageur's National Park was established on the western border, adding 365,000 acres creating a contiguous wilderness comprising more than 2.5 million acres. Ontario created the La Verendrye Provincial Park to protect the voyageur waterways east of Quetico.

The BWCA Wilderness has been the most embattled wilderness area in the National Wilderness Preservation System. In 1977 Sigurd Olson remarked, "This is the most beautiful lake country on the continent. We can afford to cherish and protect it. Some places should be preserved from development or exploitation for they satisfy human need for solace, belonging and perspective. In the end, we turn to nature in a frenzy chaotic world, there to find silence, oneness, wholeness—spiritual release."[8]

Problems with Implementation of the Wilderness Act

The Wilderness Act charged the federal agencies with a ten-year review process to inventory their lands and make recommendations for wilderness designation. Section 3 designated a National Wilderness Preservation System with lands in the National Park Service (NPS), USFS, Fish and Wildlife Service (Wildlife Refuges), and **Bureau of Land Management (BLM)** to be considered for wilderness designation during the following ten years. The USFS Roadless Area Review and Evaluation was considered inadequate, resulting in the lawsuit *Sierra Club v. Butz;* in 1977 President Carter ordered RARE II, covering 62 million acres; this was also considered inadequate, resulting in another lawsuit, *California v. Block.* The USFS developed forest management plans for each national forest and considered lands for wilderness inclusion. No roadless areas in the East were found to be eligible. The NPS also dithered in its wilderness plans, usually drawing boundaries deep inland from park roads. This caused Sen. Frank Church to lecture the NPS in the Senate Committee on Interior and Insular Affairs in 1972. His claim was that the NPS had arbitrarily under protected certain wild areas:

> [The NPS has been] setting the boundaries of its proposed wilderness units back from the edge of roads, developed areas and the park boundaries by

"buffer" and "threshold" zones of varying widths. There is no requirement for that in the Wilderness Act. No other agency draws wilderness boundaries in this way, which has the effect of excluding the critical edge of wilderness from full statutory protection. . . . In the absence of good and substantial reasons to the contrary—and I (mean) specific, case-by-case reasons—the boundaries of wilderness areas in national parks should embrace all wild land.

Sen. Church was the primary proponent of the Sawtooth Wilderness in Idaho, and the 2.36 million acre Frank Church River of No Return Wilderness was named in his honor in March 1984. The Central Idaho Wilderness Act (Frank Church/River of No Return Wilderness) allowed landing strips in regular use at time of the act. Wilderness proposals from Glacier, Yellowstone, Big Bend, and Rocky Mountain National Parks have languished from lack of enthusiasm from NPS. In some cases, citizens took over where the federal government had left slack. For instance, the Scapecoat Wilderness Area in Montana is renowned as the first citizen-initiated wilderness. These efforts were rewarded by the Endangered American Wilderness Act, signed in 1978, which protected seventeen citizen-initiated wilderness areas covering 1.3 million acres. The **Endangered American Wilderness Act** of 1978 states that areas were not to be disqualified because there are "sights and sound" of civilization outside the areas.

The Colorado Wilderness Act established guidelines for grazing activities within wilderness that applied to USFS wilderness nationwide. The Wilderness Act permits any measures necessary to control fire, insect outbreaks, and disease in wilderness areas. The Wilderness Act allows fisheries enhancement including fish traps, stream barriers, aerial stocking, protection and propagation of rare species. However, trailside shelters should not be provided except as necessary.

Snowmobiles pose challenging impediments for wilderness protection. In Yellowstone in 2000, snowmobiles had been considered for a phase-out by 2003–2004 after 65,000 public comments, the majority stating that snowmobiles had no place in a national park. The Bush administration blocked implementation, and upwards of 70,000 trips per season can now occur.

The laggard among federal agencies in protecting wilderness was the Bureau of Land Management. The BLM lagged because most of its land was desert, thus lacking the appeal of majestic forests, lakes, or mountains. In 1976, Rep. Wayne Aspinall secured the passage of the Federal Lands Policy and Management Act that provided statutory guidance for the BLM in the Department of the Interior. Included in the bill was a requirement for BLM to inventory its roadless areas for consideration as wilderness areas.

In 1976 Congress also passed the National Forest Management Act, which directed the 155 forest supervisors in the Department of Agriculture to develop fifteen-year management plans with public consultation and impact. The forest supervisors were required to prepare a detailed assessment of the plan's impact on the environment and to take specific steps to monitor and protect wildlife. This law grew out of a successful lawsuit by the Izaac Walton League of America against clear-cut logging practices in West Virginia and Montana. These two organic acts have directed the management of the majority of the federal lands for more than a quarter century.

In 1994, Congress passed the California Desert Protection Act, which established sixty-nine BLM wildernesses over 3.5 million acres. It reserved 326,000 acres in eight wilderness study areas. It also moved Death Valley and Joshua Tree National Monuments to national park status and set aside considerable wilderness in each.

Executive Orders for Wilderness Protection

Executive orders can do much to protect wilderness. President Clinton established the **Roadless Rule**, covering 58.5 million acres of USFS land to be set aside for Congress to consider as wilderness. There were 2.5 million comments on this rule, and 70% were favorable. The Roadless Rule places 0.25% of timber that the nation produces off-limits. President George W. Bush rescinded this executive order and stated that western state governors had to petition to keep unprotected federal lands under the Roadless Rule. This exemplifies the wisdom of protecting wilderness through acts of Congress so that wilderness areas become the law of the land.

Utah's 23 million acres of BLM land have only 28,000 acres protected as wilderness, but citizen proposals advocate 9 million acres. Political appointments to the Department of the Interior and the BLM can accelerate the process of wilderness recommendations, slow them to a crawl, or block them altogether. The state of Utah initiated a lawsuit against BLM wilderness proposals, and Secretary of Interior Gale Norton negotiated an end to this lawsuit by agreeing to severely curtail any BLM action on wilderness in Utah.

Rural communities may have a deep-grained distrust of the distant federal government, and consider wilderness protection an attempt to lock up land and prevent locals from using it. The Wilderness Society and local environmental organizations need to convince the locals who love their backyard's beauty and wildness that to keep it as it is will most likely require a law for protection.

NOTES FROM THE FIELD

In December 2003 I was on sabbatical working as a legislative fellow for Sen. Hillary Rodham Clinton for nine months in Washington, D.C. I noted in The Wilderness Society's *News* that a small wilderness in the Caribbean National Forest in Puerto Rico had been proposed in the House and passed, but no one had introduced a companion bill in the U.S. Senate. At the annual Christmas party for Sen. Clinton, I asked her if I could write a companion bill for the Caribbean Wilderness in Puerto Rico. She gave me a quizzical look and asked. "Why there?" I told her that New York City had 800,000 Puerto Ricans, and she said that the bill was a great idea!

The designation had been recommended in the original Management Plan for the Caribbean National Forest, as well as in the 1997 plan revision. Approximately 10,000 acres of the Caribbean National Forest (37% of the forest's 28,000 acres) were proposed as the El Toro Wilderness Area. El Toro, named after the highest peak (3,524 feet) in the forest, would be the only tropical wilderness in the U.S. National Forest Wilderness System. The Spanish Crown proclaimed much of the current Caribbean National Forest as a forest reserve in 1824, and President Theodore Roosevelt designated the area as a national forest. It is located 25 miles east of San Juan on the western side of the Luquillo Mountain Range. The forest is also a biosphere reserve, an internationally designated protected area managed to demonstrate the values of conservation.

The forest features the largest number of species of native trees (240) in the USFS, and contains fifty varieties of orchids and more than 150 species of ferns. The forest also provides a valuable water source for thousands of Puerto Rican residents. The area is also rich in wildlife, with more than 100 species of vertebrates, including the endangered Puerto Rican parrot. The area has spectacular scenery and the grandeur of the tropical vegetation can be appreciated from peaks both within and outside the area. El Toro can be seen from many vistas around the island, by sailors traveling the North Atlantic Ocean and the Caribbean Sea, as well as inhabitants of neighboring islands. The area features dense vegetation with a mixed evergreen forest ranging from one thousand meters in height on the peaks to 30 meters at lower elevations. There are cultural or historical features including Native American Taino petroglyphs.

A companion House bill was introduced by Puerto Rico's Resident Commissioner, Abibel Acevedo Vila. In a House hearing the previous summer, the USFS had stated its support for the designation of the El Toro Wilderness Area. The House bill had twenty-four co-sponsors, including the endorsement of the Hispanic Caucus. The bill was endorsed by The Wilderness Society, Sierra Club, National Wildlife Federation, and the National Hispanic Coalition Council. The wilderness area had local political support, with a resolution of support passing the Puerto Rican Senate. Rep. Nydia Velasquez was a co-sponsor from New York.

Rep. Jose Serrano stated he would be voting in favor. There were no private inholdings in the wilderness, and no competing or opposing interests.

I worked on the congressional writing of the bill, meeting with legislative aides from the House, and obtained approval from Sen. Clinton's legislative aide, Dan Utech, and director. They suggested co-sponsorship by New York's senior senator, Charles Schumer, and we obtained this. Next was delivery to the Senate cloakroom. But then the Senate adjourned, and we had to start all over again in the next Congress. The bill was introduced again in the fall of 2004 and passed. In December 2005, President Bush signed the El Toro Wilderness Act into law.

I visited Puerto Rico in Spring 2005 and hiked through the rainy tropical forest to the summit of El Toro. (See Figure 13.3.) It was a spectacular misty view, but I saw no Puerto Rican parrots. Notably, I didn't see a human soul on the 3-mile hike! About 850,000 visitors enjoy the Caribbean National Forest each year, mostly near the El Yunque Mountain and nearby hiking trails. Sen. Clinton's gift to me was a framed version of the bill's cover!

FIGURE 13.3   Caribbean National Forest wild and scenic rivers and El Toro Wilderness Area

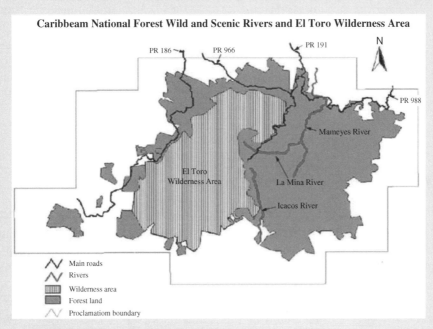

Source: Reprinted with permission from the U.S. Forest Service.

The principles of wilderness stewardship are to attain the highest level of purity in wilderness within legal restraints. The Wilderness Act specifies that administrators protect the character of wilderness. It is important to preserve air and water quality. Solitude must be protected. There needs to be a priority to favor wilderness-dependent activities. It is necessary to develop specific management objectives in concert with the public. Howard Zahniser, author of the Wilderness Act, emphasized the "wilderness philosophy of protecting areas at their boundaries and trying to let natural forces operate within the wilderness untrammeled by man."[6]

The nondegradation principle inherent in the law requires that whatever the ecological "purity" of an area when it was designated, it is to be administered thence forward toward the wilderness ideal. To train managers as stewards from all four federal wilderness management agencies, the Arthur Carhart National Wilderness Training Center, and the Aldo Leopold Wilderness Research Institute were established in Missoula, Montana, in 1993.

To protect wilderness, environmentalists often would recommend buffer zones outside of a wilderness area, whereas federal bureaucrats would draw the buffers inside the wilderness to protect against roads on the edge. Congress stated its intent against buffer zones when establishing wilderness; instead they drew the lines right to the edge of a road or development to take the place of buffer zones. Inholdings of private land within wilderness areas create a potential conflict since private individuals must be given access to their properties. The affected agency can negotiate a land swap or a purchase from those willing to do so. The Wilderness Land Trust was organized in 1992 just to obtain inholdings until the affected agency has the funds to purchase it. The Trust for Public Land and the Nature Conservancy perform similar national functions.

Current Wilderness Legislation

Sen. Jeff Bingaman (D-NM) introduced the **Omnibus Public Lands Management Act** of 2009, which included sixteen separate wilderness bills, totaling more than 2 million acres across nine states. The Senate met in a special Sunday session to overcome a threatened filibuster that had hobnailed the Senate. Key components of this bill included:

- The California Desert and Mountain Heritage Act, designating 190,000 acres of wilderness in Joshua Tree National Park

- 470,000 acres of the Eastern Sierra and Northern San Gabriel Heritage Act, protecting High Sierra and glacial valleys where the world's oldest tree, the bristlecone pine, lives
- The Sequoia and Kings Canyon National Parks Wilderness Act, designating 90,000 acres of wilderness, including the largest stand of Giant Sequoias trees in the redwood Mountain Grove
- The Dominguez–Escalante National Conservation Area of 210,000 acres and the 66,000 acre Dominguez Canyon Wilderness, preserving red rock cliffs and ancient petroglyphs and dwellings
- The 250,000-acre Rocky Mountain National Park Wilderness, providing world-class hiking and rock climbing with spectacular views of the Rocky Mountains
- The Owyhee Public Lands Management Act for wild and scenic river designation for Idaho's high desert Owyhee River and also provided more than a half-million acres of wilderness and range management in a local, consensus-driven process
- 23,000 acres in Oregon's Cascade-Siskiyou National Monument that resolved grazing permit issues
- The Copper Salmon Wilderness, protecting 13,000 acres of old growth and cedar forests in the headwaters of the Elk River in Oregon
- The Lewis and Clark Mt. Hood Wilderness, designating 130,000 acres of wilderness, including the towering Mt. Hood
- 30,000 acres of Oregon Badlands as wilderness, protecting lava flows, numerous Native American pictographs, and ancient juniper trees
- 8,600 acres of wilderness in Oregon's John Day River
- 37,000 acres in West Virginia's Monongahela National Forest
- 40,000 acres in Virginia's Jefferson National Forest
- 11,000 acres within the Pictured Rocks National Lakeshore along Michigan's coast of Lake Superior
- 235,000 acres of wilderness in and around Zion National Park in Washington County in Utah

It also provided for a land exchange in the Izembek National Wildlife Refuge that unfortunately allowed a road to bisect the refuge.

This bill also codified the National Landscape Conservation System, which is a 26 million-acre collection of national monuments, wilderness areas, scenic rivers, trails, and historic sites in the Bureau of Land Management. The conservation system is focused on preserving intact western landscapes with historical antiquities in their original settings.

LIVERPOOL JOHN MOORES UNIVERSITY
LEARNING SERVICES

The Land and Water Conservation Fund and the Forest Legacy Program

The **Land and Water Conservation Fund** was created in 1964 to provide a source of money to acquire at-risk places inside or close by national forests, parks, and other public lands. It was to be funded at $900 million from off-shore oil and gas royalties. The fund has provided $3.5 billion for 40,000 projects on 4.7 million acres. It has provided critical support for Redwoods National Park, Everglades National Park, Denali National Park, and the Appalachian Trail to purchase inholdings. However, there has been a 72% decline in funding the past decade, and the full amount has been appropriated only twice in the four decades of existence. Only 16% of the $900 million is going for its stated purpose, and the 2008 budget proposed only 6%. In August 2010 the U.S. House passed H.R. 3534, the Consolidated Land, Energy, and Aquatic Resources (CLEAR) Act, which included full funding for the Land and Water Conservation Fund at $900 million. The bill included many provisions to facilitate the cleanup and restoration of the Gulf of Mexico in the wake of the Deepwater oil disaster.

Similar to the Land and Water Conservation Fund, the **Forest Legacy Program** was created to help states protect private forest lands from development, primarily through purchase of conservation easements; to date it has funded $221.7 million for 1 million acres of protection in national forests. However, it has also suffered from budgetary constraints, with only $57.3 million appropriated in 2007 and $29 million budgeted in 2008. The program when it was created authorized $100 million per year.

National Wild and Scenic Rivers Act

In order to protect the nation's rivers, the National **Wild and Scenic Rivers Act** of 1968 was enacted. It serves to protect designated free-flowing rivers that have "outstanding remarkable scenic, recreational, geologic, fish and wildlife, historic, cultural and other similar values." The act says these rivers "shall be preserved in the free-flowing condition, and that they and their immediate environments shall be protected for the benefit and enjoyment of present and future generations."

As of 2008, the national system protects more than 11,000 miles of 166 rivers in thirty-eight states and the Commonwealth of Puerto Rico (out of 3.5 million U.S. river miles); this is little more than one-quarter of 1% of the nation's rivers. By comparison, more than 75,000 large dams across the country have modified at least 600,000 miles, or about 17% of U.S. rivers. Rivers may be designated by Congress or, if certain requirements are met, by the Secretary of the Interior. Each river is administered by either a federal or state agency. Designated segments need not include the entire river and may include tributaries. For federally administered rivers, the designated boundaries generally average one-quarter mile on either bank in the lower forty-eight states and one-half mile on rivers outside national parks in Alaska in order to protect river-related values.

Rivers are classified as wild, scenic, or recreational. Wild river areas are those rivers or sections of rivers that are free of impoundments and generally inaccessible except by trail, with watersheds or shorelines essentially primitive and waters unpolluted. These represent vestiges of primitive America. Scenic river areas are those rivers or sections of rivers that are free of impoundments, with shorelines or watersheds still largely primitive and shorelines largely undeveloped but accessible in places by roads. Recreational river areas are those rivers or sections of rivers that are readily accessible by road or railroad, that may have some development along their shorelines, and that may have undergone some impoundment or diversion in the past. Protection by this law does not impede development on private property within the designated wild or scenic river.

The Endangered Species Act

The **Endangered Species Act** (ESA) of 1973 created a program for the conservation of threatened and endangered plants and animals and the habitats in which they are found. The law prohibits "taking" an endangered or listed species or any activity adversely affecting its habitat. *Critical habitat* is defined as sufficiently large tracts of old growth forest for the spotted owl or adequate water flow in the Little Tennessee River for the snail darter, which may adversely affect the plans for a dam. The act called upon every department and agency of the federal government to work explicitly toward protecting endangered and threatened species. It required the federal government to cooperate with state governments and it pledged the United States to live up to international treaties whose purpose is to conserve species facing extinction. The act makes it illegal to destroy critical habitat, even on private land. The act has a Safe Harbor clause whereby landowners agree to protect habitat in exchange for assurances that more restrictive limits will not be imposed on their property.

The main federal agency involved in enforcing this act is the U.S. Fish and Wildlife Service (FWS). This organization has listed 1,370 endangered species under the act. Only thirty-nine have been removed from the threatened or endangered list; this included nine who went extinct. Sixteen were removed when it was discovered they really were not imperiled; only fourteen have recovered enough to be delisted. These low numbers probably reflect the fact that the act has encountered considerable political and economic inertia. The Yellowstone grizzly bears and Western Great Lakes gray wolf (timberwolf) were recently delisted. Polar bears have been proposed as "threatened." There are 309 species listed as threatened or likely to become endangered in the foreseeable future. Critical habitat has been designated for only 520 species.

A species candidate for listing must undergo a scientific review and a public comment period. A review of U.S. Fish and Wildlife Service and Marine Fisheries Service listings showed that the longer species were listed, the more likely they were to be improving and the less likely to be declining.[9] Species with critical habitat for two or more years appeared to be more likely to be improving and less likely to be declining than species without.[9] Dedicated recovery plans assisted species recovery; multispecies recovery plans were less effective; listing and regulation of any takings (trapping, hunting, any kind of harvesting) assisted in species recovery; ESA protections did not favor animals over plants; and endangered species showed less recovery than threatened species.

The cause celebré for the Endangered Species Act was the bald eagle, the U.S. national symbol. Currently the bald eagle has made such a dramatic comeback from being threatened that it is being studied for delisting. In 1963, there were 417 breeding pairs due to egg thinning caused by the pesticide DDT. In 2000, there were 6,471 breeding pairs in the lower forty-eight states. Finally, in 2007 there were about 10,000 breeding pairs, and the bald eagle was delisted. The 1940 Eagle Act prohibited disturbing eagles, and the Fish and Wildlife Service had issued rules defining disturbances in implementing the Act. They issued a draft environmental assessment rather than an environmental impact statement, because defining *disturb* did not constitute a major federal action.

The FWS prepares biennial reports on the Endangered Species Act and recently scored 1,095 species as still declining, stable, or improving. Recovery plans are critical. During the final weeks of the Bush administration, the Department of the Interior issued a rule that largely freed federal agencies such as the Army Corps of Engineers and the Federal Highway Administration from their obligation to consult independent wildlife biologists or fisheries specialists before they build dams or highways, permit construction of transmission towers, housing developments, or other projects that might harm federally protected wildlife. This rule was immediately challenged in court by environmental organizations.

Summary

Wilderness environmental policy involves federal agencies in the Departments of Interior (National Parks Service, Fish and Wildlife Service, Bureau of Land Management) and Agriculture (U.S. Forest Service). There are inherent conflicts between these agencies, for example, forestry practice is to develop sustained yield and multiple uses of forests, creating a less advantageous environment for the protection of wilderness, whereas the National Park Service has protection of the environment as its primary mission. The Bureau of Land Management is the laggard in protecting wilderness among federal agencies. The Wilderness Act codified the protection of wilderness. A federal wilderness area receives the highest level of protection. The courts are involved in defining statutes and intent of Congress. The Supreme Court occasionally has a wilderness case to hear. Last, the executive agencies have considerable leeway in management decisions that could affect wilderness, particularly in those areas not yet protected. Vigilance by the public is everlasting.

Key Terms

Adirondack Park Act

Bureau of Land Management

Conservation easements

Eastern Wilderness Act

Endangered American Wilderness Act

Endangered Species Act

Forest Legacy Program

Land and Water Conservation Fund

Multiple land use

Omnibus Public Lands Management Act

Purity theory

Roadless Rule

U.S. Forest Service

Wild and Scenic Rivers Act

Wilderness Act

Discussion Questions

1. How does the wilderness contribute to public health?
2. Describe the Wilderness Act.
3. What were some of the challenges made to the Wilderness Act?
4. What are some current problems facing those who wish to protect wilderness?

5. Create an outline of New York's wilderness protection history.
6. What are some of the political and economic forces that affect wilderness protection in New York?
7. How is New York's wilderness currently being protected?
8. What are some measures that could be taken in the future to expand and protect New York's wilderness?
9. Discuss some of the current legislation that exists regarding wilderness protection.
10. Describe the Land and Water Conservation Fund.
11. How successful has the Endangered Species Act been?

CHAPTER 14

ENVIRONMENTAL POLICY AND ADVOCACY GROUPS

The Wilderness Society: A Case Study

William H. Meadows

LEARNING OBJECTIVES

- To understand the important role that environmental advocacy groups play in environmental policy
- To become familiar with the goals and actions of the Wilderness Society
- To understand the roles of the different branches of government in protecting the wilderness
- To become familiar with the laws that dictate wilderness protection

One might say the wilderness movement is the progeny of the negative side of President Franklin Delano Roosevelt's New Deal. While many of the public works projects created by the New Deal served useful ends, others resulted in irreversible damage to the land by pushing new roads into the hinterlands. In 1935, eight men—three of them professional foresters—concerned about the metastasizing invasion of roads and machines into the last remnants of wild country, decided to put a stop to the degradation and formed the **Wilderness Society**.

One of the founders was Bob Marshall, a frenetic hiker and tireless advocate for land preservation, who asserted that "there is just one hope of repulsing the tyrannical ambition of civilization to conquer every niche of the whole earth. That hope is the organization of spirited people who will fight for the freedom of the wilderness." This spirit of informed activism still drives the Wilderness Society today as it fulfills its mission to protect wilderness and inspire the American people to care for their nation's fast-disappearing wild places.

Federal Public Lands and Wilderness

The Wilderness Society has played a unique and significant role in the history and stewardship of the federal public lands, a rich and extensive system encompassing 623 million acres of deserts, mountains, forests, rivers, and wetlands. This system includes all of the nation's national parks, national forests, wild and scenic rivers, and national wildlife refuges along with the vast Western territories overseen by the Bureau of Land Management (BLM). Some of the wildest, untouched portions of these federal land units comprise the **National Wilderness Preservation System (NWPS)**, which boasts a total of 109 million acres of designated wilderness.

Wilderness is the highest form of land protection in the world. Here, nature is left to its own devices and people are merely the visitors who do not remain. Created through specific acts of Congress, wilderness areas must forever remain free from roads, mechanical devices, or human structures of any kind. The extra layer of security afforded a piece of land via the designation process is there to ensure that its values will endure in perpetuity.

The driving force guiding the Wilderness Society is a fundamental commitment to the principle that the United States needs a well-governed system of public lands accessible to all citizens, as well as more designated wilderness to benefit those same citizens. To that end, it continually grapples with the notion of what deserves wilderness protection and what may need protection of another type. In addition, its job is to make certain that the nation's most pristine wild lands are not compromised before Congress has a chance to act to make them part of the NWPS.

For more than seven decades, the Wilderness Society has been a leader in the conservation world in three key areas: (1) monitoring the policies and practices that affect the long-term viability of the federal public land system, (2) influencing governmental decisions about which activities will be allowed to occur within the system's borders, and (3) pushing Congress to enact wilderness and other types of protective legislation. Conservationists by trade take a far-sighted approach to the land and continually seek ways to coalesce the people, policies, and politics around the vision of achieving a healthy and sustainable planet.

Why Wilderness?

Public lands and wilderness play a significant, if largely unseen, role in the health of local communities and the country as a whole. The ecosystem services that flow from U.S. public lands for the most part are uncounted national assets, which nevertheless directly benefit the taxpayers who own them. Natural filtration systems clean the air and purify the headwaters from which cities downstream eventually drink. Federal landscapes will also play an expanded role in meeting the nation's need for renewable energy and addressing the impacts of global warming.

The National Forest System alone, a diverse and complex land base managed by the **U.S. Forest Service** under the auspices of the Department of Agriculture, encompasses a total of 193 million acres of native forests and grasslands. With the oxygen these woodlands emit and carbon dioxide they absorb and sequester, national forests are a functioning and very vital component of the United States' "lungs."

When the idea of creating the first national parks was originally promoted at the end of the nineteenth century, parklands were recognized for their intrinsic value and were not expected to carry any economic weight. Rather, the taxpayers would carry the cost—because parks benefitted the citizenry. The irony is that since that idealistic beginning, the United States generally has devalued most of what our public lands add to the health and well-being of the country.

The wilderness areas found within the National Wilderness Preservation System, which jewel our public lands, serve an additional purpose. Unaltered by human intervention, these special places remain safe havens—sometimes the only untouched habitat left—for a plethora of species. As such, they are repositories of biodiversity and offer a wealth of opportunity for future scientific discoveries.

Not to be overlooked are the health benefits derived from the mere presence of wild lands across the country where families can get outside and recreate. The federal public lands, open to all, offer an attractive alternative to the sedentary

WILDERNESS AND HEALTH: TAXOL

The story of the drug Taxol® is a prime example of the kinds of rich and diverse biological surprises still awaiting recognition in the twenty-first century. A historical marker commemorates the general area in the Gifford Pinchot National Forest of Washington state where in 1963 a team of botanists collected bark from the Pacific yew tree, a species found in old-growth forests. (The overwhelming majority of the ancient forests still extant in this country—trees ranging from about 150 to more than 800 years old—subsist only on public lands.) The discovery of a natural product produced from the Pacific yew led to the anti-cancer compound, Taxol, now used to treat refractory ovarian cancer, breast and lung cancers, and Kaposi's sarcoma. Wilderness areas may prove to be this country's most valuable untapped source of future pharmacological discoveries and other innovative products—many of them derived from species surviving exclusively within an ever-shrinking pool of undisturbed habitat.

American lifestyle and one possible answer to how the nation might begin addressing its burgeoning obesity epidemic.

The spiritual value of wilderness in our stressed-out, overly mechanized twenty-first-century world cannot be overstated either. In his seminal "Wilderness Letter," celebrated author Wallace Stegner called wilderness the "geography of hope" and posited that it was important simply because it existed. "The reminder and reassurance that it is still there," he said, "is good for our spiritual health even if we never once in ten years set foot in it."[1]

One might begin to understand the inexorable pull of wild places on people and the innate ability of the land to feed the human spirit by considering the enormous impact a relatively small patch of green called Central Park has on the city of New York. A shift in energy seems to occur just by walking a few steps off the sidewalk from the frenzy of the urban jungle into the park's grassy meadows. Wilderness offers this same kind of respite on a grander, national scale—from the smallest wilderness area, the Rock and Islands Wilderness in Northern California (5 acres), to the largest one in the entire system, Alaska's Wrangell-St. Elias Wilderness at 9,078,675 acres.

Political Framework

Guiding the direction and day-to-day management of the federal public land system is a multilayered and diverse array of congressional committees, federal agencies, statutes, and administrative regulations. Two cabinet-level departments—Interior and Agriculture—have jurisdiction over the four major land management agencies: the U.S. Forest Service, the U.S. Fish and Wildlife Service, the National Park Service, and the Bureau of Land Management. Each agency, in turn, is governed by an organic act or similar statute, which delineates that agency's mission and legal responsibilities. All of these have headquarters in Washington, D.C., as well as unique regional, district, or state structures.

Nongovernmental organizations (**NGOs**) like the Wilderness Society must be cognizant of every layer of authority and be prepared to influence the decision making that occurs up and down the hierarchical ladder. It is incumbent on us to be primed to intercede if and when decisions on any rung of this ladder might adversely affect specific wild places or the public land system as a whole.

The ideal and most effective advocate in the fast-moving political arena has a deep understanding of the processes involved in shaping good policy and can provide some oversight to its implementation. The advocacy process involves cultivating solid, bipartisan relationships with government officials as well as producing irrefutable data to bolster the case for land protection. Conservationists must be able to interact competently with every decision maker who has relevance on land use issues, including members of Congress and their staffs on Capitol Hill, the federal agencies at the national and local levels, and even state governments. (Governors usually have well-honed political skills and operate very cognizant of what happens to the federal lands within their states' borders.)

The tension in a democracy is for the decision makers to find the right balance between being responsive to individual citizens and interest groups and at the same time crafting policies that will afford the greatest good to the greatest number. The Wilderness Society's role is to help these leaders act as honest brokers on issues related to the public lands and wilderness.

In general, the management of the public lands—especially the landscapes overseen by the Bureau of Land Management and the U.S. Forest Service—has been guided by two major principles: **multiple use** and **sustainable yield**. The constant tug of war is over what exactly will be allowed to happen on the ground under these standards. Timber, mining, oil and gas, motorized recreation, and other industries look to the public lands as a source of development and profits. At the same time, hunters, anglers, hikers, and campers seek solitude, the opportunity to experience nature, and wildlife protection. Added to the mix are wilderness proponents who want to preserve more acreage in its natural condition—often in many of the same areas coveted by the extractive industries. The question then becomes, What is the best use of the nation's wild lands now and in the future? Parsing the difference between sustaining the land's ecological and more spiritual values versus exploiting its economic value falls to the legislators and administrative rule makers.

Historically, the unequal amount of power and influence wielded by groups with access to corporate money often left private citizens with little say about what played out on their public lands. Espousing the principle that conservation values should weigh heavily in every land use decision, advocacy organizations began to change that equation in the 1970s by gathering together citizen activists and combining forces to effect large-scale change.

NGOs such as the Environmental Defense Fund (>500,000 members), the Natural Resources Defense Council (1,200,000 members), the Sierra Club (1,300,000 members), and the Wilderness Society (400,000 members) represent hundreds of thousands of like-minded individuals from every corner of the country. Members have entrusted these organizations with the job of holding the government accountable to a conservation perspective. In addition, these groups provide information and expertise in support of the "green" perspective and help codify it into law. Stuart Brandborg, who served as the Wilderness Society's president from 1964 through 1976, described this phenomenon as tapping into the "strength of determined citizens who have realized their own power."

The Wilderness Society and Public Policy

Advocacy groups play a pivotal role when laws are passed and policies enacted. The Wilderness Society intersects with public policy on three fronts: (1) Congress, where the laws get written and federal dollars are appropriated; (2) the administration, which includes institutions such as the White House, the four federal land management agencies, and the Council on Environmental Quality; and (3) the courts.

Congress

Times have changed radically since Howard Zahniser, author of the Wilderness Act of 1964, spent eight long years midwifing every word of the statute and promoting it to both friend and foe in Congress. The notion that a single individual would author most of the text for a potential piece of legislation is an anathema today. In fact, when e-mails were uncovered during President George W. Bush's tenure revealing that the text of a piece of legislation was written by industry, it caused a firestorm in the press.

Developing policy was much less complex and rallied far fewer interest groups in Zahniser's day. He had direct access to a less formal way of doing business on Capitol Hill. Significantly, the "sunshine" laws passed in the 1970s, which were designed to increase public disclosure of governmental agencies following the Watergate scandal, were not in place at that time. There was no specific requirement to provide public access to information on the special interest groups that may have influenced lawmakers before a bill reached the floor.

The overall role of the **policy advocate** has grown during the past few decades. National conservation groups today boast an enormous amount of professional expertise, partially because the individuals who staff congressional offices and the federal agencies are experts in their own rights. Laws get written and policies change when pressure is brought to bear on Capitol Hill. But before anyone will listen to us, we need to establish our bona fides and prove our credibility to a continually shifting set of decision makers. That means maintaining a sterling reputation for integrity and unwavering commitment to the facts. As a counterweight, nearly every industry employs highly skilled lobbyists who know the issues inside out and will usually add a contrary but valid perspective to the dialogue. Some of the best, most representative laws passed by Congress emerge from this messy but creative cauldron of competing ideas and conflicting viewpoints.

The key to creating good national policy legislatively is to find a core group of congressional backers who will champion an issue. Those champions, in turn, rely heavily on their staffs, who must be well informed about the broad array of questions involved and convinced that the cost of backing a particular piece of legislation will be worth the political capital expended. To that end, groups like the Wilderness Society must present the most compelling case possible for land protection while also demonstrating that constituents from the member's local district understand, believe in, and actively support the proposed solutions.

What is clear today is that the sheer volume and breathtaking range of policy issues in play at any given moment on Capitol Hill is staggering. It is almost impossible for any single member of Congress to be thoroughly grounded in every issue in order to make smart decisions about complex policy areas. For example, in most cases a senator or representative will not understand the particular place, unique ecology, or long-term impact of development on a certain type of landscape. But teams of scientists working on the ground for conservation organizations do. Policy advocates must package and disseminate research findings in a way that clearly explains the issue in question, builds an airtight case for preservation, and provides members of Congress with the tools to convince their colleagues.

Public Land Legislation

A suite of laws passed over the past thirty-plus years describes the missions of the four federal land management agencies and outlines what can and should occur on U.S. public lands. The Wilderness Society continually monitors what is happening within the boundaries of the public land system, contests inappropriate activities, and proposes sustainable solutions to land use problems. Several important laws govern agency actions and provide the basis for the Wilderness Society's activism. We discuss three of these acts.

The Federal Land Policy and Management Act Passed in 1976, the **Federal Land Policy and Management Act (FLPMA)** repealed the archaic public land disposal laws (except for the General Mining Law of 1872) and became the governing statute for the millions of acres of Western wild lands overseen by the **Bureau of Land Management (BLM)**. The act stated that these lands were to be retained for the long-term use of the American people unless "it is determined that disposal of a particular parcel will serve the national interest." It also made the process of land use planning the cornerstone of how the agency managed the land. FLPMA stipulated that the "United States receive fair market value of the use of the public lands and their resources," and that the government "give priority to the designation and protection of areas of critical environmental concern" to preserve historic, cultural and natural values.

As one can imagine, vexing questions could arise from many possible—and extremely broad—interpretations of this law. Which areas are actually of critical environmental concern? What amount of resource extraction should be allowed to occur before it will detrimentally affect the long-term use of the land by the American people?

Stewardship of all 258 million acres of BLM land is rooted in the public processes established by FLPMA, and Wilderness Society staff regularly comment on every stage of the agency's land use planning process to raise issues of concern as those plans evolve. Part of that job involves generating scientific research and submitting information for inclusion in the public record. It is equally essential to rally public support to add an even stronger voice for the conservation perspective to the debate. The desired outcome is ecologically sound land use plans to guide the BLM as it moves forward.

Of direct interest to the Wilderness Society's organization is how much of its land the BLM will set aside in the plans to protect as potential wilderness during the period before Congress can act to designate it. Establishing such interim protection is a vital step in the movement toward official wilderness designation, since wilderness values are easily compromised by activities such as off-road vehicle abuse, oil and gas drilling, hard rock mining, road construction, logging, and other types of development.

A large segment of the Wilderness Society's conservation portfolio involves monitoring the BLM's responses to a growing menu of requests for access to the land from industry and other interest groups, requests that emerge outside of the land use planning process. For example, from 2001 through 2007 the BLM issued more permits for oil and gas exploration and drilling than at any other time in its history, many of the potential leases in fragile, wilderness-quality landscapes. Under the federal multiple use mandate, energy development is allowed on the public lands. But the core conundrum is how to strike the correct balance between that use and others, including the preservation of biodiversity and solitude. Where and how much energy development should occur?

A similar and no less significant problem is the proliferation of powerful off-road vehicles that inevitably tear up the backcountry. In states such as Utah, and increasingly all over the West, off-road vehicle abuse by all-terrain vehicles (ATVs) and dirt bikes arguably has become the single greatest threat to wild land viability. This problem begs the question of how much and what kind of recreation should be allowed to occur on our public lands—and where. If the conservation community cannot halt the improper use of the land under FLPMA through legislative or administrative means, they may seek satisfaction through the courts.

National Wildlife Refuge System Improvement Act   For almost a century, the **U.S. Fish and Wildlife Service** managed the 150-million-acre National Wildlife Refuge System under a variety of laws—without an "organic act" or comprehensive piece of legislation spelling out how it ought to be managed and used by the public. But in October 1997 that statutory hole was filled. President Bill Clinton signed the **National Wildlife Refuge System Improvement Act (NWRSIA)** to ensure that the refuge system would be managed as a national system of related lands, waters, and interests for the protection and conservation of the nation's wildlife resources. As the only system devoted

THE BLM AND FLPMA

Two seminal moments in the history of the BLM stand out. The first was the passage of FLPMA, which directed an agency previously labeled by some with the moniker "Bureau of Livestock and Mining" toward a mission that recognized the importance of conservation on the land it manages. The second saw the expression of that mission in the form of a national system of conservation lands, when more than thirty years later, in March 2009, Congress made the National Landscape Conservation System permanent. For the first time the BLM became the overseer of a permanent system of protected areas set aside primarily for conservation purposes, much like the lands managed by the Park Service and Fish and Wildlife Service. This watershed act may forever transform the way this agency sees itself and how it approaches the landscapes it manages.

specifically to wildlife, it supports a network of diverse and strategically located habitats in every state of the union: 549 refuges in all.

The refuge organic act defines a strong and singular wildlife conservation mission for the nation's wildlife refuges and directs the Secretary of the Interior to maintain the biological integrity, diversity, and environmental health of the system. It also requires each refuge to prepare a comprehensive conservation plan. In addition, the act established a new process for determining which activities would be considered "compatible uses" for refuge lands.

NWRSIA provides guidance and legal boundaries for both the Fish and Wildlife Service and outside interest groups advocating a particular perspective on how refuge landscapes should be managed. For instance, compatible use is the seminal issue in the ongoing debate over whether to build a road through the Izembek National Wildlife Refuge in Alaska to link the tiny communities of Kings Cove and Cold Bay. The entire world population of Pacific black brant stops to feed at the Izembek Refuge, and virtually all of the world's emperor goose population passes through. Besides millions more birds, this habitat supports brown bear, wolves, wolverines, tundra hares, sea otters, salmon, and thousands of harbor seals. The central land use question revolves around whether a road would undermine the reason the refuge was created in the first place. Conservationists believe it would.

National Forest Management Act   Created in 1976, partially out of the confusion surrounding the policies then governing America's national forests, the National Forest Management Act (NFMA) was the single most far-reaching piece of forest legislation since the Forest Service was established in 1905. Ostensibly its purpose was to define forest management policies that both the timber industry and the public could understand.

While NFMA did not ban clear-cutting trees outright, it did severely limit that application and instructed the Forest Service to maintain species diversity— not just maximize the growth of those trees that are useful for commercial purposes. Further, the act stated that if all multiple use objectives are met, the sale of timber from each forest must be limited to a quantity equal to or less than that which the forest could replace on a sustained yield basis. Finally, NFMA required the development of land use plans—one plan to a forest—that would lay out in detail all the uses of the forest. These comprehensive plans would be subject to public review, possibly one of the act's most significant provisions.

Administrative Actions

Congress passes public land legislation and delegates its execution to the four federal land management agencies. Charged with implementing the law on the

CASE STUDY: NATIONAL FOREST MANAGEMENT ACT AND SPOTTED OWLS

The fact that ancient forests still inhabit portions of the Pacific Northwest is in part a testament to the impact and reach of the **National Forest Management Act (NFMA)**. The statute's requirement that every national forest develop a comprehensive, integrated land and resource management plan kicked off a nationwide planning process in the early 1980s. Planning started with the eastern woodlands, then moved west, finally reaching the Pacific Northwest mid-decade. It did not take the Forest Service long to realize that if logging were to continue in that region, the agency would have problems complying with NFMA's species diversity requirement. Its own regulations were even tougher than what was outlined in NFMA. Forest Service rules required more than just maintaining plant and animal communities; it had to ensure *viable populations of all native vertebrate species* found in the forest.

In the meantime, biologists and other experts from throughout the conservation community had strong and growing evidence that old-growth forests comprised unique habitat values, and that many species, including the northern spotted owl, required this type of habitat to maintain their viability. If ancient forests disappeared, so would the species. The issue came to a head when the Forest Service released land use plans for all the national forests in Oregon, Washington, and northwest California anyway—plans that included extensive areas where old-growth logging would still occur. The environmental community sued, and thus began a series of lawsuits and appeals that eventually resulted in court injunctions to halt the logging of old-growth habitat until the agency complied with the law.

It was not until President Clinton came to office in 1993 that the situation turned the corner. After a considerable amount of dialogue among timber workers, scientists, the green community, and the new administration, the White House decided to amend the original forest plans with an overarching plan to protect the old-growth forest ecosystem. It brought together a number of federal agencies with jurisdiction in the region to design and implement a scientifically credible blueprint for all of the national forests within the range of the northern spotted owl. The Northwest Forest Plan adopted in 1994 is an extraordinary example of success by conservation advocates after a tortuous journey that began with the passage of NFMA and ended nearly two decades later in a far-reaching and very positive outcome on the ground.

The hard-won lesson born of the spotted owl controversy was the importance and impact of science on public policy. Environmentalists must continually challenge the federal agencies to use the best possible science—and produce the needed research for those same agencies if they do not have the budget or expertise to complete it. In fact, agencies often learn a new way of looking at the world from the information presented in the comments during their land use planning processes. Facts about economic considerations, habitat fragmentation, migration corridors, and water quality are just a few examples of the data our community will bring to the table—subjects the land use plans might need to address to stay within the confines of the law.

ground, these agencies propose rules and regulations that outline how a given statute will be expressed on the land. The strictures and directives established by the rule-making process will guide an agency's day-to-day decisions and activities.

It is no longer enough for environmental organizations like the Wilderness Society to understand the innermost details of a particular issue; they must also have extensive expertise in how to navigate the complex regulatory system as mandated by law. To successfully affect land use practices and maintain the health of the land, interest groups must respect the constraints the federal agencies work under while at the same time recognizing the discretion they have to design solutions.

RULE MAKING

Regulations affecting the federal public lands do not originate exclusively through the Forest Service, Fish and Wildlife Service, Park Service, or Bureau of Land Management. Rules established and implemented by other federal agencies may also have an impact on the land. For example, in 1999 the Environmental Protection Agency (EPA) was responsible for a powerful rule—backed by solid public support—targeting the effect of air pollution on natural areas sometimes hundreds of miles away from the pollution's source. Prompted by the rapid decline in air quality and growing loss of "viewsheds" within some iconic parks, the EPA issued the Regional Haze Rule under the premise that it had a legal obligation to protect Class 1 natural areas.

The rule calls for state and federal agencies to work together to improve visibility in 156 national parks and wilderness areas such as the Grand Canyon, Yosemite, the Great Smokies, and Shenandoah. Its wide-ranging effect was to regulate industry emissions into the atmosphere for their longer-term environmental impact downwind. The new standard stipulated for the first time that industry must not only consider the effects of its pollution on city dwellers living within the immediate area of a smokestack but also on the health of the nation's natural resources writ large.

The other side of the rule-making coin is exemplified by a last-minute regulation finalized during the waning days of President George W. Bush's tenure in office. That rule allowed federal agencies to ignore the input of government scientists and decide for themselves whether highways, dams, mines, and other construction projects might harm endangered animals and plants. The new approach essentially eliminated the mandatory, independent reviews government scientists had performed for thirty-five years. In addition, the regulation prohibited federal agencies from assessing whether a development project contributed to global warming while evaluating the project's effect on species. This decision was an extreme blow to the conservation community and a potential death knell for any species on the edge of extinction.

The formal federal rule-making process, established by the Administrative Procedures Act, obligates a land management agency to take the will of the people into account before any proposed rule becomes the government's official policy. This directive, which requires agencies to request and consider public comments, offers the conservation community an extraordinary opportunity to add substance to the official record as well as give a voice to their members and other critical stakeholders before the final decision is made. The process also allows these same stakeholders to appeal a decision if it appears the agency has ignored crucial data or would violate the law by continuing down the course it is setting with the new rule.

Actions by the federal agencies are not entirely bound up in the regulatory structure. Since the 1990s, the norm has become for government officials to use other, less formal administrative tools to try to change the approach to land management. For example, the Secretaries of the Interior and Agriculture are free to issue to their staffs "instructional memoranda" that outline how an agency will deal with specific situations going forward.

While not as widely recognized as legislation or rule making, these kinds of internal actions—almost by fiat—can be some of the most potent tools an administration has at its disposal for instituting changes to public policies without any input from the American people. Unlike new regulations, which require an open public process to institute, or passing a law, which demands congressional support and action, the head of a federal agency can, with a single stroke of a pen, direct his or her staff to change the way they do business on the ground. Because this process can be misused, part of our job is to make certain the secretaries' authority to act is not improperly substituted for the regulatory process.

In 2003, the Wilderness Society experienced the repercussions of such a memo firsthand when then Secretary of the Interior, Gale Norton, issued a new instructional memo to field staff based on her reading and interpretation of the FLPMA statute. The memo ordered them to stop inventorying or protecting any more wilderness-quality lands. Short of convincing Congress to override her instructions through legislation, the conservation community had little recourse against the decision. Wilderness proponents spent the next five years in a defensive mode, trying to protect the land from a host of potential hazards before it fell victim to incursions from oil and gas development or unfettered off-road vehicle abuse.

Administrative Appeals and the Courts

Another leg of the public policy stool involves appealing to a higher authority when a federal agency violates environmental statutes or its own regulations, actions that may result in damage to the land. Through the land use planning processes and laws such as the National Environmental Policy Act (NEPA), Congress opened the way for the public to be able to comment on an agency's proposed plans and activities, appeal its decisions if warranted, and subject them to judicial review.

Most often, an administrative appeal will be presented to an appeals review board, normally comprised of impartial staff within a federal agency. Their charge is to take a fresh look at the dispute. If an internal appeal does not work and there is no higher authority to intercede, it may become necessary to bring the question before a federal judge for remediation. A lawsuit with written briefs and a hearing may proceed once the court has determined that the aggrieved party has legal standing in the case.

Over the years, the environmental community has earned a reputation for causing "too many lawsuits" and "tying things up in court." What is frequently overlooked is the indispensable watchdog role the community plays in making certain that the government follows the rules the public helped create and the laws established by elected members of Congress. While it is no doubt very difficult for federal agencies to strike the correct and very delicate balance among competing interest groups, in every case they must follow the law. Administrative and judicial appeals provide the means for all sides to present arguments for or against governmental actions.

Local Advocacy

Advocacy organizations above all must be credible, and part of that credibility stems from the recognition that solutions to land use problems must work locally as well as nationally. The Wilderness Act of 1964 was a national law, yet the growth of the National Wilderness Preservation System over nearly half a century is the direct result of locally based grassroots activism. In most cases, wilderness bills succeed when local partners, including smaller conservation advocacy groups and the people living on the ground near a proposed wilderness area, buy into the notion that wilderness designation will benefit their communities.

Before members of the House or Senate will lend their names to champion a wilderness bill, they want to know that a healthy number of the constituents in their districts embrace and support the proposal. If local media and state and county officials get behind the legislation, that is even better. Sometimes the governor of the state will speak out and take a pro-wilderness stance too.

The bulk of wilderness bills are bipartisan. During the horse-trading that occurs on Capitol Hill, senators and representatives from other states normally will vote for wilderness if the delegation from the state where the new area is located wants it. Because designation involves wild lands already in the public domain, wilderness legislation does not require money to expand the public estate. These bills simply add an extra layer of protection to a portion of it.

Reaching the tipping point, the optimal level of buy-in from all the interested stakeholders, is no easy task. Conservation groups face a heavy lift whenever they want to build public support for a piece of legislation or influence federal agency decisions about what happens on the land. Broad-based public education is a process that requires time, expertise, and patience. And occasionally, with extremely polarized and contentious issues such as protecting the Arctic National Wildlife Refuge from oil and gas drilling, the process of building public awareness and support has demanded decades of work.

The conservation community cannot just tell people what they want or need in their backyards; it must construct a solid case. The process may involve conducting original research or undertaking literature searches to create the scientific underpinnings for a proposal. It may also require funding local, regional, and national polls to assess public opinion. Once the facts are in place, communications experts will pitch the story to the traditional and online media—with the hope that the press will consider the issues compelling and important enough to cover.

Meanwhile, other staff must be in the field, attending local meetings and reaching out to officials such as mayors and county commissioners in addition to building trust and dialogue with community associations, business interests, garden clubs, and faith-based groups. Conservationists must convince these groups to listen to their input and convince them of the value of their cause. Additionally, conservationists face opposition as well. Usually opponents are conducting the same kind of effort to try to convince local stakeholders that wilderness is not the best choice for the land.

If and when the "noise" around a particular land use debate from the grassroots and the media becomes loud enough for Congress or a federal agency to take notice, the issue may begin to take hold. Political power increases geometrically when individuals work together to enact change—be they the members of a national conservation organization or a rural community situated near the border of a piece of federal land.

Wilderness Future

Among the myriad reasons to continue to set aside more unspoiled wilderness in the twenty-first century, the looming crisis of global warming may be paramount.

CASE STUDY: ROADLESS AREAS

No one has yet written the complete history of the battle over national forest roadless areas, possibly the highest-profile forest issue of the twentieth century. But if it were chronicled, that saga would tell the tale of a long and winding path through land use planning, administrative actions, and the courts.

At about the same moment the new national forest planning process kicked off in the 1980s, a second major development in forest policy started to emerge, this time on the wilderness front. In 1984 Congress designated 6.8 million acres of new wilderness on national forest lands in twenty states. The lands they chose to designate had been part of a process called RARE II (roadless area review and evaluation) begun by the Forest Service a decade earlier. After Congress acted, the remainder of the RARE II lands not part of its wilderness package—another 58.5 million unroaded acres—were left in limbo and released back into individual forest planning processes. A huge unanswered question remained: What would become of these unspoiled areas? How would the agency manage them going forward?

Not willing to lose so much potential wilderness either by direct encroachment or default, the Wilderness Society invested significant organizational resources to find ways to protect the roadless areas until Congress could take a second look at them as possible wilderness candidates. We pressed the Forest Service to maintain the wilderness character of each area and deployed ecologists and economists to conduct research to prove their value to plant and animal species and human communities—as well as to demonstrate the unreasonably high cost of resource extraction. Meanwhile, the environmental community as a whole was raising public awareness about the significant benefits the nation accrued from roadless forests, heightening public concern about their possible loss.

The battle to preserve the last vestiges of unspoiled forest lands has continued for more than two decades, many times forest by forest—in a system that encompasses a total of 144 national forests and grasslands. Decades after these lands were first identified through the RARE II process, increased public awareness and growing questions about the economic sense of having the taxpayers subsidize new logging roads into pristine forests, finally led the Clinton administration to issue the Roadless Area Conservation Rule, adopted in January 2001. The Roadless Rule, which generally prohibited road building and logging in all 58.5 million acres of inventoried roadless areas, garnered 1.7 million public comments, becoming the most extensive public involvement process in the history of federal rule making.

Despite the Roadless Rule's obvious and historic level of public support, the rule ran into immediate trouble when President George W. Bush took office. Because the new administration did not believe in the rule, it handicapped the Clinton-era regulation by repeatedly undercutting its provisions and failing to defend it against legal challenges in court. In 2005, the Bush administration attempted to replace the national rule with a state petition process, a procedure that would allow individual states to decide what happened to roadless lands on federal property. Conflicting decisions and injunctions have been issued for and against the rule in courts in California and Wyoming over the past several years, with appeals pending.

Remarkably, almost all the roadless areas emerged unscathed from the Bush administration's eight-year assault. As of early 2009, only 7 miles of road building and 600 acres of logging have occurred within almost 60 million acres of inventoried national forest roadless areas. But this story is not over yet. Pressures for resource exploitation continue to threaten roadless areas across the nation, from phosphate mining in Idaho near Yellowstone National Park to logging in New Hampshire's White Mountains. Conservationists are committed to finding a way to protect national forest roadless areas in perpetuity. Since administrative rules are subject to the vagaries of politics, the long-term solution—if not through formal wilderness designation—would most likely be another type of legislative fix.

Alaska's coastlines are eroding at a precipitous pace; birds have begun to winter farther north; the proliferation of insect infestations is felling trees and in the process fueling catastrophic wildfires; iconic wildlife species have changed their migration patterns or are disappearing altogether.

America's public lands comprise the largest and most comprehensive wild land system in this country, and wilderness represents some of the only large, intact habitat left anywhere in the United States. No one yet knows what will be needed for species adaptation as the climate continues to change. Sustaining the wild open spaces we own in common offers us maximum flexibility in uncertain times. Where will native creatures go when their habitats shrink or vanish if we have not set aside enough space for them to migrate and thrive?

By some estimates there are at least 200 million more acres of possible wilderness within the lower forty-eight states and Alaska. The Wilderness Society has those potential acres in its sights to achieve the long-term vision for the United States our founders saw. As important as these landscapes are, however, the Wilderness Society also recognizes that federally designated wilderness alone will never be enough to preserve the full complement of diverse species and life-sustaining processes necessary to maintain our nation under the new world order.

Both citizens and politicians alike must begin to think more broadly and approach the climate problem with new and creative solutions. The answer may involve linking state and private lands to the federal estate to form additional migration corridors. It may mean investing significantly more dollars in the federal land management agencies to provide the resources necessary for them to manage the land for global warming and safeguard critical ecosystems and watersheds. It undoubtedly will require all of us to erase the human-made borders in our minds that stop us from seeing nature's processes in their totality and wholeness.

The secondary challenge is for us to shepherd in this new era of greenhouse gas reduction and powering up renewable energy sources in an eco-friendly manner. It would be a grave mistake to trade one environmental problem for another by developing the infrastructure for renewable energy—transmission lines, wind towers, and other facilities—in a way that damages fragile, wild landscapes. Sustainability must become the guiding principle of a new land ethic that will manifest in our policies, laws, and activities on the ground.

The future of our wildest places is bright with possibility if we remain committed, smart, and willing to approach the natural world with humility and care.

Summary

Environmental advocacy groups are nonprofit and present information about the environment to protect the public health. This includes air, water, and land. The Wilderness Society has a focus on land issues, particularly wilderness. More than 100 million acres have been protected, and 200 million remain. The activities of these groups focus on making environmental policy through legislation in Congress, through executive agencies' policies, and through the courts when an agency of the federal government appears to be violating the law. Environmental groups have access to congressional staffs and members, staff and political appointees of the executive branch, and can sue or join as friends of the court in federal lawsuits. They have large memberships who can directly influence opinion from letters, through newspapers, funding research initiatives by the nonprofits, and advocating locally for a wilderness area or environmental solution. They are the grass roots of activism. Last, their members vote in large numbers.

Key Terms

Bureau of Land Management (BLM)

Federal Land Policy and Management Act (FLPMA)

Multiple use

National Forest Management Act (NFMA)

National Wilderness Preservation System (NWPS)

National Wildlife Refuge System Improvement Act (NWRSIA)

Nongovernmental organizations (NGOs)

Policy advocate

Sustainable yield

U.S. Fish and Wildlife Service

U.S. Forest Service

The Wilderness Society

Discussion Questions

1. How does wilderness contribute to human and environmental health?
2. What are some of the goals of the Wilderness Society?
3. Discuss the role of each branch of government in wilderness protection.
4. Discuss some of the major laws regarding wilderness protection.
5. What is the main role of the citizenry in protecting the wilderness?

CHAPTER 15

ALASKA

America's Wilderness Frontier: A Case Study

LEARNING OBJECTIVES

- To learn about the Arctic National Wildlife Refuge
- To understand the difficulties of passage of the Alaska National Interest Lands Conservation Act

Alaska contains the greatest amount of roadless and wild lands in the United States, but its history of land protection and commercial development interests mirrors the democratic processes in the lower forty-eight states. While Alaska's politicians have favored development, the nation's environmental groups and the federal government have led the fight to protect these vital lands. Congress has enacted legislation that creates national parks, wildlife refuges, national monuments, and wilderness areas.

Arctic National Wildlife Refuge

On December 6, 1960, the Secretary of the Interior created the **Arctic National Wildlife Refuge (ANWR)** under Public Lands Order 2214, which reserved 8.9 million acres as the Arctic National Wildlife Range. Inspired by the Tanana Valley (Alaska) Sportsmen's Association in 1959, which proposed a national wildlife refuge in recognition of the many game species found in the area, the ANWR allowed hunting and trapping. National Park Service scientist Lowell Summer stated, "ANWR symbolizes freedom . . . freedom to continue, unhindered and forever if we are willing, the particular story of Planet Earth unfolding here . . . where its native creatures can still have freedom to pursue their future, so distant, mysterious . . . ." George Leroy Collins, an advocate for Alaska working for the National Park service, stated, "This area offers what is virtually America's last chance to preserve an adequate sample of the pioneer frontier, the stateside counterpart of which has vanished." In 1957, Margaret (Mardy) Murie related after traversing the Sheenjek Valley in ANWR with her naturalist husband, "I feel that, if we are big enough to save this bit of loveliness on our earth, the future citizens of Alaska and of all the world will be deeply grateful. This is a time for a long look ahead." (See Figure 15.1.) Her husband Olaus Murie added in 1961, "A wilderness area is a little portion of our planet left alone." Supreme Court Justice and prolific outdoor writer and adventurist William O. Douglas said in 1960, "This last American living wilderness must remain sacrosanct. This is the place for man turned scientist and explorer, poet and artist. Here he can experience a reverence for life that is outside his own and yet a vital and joyous part of it."

In ANWR, there are forty species of land and marine mammals and thirty-six fish species. Polar, grizzly, and black bears, along with wolf, wolverine, Dall sheep, moose, musk ox, and caribou are abundant. In 2002 there were less than 350 musk oxen left in ANWR, and the grizzlies had doubled their musk ox kill rate. The U.S. Geological Survey (USGS) had concluded that musk oxen on the Arctic Range were vulnerable to disturbance from activities associated with petroleum exploration because of their year-round residency, their small population numbers, and

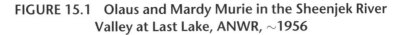

FIGURE 15.1   Olaus and Mardy Murie in the Sheenjek River
Valley at Last Lake, ANWR, ~1956

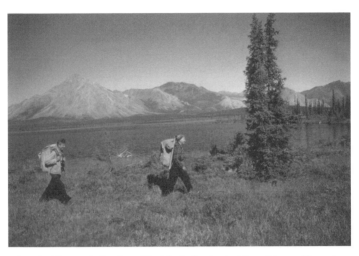

Source: Reprinted with permission from The Murie Center Archives, Moose, Wyoming.

their need to conserve energy for the nine months of the winter if they are to successfully reproduce. Across the Coastal Plain are countless ponds, wetlands, creeks, rivers, and coastal lagoons where vast flocks of birds, ducks, and geese hatch their summer families. They migrate from every state in the United States (except Hawaii) and from distant parts of Asia and South America. Additionally, 180 bird species nest in ANWR, including the Savanna sparrow, the rough-legged hawk (which has legs that are fully feathered down to the toes), and the Arctic peregrine falcon, which may migrate to the Atlantic coast, including New York City.

Sarah James, a Gwich'in Native Athabaskan living in Arctic Village, said, "For generations spanning 20,000 years we have hunted the Porcupine Caribou herd for food and clothing. But the land and the caribou mean much more to us than the subsistence they provide. They are sacred to us and are part of our culture and way of life."[1] Parks and wildlife refuges in Alaska are part of the Native culture, with the Gwich'in ardently fighting to protect ANWR against oil development.

Alaska National Interest Lands Conservation Act: National Parks, Wildlife Refuges, and Wilderness

In 1963, The Wilderness Society held its annual meeting in Alaska at Camp Denali, outside the boundary of Mt. McKinley National Park. The purpose was

NOTES FROM THE FIELD

In the summer of 1972 I was headed north with my younger brother Roger to visit the ANWR in northeastern Alaska. We flew to Anchorage and traveled by train to Fairbanks and on to Fort Yukon on the Yukon River. There we boarded a twin Beech aircraft for our flight into the dirt strip runway at Arctic Village on the border of ANWR. Here we first saw the Brooks Range towering above us but covered in an afternoon haze. We walked through the village playing hide-and-seek with the Gwich'in Athabaskan Native children. The Gwich'in tribe lives off caribou, small game, and salmon in the rivers. Their lives are intertwined with nature and they are stalwarts in protection of ANWR against oil drilling or other developments that might disturb the rhythm of the land.

Our bush pilot loaded our packs into a Cessna 185 on floats for the flight through the ANWR and loaned us a rifle for protection as well. We flew over to the Sheenjek River and marveled at the verdant greens below us. It was July, and the Arctic flora was in full rapid bloom for the short growing season. Clouds bracketed the horizons and descended to the tops of the Brooks Range. We flew next to the cloud bank, searching for a route to the Arctic plain. Finding no breaks in the clouds, our pilot changed course, flying back down the Sheenjek River to Last Lake for a short landing. We bounced right up on the opposite shore. The pilot handed our packs to us, said he would pick us up on Shrader Lake in two weeks weather permitting, and good luck! We had more than 150 miles of sheer wilderness ahead to reach Shrader Lake and the Arctic plain.

We hiked along the river bank, occasionally treading on the braided gravel beds for easy walking. The challenge of the riverbed was the continually dividing river, which required wading across one of the branches, but the high riverbank was no relief since the tussocks would not enable one to walk with ease. Tussocks of grass are too narrow to walk along the tops, and the space in between was too narrow for a hiking boot—and frequently the tundra had melted, leaving muck behind. Carrying a backpack made walking on the tussocks a significant challenge. As we hiked northward we saw small herds of caribou coveting the last ice fields on the river, where they could escape the incessant mosquitoes with the cold air. As we searched the mountains around us, we could spot three to six Dall sheep in single file. They were always near the summits, probably for safety from wolves.

We hiked for several days, getting used to our freeze-dried food but realizing we had underestimated our caloric needs considerably for carrying heavy packs all day long. The river began to shrink as the banks became steeper nearer to the Arctic Divide. All of the peaks surrounding us now had glaciers drooping into the passes between the mountains. We ascended the glacier on our left and joyously saw the Hulahula River disappearing north into the Arctic clouds. There were no trails to follow, and we never saw a footprint or sign of any previous hikers. We reached the headwaters of the Hulahula and caught a few small trout to supplement our freeze-dried food. We reached the halfway point down the Hulahula, spotting the low divide that we needed to head toward in order to reach Shrader Lake. We ascended this pass and were impressed with all of the red and purple lichens and Arctic plants.

As we crossed toward Peters and Shrader lakes, we were met by a deep chasm with a roaring river at its base that was too dangerous to cross. This was the benignly labeled "Katak Creek" on the map. We decided there was no choice but to hike up the valley to the source to find a narrow place to cross. The hike was a challenge, with rocky cliffs descending to the creek below. We hiked all day to the glacier where the Katak boiled out of the ice. The creek was still 10 meters across, and the water was gushing in full force. We saw a beach for our camp across the river and changed into jogging shoes to wade across the frigid stream. We carefully crossed with a rope between us.

In the morning I emerged from our tent to photograph the raging torrent to discover it was a mere trickle. It had swollen from the day's glacial melt—we had learned the hard way that the time for river crossings was the early morning when one is downstream of glacial-born streams. A young caribou walked through our camp; we took our day hike to Shrader Lake. From our tent site we could see across the barren Arctic plain. This was the birthing grounds of the Porcupine caribou herd, numbering from 125,000 to 175,000, although their numbers have steadily declined over the past decade. In the early spring the herd migrates 400 miles north and west to the Arctic plain of ANWR to give birth to its calves. Here the Arctic grasses and plants burst forth full of energy for rapid growth and nourishment of the young caribou. It is also relatively safe from the wolves since the herd is densely packed. Grizzly bears, wolves, and golden eagles are more common in the Brooks Range mountains, making the coastal plain the safest place for a calving grounds. The herd calves in different quadrants of the plain every year such that there would be no isolated place for oil development on the Arctic plain.

Roger and I hiked to the flanks of Mt. Chamberlain, where we enjoyed the Arctic mountain beauty. The ANWR experience was an adventure in the wild where we met a pristine Arctic environment and the challenges of a remote wilderness. There are few opportunities to witness a scale of magnificent beauty such as ANWR, the wildest of America's wildernesses.

to raise awareness of Alaska conservation issues for national environmental organizations. Delegates produced a statement calling on state and federal officials to make sure that wilderness areas were preserved in any plans for future land use. Alaskans were resistant to this idea, but one group, the Federal Field Committee, developed a report calling for land planning in Alaska, including identifying areas as conservation units. Realizing that congressional action would be the only way to protect any wilderness in Alaska, in early 1971 a number of national conservation groups met together to lobby in Washington, D.C., to include conservation withdrawals in the Alaska Native Claims Settlement Bill. They called themselves the Alaska Coalition, which grew to more than 1,000 conservation, sporting, religious, and labor groups working to protect public lands in Alaska.

In 1980, Congress passed the Alaska National Interest Lands Conservation Act. This law is probably the most significant land conservation measure in the history of the United States. To make this happen, a Native claims settlement needed to be worked out first. When Alaska was granted statehood in 1959, the Statehood Act granted the state of Alaska the right to select 104 million acres of land that it could manage as a revenue base. During the first eight years of statehood, Alaska identified 26 million aces for selection, but going forward, the state began staking out more and more land that encroached on the Alaskan Natives' traditional lands. Consequently, the Native community argued that, without a treaty or an act of Congress extinguishing Native title, the state should not make any more selections. Stewart Udall, the Secretary of the Interior at the time, agreed and declared a freeze on any additional state land selections. Even with the support of the Department of the Interior, the Native community would have been hard pressed to obtain a lands claim settlement in the Congress if it hadn't been for the discovery of oil at Prudhoe Bay in 1968. Because of the land freeze, however, the state couldn't proceed with development. Suddenly, the oil industry, the administration of President Richard Nixon, and the state of Alaska were advocating on behalf of the Natives.

Enacted in 1971, the Alaska Native Claims Settlement Act (ANCSA) created twelve Native-owned regional corporations, granted $963 million in seed money, and authorized the Native corporations to select 44 million acres of federal lands in Alaska. Of the approximately 80,000 Natives enrolled under ANCSA, those living in villages (approximately two-thirds of the total) would receive 100 shares in both a village ($n = 200$) and regional ($n = 12$) corporation. The environmental community—concerned that Alaska was being carved up with too much emphasis on development—was also involved in the ANCSA debate. Its efforts are reflected in Section 17 (d)(2) of the act, which directs the Secretary of the Interior to withdraw 80 million acres of significant federal lands from development. These lands, referred to as "d-2" lands, were to be available for potential congressional designation as national parks, wildlife refuges, wild and scenic rivers, or national forests.

Most important, the d-2 provision of ANCSA set a deadline for Congress to respond; if it did not act to designate these lands earmarked for special protections by 1978, the withdrawal would expire and the lands would be reopened to development. The intent of Congress was to preserve unrivaled scenic and geological values associated with natural landscapes, to provide for maintenance of sound populations of wildlife, including species dependent on vast, relatively undeveloped areas, and to preserve in their natural state extensive unaltered Arctic tundra, boreal forest, and coastal rainforest ecosystems.

In March 1972, Secretary of Interior Rogers C. B. Morton withdrew the 80 million acres in areas that the conservation lobby and officials in the Park Service, Fish and Wildlife Service, and Bureau of Land Management had recommended. He also set aside 45 million acres for study, for possible future conservation units, 40 million acres around villages and in traditional areas for Native selection, and an additional 3 million acres from which Natives could select "make-up lands" if any of the conservation withdrawals took traditional Native lands. Finally, the secretary designated 35 million acres for the state to select. Further state selections would have to wait until the conservation and Native selections were complete. This was more than the conservationists had hoped for, and it was in line with ANCSA.

This action by the federal government seemed to freeze Alaskans out of the process and made many Alaskans angry. Rep. Nick Begich (D) called it a "massive land grab." Soon afterward the state filed a suit challenging the federal withdrawals. In the meantime, the Joint Federal-State Land Use Planning Commission established under ANCSA 17(a) began its work, taking testimony that recommended resolution of a number of federal/state conflicts. Federal and state negotiators also worked independently of the commission. The state then withdrew its lawsuit in exchange for the right to make some immediate selections in areas that had been set aside for conservation. Three months later, in December 1973, the secretary forwarded his final recommendation for conservation withdrawals—more than 83 million acres—to Congress. Conservationists were not pleased, for they had hoped for a lot more acreage, and they wanted much of the withdrawn land classified as wilderness. That meant it would not be open to mining, hunting, fishing, motorized boats or vehicles, or other imprints of man.

Because of the Watergate drama of 1973–1974, the Alaska lands bill slipped from congressional attention. But Jimmy Carter made conservation in Alaska a major campaign initiative in his run for president. When he was elected president in 1976, he expected Congress to act before the old eight-year deadline for land selection in 1978. On the first day of the new Congress in 1977, Rep. Morris Udall (D) of Arizona introduced a bill calling for 115 million acres of Alaska conservation reserves, much more than provided in ANCSA. The bill was named H.R. 39 and would become famous in Alaska by that name. The bill would protect the environmental "crown jewels of Alaska," Udall said, a phrase that would be heard often in the d-2 debate. The crown jewels were Alaska's "most spectacular natural environments, recreation areas, and wildlife habitats." The bill would create ten new national parks and expand existing ones, create fourteen new wildlife refuges, twenty-three wild and scenic rivers and would enlarge the two national forests where there were mineral deposits. The national wilderness system created by the 1964 Wilderness Act would be doubled.

The House assigned the bill to a subcommittee for General Oversight and Alaska Lands. The Alaska Coalition publicized the subcommittee hearings widely before the representatives arrived at them. As a result, more than 2,000 people testified, with almost all of them speaking in favor of the bill and for wilderness in Alaska. Although the tide seemed to be running with the environmentalists' drive for a strong environmental bill, the U.S. Senate has a tradition of not passing any bill that affects a particular state when the senators from that state have strong objections. This gave Alaska's senators, Ted Stevens (R) and Mike Gravel (D) leverage, and instead of taking up the House bill, they persuaded the Senate to mark up its own bill. The tactic was to use every opportunity to delay the bill so that the deadline of December 1978 would pass before Congress could produce a bill.

Sen. Stevens recognized that a compromise was probably necessary, because if Congress did not produce a bill, Alaska would be left in limbo. Sen. Gravel, on the other hand, had said from the beginning, when Udall introduced H.R. 39, that he would filibuster and kill any bill he did not like. As the Senate dithered over its Alaska bill for months, environmentalists became more and more concerned. Some began to think that Stevens and Gravel would be able to sidetrack the whole process and six years of work would go up in smoke. When negotiations collapsed, Secretary of the Interior Cecil Andrus made it clear that he would use any means he had to withdraw all the lands under discussion if Congress failed to produce legislation. Meanwhile, in the last hours of the 95th Congress, Gravel took to the Senate floor to filibuster a joint resolution to extend the deadline for two years. On October 14, 1978, the session expired with no Alaska bill.

In early November, the state of Alaska did not wait and filed an application with the BLM for 41 million acres. Nearly one-quarter of the selections were in proposed new federal conservation units! Two days later, Secretary Cecil Andrus withdrew nearly 111 million acres of Alaska land, using the authority of the Federal Land Policy and Management Act of 1976. Andrus named 40 million of the withdrawn land as study areas, preventing mineral or other commercial activity. At the request of the Agriculture Secretary, President Carter suspended the operation of public land laws on 11 million acres of the existing Tongass National Forest. Then, two weeks later, President Carter withdrew 56 million more acres in Alaska, using the authority of the 1906 Antiquities Act, placing the land in seventeen new national monuments. This brought the total Carter administration withdrawals to 154 million acres. Without a doubt it was the most dramatic and sweeping withdrawal of public lands in the history of the nation, and it left Alaskans in a state of confusion. Charles Clusen, executive director of the Alaska Coalition, noted, "President Carter has now replaced Teddy Roosevelt as the greatest conservation president of all time."

Carter's and Andrus's actions did indeed produce an Alaska lands act before the end of the next Congress. At the beginning of the 96th Congress, Morris Udall again introduced H.R. 39, but this version was a stronger environmental bill, without many of the compromises of the original one. In the meantime, Sen. Stevens guided a compromise bill through the legislative process. It would set aside only 104 million acres of new reserves, 15% less than Udall's House bill. The bill included more than 56 million acres of new wilderness lands. The Senate passed the bill in August. Stevens warned the House environmentalists that the Senate bill was a "take it or leave it" proposal. Neither he nor Sen. Gravel would accept any amendments. In the House, Rep. Udall prepared to stand firm. There matters stood as the country went to the polls in November 1980. It would be the American people who would resolve this impasse and make the decision on Alaska lands.

In the 1980 elections, voters elected Ronald Reagan president and sent a Republican majority to the Senate. When the new Congress took office in January, there were fewer delegates in favor of a strong environmental bill than there were in the 96th Congress. There was now no chance of getting approval of Udall's H.R. 39. Accepting this reality, two weeks after the election Udall asked the House to approve the Senate bill. They did so by voice vote. On December 2, 1980, President Carter signed into law the Alaska National Interest Lands Conservation Act.

In Washington, D.C., President Carter said of the act, "It is a victory in the long struggle to resolve this issue, and is truly an historic moment in our nation's history." Sen. Paul Tsongas (D-MA), a steady conservation supporter, said that the bill was "a victory for the Administration and for those of us in Congress who have worked for so many years to protect the staggering beauty and abundant natural resources, and wildlife of the Alaska wilderness." "No single piece of legislation in our history," he said, "surpasses this act." ANILCA set aside 104 million acres of Alaska land in a variety of new conservation units; 56.4 million were classified as wilderness. It provided national park protection to ten new areas and made additions to three existing ones. It added 1.3 million acres to the Tongass Forests, naming 5.4 million of them wilderness. In the creation of a vast area of reserves across the south flank of the Brooks Range south to the Yukon River, ANILCA brought protection to a significant area of the state previously open to mining and other kinds of entry. These units included the Gates of the Arctic and Kobuk Valley national parks, the Cape Krusenstern National Monument, Noatak National Preserve, and four wildlife refuges. West of the Canada border, the act created the vast Wrangell-St. Elias National Park and Preserve, together with the Tetlin National Wildlife Refuge. On the upper Yukon River, ANILCA set up the Yukon-Charley Rivers National Preserve, together with the Yukon Flats National Wildlife Refuge, and on BLM land, the Steese National Conservation Area and the White Mountains National Recreation Area. Though the name of Mt. McKinley remained, the park was renamed Denali National Park and expanded.

Near the Alaska Peninsula, ANILCA created the Lake Clark and Katmai National Park and Preserves and the Aniakchak National Monument and Preserve. In all of these areas, wildlife, water, and land resources would be more fully protected than ever before. Conservationists in America were happy at first, even though they did not get many of the areas they wanted to protect into the bill. As they began to carefully review the bill some became even more disappointed, for what at first seemed to be protection instead was very confusing. Senators Stevens and Gravel and Rep. Don Young (R) had been able to write a great many exceptions into the act. Some of the exceptions drew boundaries of one sort or another around lands of economic potential, excluding them from the conservation units. The Alaska Coalition had wanted whole ecosystems preserved, but in many instances, the ecosystems were cut up or incomplete. A number of units that the conservationists had wanted named as parks had instead been given a new conservation classification: preserve. This meant that sport hunting and other kinds of activities were permitted in them—these activities were banned from lower forty-eight parks. Snow machines, motorboats, and floatplanes, as well as high-powered rifles, chain saws, and even cabins would be allowed in areas called "wilderness." The act allowed prospecting on most land known to have mineral or oil potential, including such areas as Glacier Bay National Monument (where a rich nickel-copper deposit was found in the 1950s) and a bornite (a sulfide of copper) deposit in the Kobuk River drainage. Areas specifically excluded from the act included a world-class lead and zinc deposit, Red Dog, on the Arctic coast north of Kotzebue, a molybdenum deposit at Quartz Hill in the Misty Fjords National Monument near Ketchikan, a silver and lead deposit at Greens Creek near Juneau, and a gold deposit at Golden Zone. In the Tongass National Forest, where two pulp mills operated in Ketchikan and Sitka, the act provided a $40 million annual subsidy for the U.S. Forest Service: Alaska Region. This was to make sure that timber lease sales, together with forest roads, would allow 4.5 million board feet of timber to be cut annually, a 35% increase in the average annual cut from the past. No other forest region in the country was supported like this for timber lease sales.

Conservationists considered many of these exceptions as serious flaws in the act. Areas can be closed if the guaranteed access caused negative impacts on resources. Access was guaranteed to inholdings in the national parks and refuges. Access was also to be protected to state lands and waters that lie within federal units or are surrounded by them. In addition, the Secretary of the Interior was to assess the potential for oil development in the coastal plain of the Arctic National Wildlife Refuge. After review of all the exceptions, some critics wondered if it could be called a conservation act at all. Yet most recognized that even though there would be much controversy as the act was implemented, it did provide a framework for preservation in Alaska. President Carter, writing fifteen years after ANILCA, said that it was "one of my proudest accomplishments as President," an assessment most Americans agreed with.

Implementation of ANILCA was challenging for the Department of Interior: they had a hostile local population; there were many types of inholdings and competing uses; they had to establish day-to-day operations in the new conservation agencies; they had to deal with the state of Alaska, Natives, and the ANILCA-mandated Alaska Land Use Council; last, they had to prepare nearly 100 separate sets of regulations, reports, and studies. ANILCA required the National Park Service to prepare general management plans with appropriate environmental compliance documents for all new park areas within five years and conduct wilderness reviews of all lands within the park system not designated as wilderness. The NPS requested $11.4 million to do the job, but only $3 million was appropriated, making budget shortfalls one of the greatest challenges facing wilderness management. Fortunately, isolation and lack of development pressures left most of the Alaska conservation parklands intact.

Oil Versus Wilderness on the ANWR

The **Alaska National Interest Lands Conservation Act (ANILCA)** of 1980 renamed the Arctic Range the Arctic National Wildlife Refuge and expanded the refuge southward and westward to include an additional 9.2 million acres (total area 19.6 million acres). The Sheenjek, Wind, and Ivishak rivers were designated wild rivers. Section 702(3) of the ANILCA designated much of the original refuge—but not the coastal plain—as a wilderness area. Congress postponed decisions on the development or further protection of the coastal plain. Section 1002 of the ANILCA directed a study of ANWR's coastal plain and its resources to be completed after five years and nine months of enactment. The resulting 1987

NOTES FROM THE FIELD

Climbing Bob Marshall's mountain proved to be a superlative wilderness adventure deep in the Gates of the Arctic National Park in the Brooks Range. Robert Marshall, a founder of The Wilderness Society, explored the Brooks Range for 510 days during 1929, 1930–1931, 1938, and 1939. An indefatigable hiker and explorer, he climbed twenty-eight peaks in the Arctic Divide region of the North Fork of the Koyukuk River and mapped the rivers and peaks covering 12,000 square miles of blank space on the map. Despite this success, he was frustrated from his goal of climbing the domineering peak of the central Brooks Range, Mt. Doonerak. He likened it to the "Matterhorn of the Arctic" and considered it to be more than 10,000 feet (actually, at 7,457, several other peaks in the Brooks Range are higher). Named Doonerak by Marshall after the local Inuit's name, they told him that dooneraks or "spirits" were everywhere in their lives and frequently played tricks on them. Marshall's legacy has been his writings on the spirit of wilderness and adventure.

> The sheer stupendousness of the wilderness gives it a quality of intangibility which is unknown in ordinary manifestations of ocular beauty. . . . Another singular aspect of the wilderness is that it gratifies every tone of the senses. . . . In the wilderness, with its entire freedom from the manifestations of human will, that perfect objectivity which is essential for pure aesthetic rapture can probably be achieved more readily than among any other forms of beauty. Adventure, whether physical or mental implies breaking into unpenetrated ground, venturing beyond the boundary of normal aptitude, extending oneself to the limit of capacity, courageously facing peril. Life without the chance for such exertions would be for many persons a dreary game, scarcely bearable in its horrible banality. . . . My own belief which I realize the majority do not share, is that most exploration today is not of material value to the human race in general but is of immense value to the person who does it.[2]

He advocated the wilderness preservation of all of northern Alaska above the Yukon except for a small developed portion near Nome.

In June 1992 I yearned to explore this wilderness extraordinaire up in the North Fork of the Koyukuk and climb Mt. Doonerak. My climbing partner, Dan Luchtel, an environmental scientist at the University of Washington, and I met Don Glaser, our bush pilot in Bettles, who flew us in a Turbo Beaver on floats toward the Gates: Frigid Crags on the left and Boreal Mountain on the right. We turned right to fly up the North Fork of the Koyukuk and came upon a peak with a sheer 2,000-foot face that rose even higher than the plane—that was Doonerak! We passed a deep canyon 1,000 feet below and suddenly we were on the Arctic Divide, landing on Summit Lake. We unloaded our heavy packs and the plane took off, leaving us all alone.

The following morning we hiked along the mountain bases in soft moss, lugging our 75-pound packs. An occasional caribou antler disappeared into the encroaching moss. We were in a verdant high Arctic paradise with three of four lakes glistening behind us, the incipient North Fork gurgling to our right, and high barren peaks providing the backdrop to our amphitheater. We enjoyed lunches of sausage, cheese, crackers, candy bars, and lemonade, made with crystal-clear, ice-cold Koyukuk water. Figure 15.2 shows Mt. Doonerak looming above us. We took off our boots and put on tennis shoes to wade across Alinement Creek. Continuing downriver, we reached a level plateau where we could see Amawk Creek descending from the mountains. We made a beeline across the plateau and had our first fierce encounter with the Arctic's infamous sedge tussocks. Above the permafrost, the Arctic grasses bunch and clump together to build a foot-high tuft that densely compacts the vegetation to produce a stool that can almost hold up a person. We ascended the steep Amawk River to a high alpine meadow with Arctic poppies and dryas where we replenished our water bottles at the edge of St. Patrick's Lake.

The next morning we took our climbing gear for the ascent of Mt. Doonerak. We hiked downward past several canyons to the gully leading up to Midnight Pass, where we could see down a scree slope to a high rock-ribbed valley below Hanging Glacier Mountain and the west side of Doonerak. At the bottom we could see a

FIGURE 15.2 Author in the North Koyukuk River Valley with Mt. Doonerak towering above

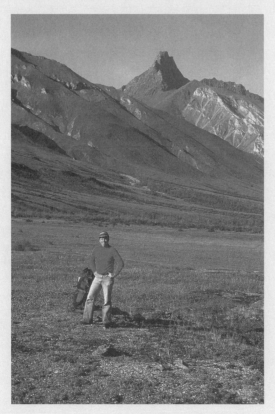

Source: Dr. William Rom.

corner of Marshall Lake; it was free of ice. It was open water in contrast to Marshall's sighting on July 5, 1930. Beyond us was a mile of ridgeline. We roped up and carefully crossed the knife edge to traverse above the last remaining glacier above Doonerak. We bypassed a 200-meter sheer rock face to descend and climb back up to a glacial couloir below the face of Doonerak. Above us was the full final summit pyramid of Doonerak. Fifteen hundred feet of near-vertical granite loomed above us. Below it dropped another 2,000 feet on both sides. Our tiny ridge of rock scree led to the slopes at the base of summit pyramid. An 800-foot vertical chimney characterized the right side. We could follow a route of broken rock up a fourth of the mountain, then exposed faces up to a broad band crossing the middle of the peak, leading to the left where there was a crack and gully heading up a steep face to the summit. We found the lower stretches easy going, then found footholds and handholds up toward the broad band. Ahead were the vertical cliffs of the west face. We carefully began to cross the band. It was wide, good rock and the going was steady. We were both climbing well with upwards, traverses, belays, until finally—summit!

We found the summit to have a large flat area where we could take pictures, eat our snacks, and enjoy the countless unnamed peaks to the north, west, and east. We unfurled our Explorer's Club flag for a photo (see Figure 15.3). We descended carefully in the late evening and bivouacked on the shores of Marshall Lake until 4 a.m., when shivering kept us awake. We headed back to our camp on St. Patrick's Lake. We descended to the North Fork of the Koyukuk where we found a crossing, hiked south to Ernie's Creek for further exploration, and down to Frigid Crags where our bush pilot found us on a sandbar for the flight back to Bettles. It was another great Alaskan adventure where we hadn't seen a soul.

FIGURE 15.3   Author with Explorer's Club flag on summit of Mt. Doonerak

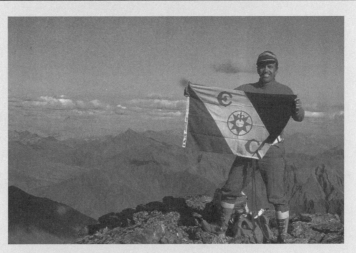

Source: Dr. William Rom.

report was called the 1002 Report or the Final Legislative Environmental Impact Statement. Section 1003 of ANILCA prohibited oil and gas development in the entire refuge, or "leasing or other development leading to production of oil and gas from the range" unless authorized by an act of Congress. Congress attempted to authorize opening of ANWR in fiscal year 1996 reconciliation bill, but President Bill Clinton vetoed the measure and it was subsequently dropped. Attempts to prevent ANWR oil drilling failed in the Senate on April 18, 2002, by a vote of forty-six yeas to fifty-four nays on a filibuster that required sixty votes.

In 2004, Sen. Barbara Boxer (D-CA) offered an amendment blocking ANWR development that passed with fifty-two yeas and forty-eight nays. The U.S. oil industry quietly decided to sit out the battle over ANWR, with Exxon-Mobil, ChevronTexaco, BP Amoco, Shell Oil, Conoco Phillips, and Anadarko Petroleum deciding to focus on other priorities in Washington, D.C. More than $7 million was appropriated by the state of Alaska since 1993 to lobby through Arctic Power for the opening of ANWR to oil development.

The most recent government study of oil and natural gas prospects in ANWR, completed in 1998 by the USGS, found that there was an excellent chance (95%) that at least 11.6 billion barrels of oil were present on federal lands in the 1002 area. There also was a small chance (5%) that 31.5 billion barrels or more were present. USGS estimated that there was an excellent chance (95%) that 4.3 billion barrels or more were technically recoverable (costs not considered), and there was a small chance (5%) that 11.8 billion barrels or more were technically recoverable. The USGS estimated that, at $24 (1996 dollars) per barrel, there was a 95% chance that 2 billion barrels or more could be economically recovered and a 5% chance of 9.4 billion barrels or more.[3] The U.S. Energy Information Administration estimated that at a relatively fast development rate, production would peak about fifteen to twenty years after the start of development, with a maximum daily production rate of roughly 0.015% of the resource. Peak production could reach 750,000 barrels per day. U.S. petroleum consumption is about 25 million barrels per day. There was likely to be natural gas also in the 1002 area, but currently there is no natural gas pipeline to bring the gas to market.

The major harm of industrial development would be to the wilderness character of the ANWR plain. There also may be harm to the Porcupine caribou calving grounds, migratory bird nesting, and polar bears. Winter exploration would disrupt polar bear dens and winter foraging by musk oxen. Oil spills would likely occur, and advanced technologies might not be mandated on ANWR lands. In a 2003 report, the National Academy of Sciences highlighted impacts of existing development at Prudhoe Bay on Arctic ecosystems.[4] Among the harmful environmental affects noted were changes in bowhead whale migration, in distribution and reproduction of caribou, and in populations of predators and scavengers that prey on birds. The 1002 area is the most biologically productive part of the Arctic Refuge for wildlife and is the center of wildlife activity. The Porcupine cows with young calves appear to be very sensitive and avoid roads and other human disturbance for distances of a mile or more. In 2000, heavy snowfall delayed cows in reaching the 1002 area, and calf survival statistics were the lowest ever recorded. In their first 1002 Report, the Fish and Wildlife Service stated that oil and gas development would cause a displacement or reduction of 20%–40% of the herd; this statement disappeared in the final report.

The 1002 area covers 1.5 million acres, and one 2,000-acre drill site with maximal lateral capability of 7 miles in any direction would cover only a small portion of the 1002 area. A limited footprint for development seems unrealistic because numerous sites dispersed around the coastal plain would obviously be necessary. Approximately 100,000 acres of Native lands are also available on the coastal plain, mostly apart of the 1002 area; currently the rules and regulations of ANWR apply to these lands. Bills in the U.S. House of Representatives (Rep. Edward Markey, D-MA) and in the Senate (Sen. Joseph Lieberman, I-CT, with twenty-four co-sponsors) have been continuously introduced to protect the 1002 area as a federal wilderness area.

Summary

Alaska presented the last great frontier for wilderness preservation. Conservationists had to work with Native communities, the state of Alaska, and their elected representatives to achieve protection of these lands. Emerging from these competing interests were two key federal laws: ANSCA provided for a Native claims settlement, and ANILCA provided 104 million acres of protected lands. National parks, monuments, wilderness areas, and wildlife refuges were created or existing ones expanded. The final bill was a Senate version that had 15% less wilderness lands and many more provisions providing access to state lands or mineral resources that could be exploited. ANILCA failed to protect the coastal plain of ANWR from oil drilling, causing Nicholas Kristof of the *New York Times* to write after his visit, "The argument that I find most compelling is that this primordial wilderness, a part of our national inheritance that is roughly the same as it was a thousand years ago, would be irretrievably lost if we drilled. The Bush administration's proposal to drill is therefore not just bad policy but also shameful, for it would casually rob our descendants forever of the chance to savor this magical coastal plain—and to be slapped in the butt by a frisky polar bear."

Key Terms

Alaska National Interest Lands Conservation Act (ANILCA)

Arctic National Wildlife Refuge (ANWR)

Discussion Questions

1. What were the main tenets of the Arctic National Wildlife Refuge?
2. What was the purpose of the Alaska National Interest Lands Conservation Act?

CHAPTER 16

THE CLEAN WATER ACT AND WATER ECOSYSTEMS

LEARNING OBJECTIVES

- To understand the political and historical factors leading to the creation of the Clean Water Act
- To understand the problems with the implementation of the Clean Water Act
- To understand the problems with keeping drinking water safe and how the government seeks to protect drinking water
- To understand water ecosystems and public health and environment

Clean water became an issue in the environmental movement with the visible pollution of lakes and streams in the 1960s and culminated in the surface fire of oil and organic pollutants on the Cuyahoga River that reached its terminus in Cleveland, Ohio, and Lake Erie. Approved much earlier, the Federal Water Pollution Control Act of 1948 was the first major U.S. law to address water pollution. Growing public awareness and concern for controlling water pollution led to sweeping amendments in 1972 and again in 1977; the law was named the Clean Water Act.

The Clean Water Act

The **Clean Water Act (CWA)** established the basic structure for regulating pollutant discharges into the waters of the United States. It gave the Environmental Protection Agency (EPA) the authority to implement pollution control programs, such as setting wastewater standards for industry; maintained existing requirements to set **water quality standards** for all contaminants in surface waters; and made it unlawful for any person to discharge any pollutant from a point source—for example, a factory site into navigable waters—unless a permit was obtained. It prohibited the discharge of pollutants in toxic amounts; funded the construction of sewage treatment plants under the construction grants program; and developed technology necessary to eliminate the discharge of pollutants into navigable waters. The Clean Water Act also recognized the need for planning to address the critical problems posed by non-point source pollution.[1] The Clean Water State Revolving Fund was established to address water quality needs by building on EPA–state partnerships. It supplies loans and grants for sewage treatment, non-point source pollution control, and estuary protection.

The Clean Water Act is the cornerstone of surface water quality protection in the United States. The statute employs a variety of regulatory and nonregulatory tools to sharply reduce direct pollutant discharges into waterways, finance municipal wastewater treatment facilities, and manage polluted runoff. These tools are employed to achieve the broader goal of restoring and maintaining the chemical, physical, and biological integrity of the nation's waters so that they can support the protection and propagation of fish, shellfish, and wildlife and recreation in and on the water. For many years following the passage of CWA in 1972, the EPA, states, and Native American tribes focused mainly on the chemical aspects of the integrity goal.

During the past decade, however, more attention has been given to physical and biological integrity. Examples of chemicals are hydrocarbons, PCBs, phosphates, and so on, and physical and biological integrity focuses on entire river ecosystems. Also, in the early decades of the act's implementation, efforts focused on regulating discharges from traditional **point source** facilities, such as municipal sewage plants and industrial facilities, with little attention paid to runoff from streets, construction sites, farms, and other "wet weather" sources. For **non-point source** runoff, including farms, voluntary programs such as cost sharing with landowners are the key tools. For wet weather point sources, like urban storm sewer systems and construction sites, the EPA employs a regulatory approach. EPA evolution of CWA programs over the past decade has shifted from a program-by-program, source-by-source, pollutant-by-pollutant approach to a more holistic **watershed-based strategy**. Under the watershed approach, equal emphasis is placed on protecting healthy waters and restoring impaired ones. Involvement of stakeholder groups in the development and implementation of strategies for achieving and maintaining state water quality and other environmental goals is the major goal.

The CWA mandated that EPA coordinate activities of other federal agencies, such as the Corps of Engineers or the Bureau of Reclamation and Federal Power Commission to manage and regulate stream flow by building or licensing dams. The CWA encourages federal, state, and interstate cooperation when watersheds cross state lines. The EPA was directed by the CWA to research and survey the results of the harmful effects of pollutants on the health or welfare of people and to set up field laboratories. Pesticides and waste oil were specifically mentioned as topics for research. Research was directed toward understanding freshwater ecosystems, including river study centers partnering among states and environmental stakeholders. Sewage treatment was to be integrated with waste treatment management and recycling combined; both industrial and municipal wastes, including but not limited to solid waste and waste heat and thermal discharges, were to be integrated. Cost sharing was part of the waste treatment construction, beginning with a 75% federal share and dropping eventually to a 55% share. Certain innovative grants could achieve a higher federal percentage.

The EPA was directed by the CWA to assist and support the implementation of a Comprehensive Conservation and Management Plan for Long Island Sound. The western portion of the Sound has a severe eutrophication problem due to high nutrient runoff and slow tidal action, which is slow to flush out the runoff. The excess nutrients stimulate algal and phytoplankton growth (eutrophication) resulting in reduced oxygen in the ecosystem. Summer hypoxia causes massive die-offs of fish and other forms of aquatic life. It disrupts the natural marine ecosystem, and it is costly to commercial fishing, aquatic recreational activities, and even sunbathing on the Sound's public and private beaches. New York and Connecticut agreed on achieving a 61.5% nitrogen

CASE STUDY: EPA FUNDS TERTIARY SEWAGE TREATMENT TO PROTECT FEDERAL WILDERNESS IN ELY, MINNESOTA

A $2.3 million demonstration grant was made to Ely, Minnesota, to treat municipal waste, with a tertiary treatment to reduce phosphates by more than 80%–85% from entering Shagawa Lake; this lake drains into the federal Boundary Waters Canoe Area Wilderness. The phosphates contributed to toxic algal blooms from July to September that had been treated with copper sulfate; these treatments were from a boat criss-crossing the entire lake. The tertiary treatment took more than two decades to show results in reduced algal blooms. Tank models predicted a drop from 51 to 12 micrograms per liter of phosphorus, but the level dropped only to 29 micrograms. The only noticeable biological change was a drop in chlorophyll concentration by half during May and June. Problems with blue-green algal blooms continued in the late summer and into the 1980s.

Phosphorus was identified as the key nutrient that caused algal blooms rather than nitrogen from studies in Ontario's Experimental Lakes Area. Scientists divided a study lake in half by a plastic curtain. Phosphorus was added to one side, and the resulting algal bloom was impressive causing policymakers to phase out phosphorus from detergents.[2]

Subsequent laws that have affected parts of the Clean Water Act include Title I of the Great Lakes Critical Programs Act of 1990. This law implemented the Great Lakes Water Quality Agreement of 1978, signed by the United States and Canada, where the two nations agreed to reduce certain toxic pollutants in the Great Lakes. EPA was required to establish water quality criteria for the Great Lakes, addressing twenty-nine toxic pollutants with maximum levels that are safe for humans, wildlife, and aquatic life. It also required EPA to help the states implement the criteria on a specific schedule. A wastewater management program was to be developed for the rehabilitation and repair of Lake Erie.

EPA was to conduct a study of the Tahoe Basin ecosystem in order to preserve the fragile ecology of Lake Tahoe. A Chesapeake Bay Program was authorized to implement and coordinate science and to improve the water quality and living resources in the Chesapeake Bay ecosystem. The National Coastal Water Program coordinates the Chesapeake Bay Program, Great Lakes Program, and Gulf of Mexico Program. The Coastal Zone Management Act Reauthorization Amendments of 1990 required the twenty-nine coastal states with federally approved coastal zone management plans to develop and submit coastal non-point source pollution control programs for approval by the National Oceanic and Atmospheric Administration and EPA. States were required to issue management measures for certain categories of runoff and erosion, and to evaluate non-point sources and identify coastal areas that would be negatively affected by specified land uses.

The Ocean Dumping Act in 1972 prohibited ocean dumping without a permit in any ocean waters under U.S. jurisdiction by any U.S. ship sailing from a U.S. port. The law also has provisions related to the creation of marine sanctuaries, conducting ocean disposal research, and monitoring coastal water quality.

reduction from point and non-point sources of pollution, with a **total maximum daily load (TMDL)** to be reduced from 4,552 pounds to 1,768 pounds per day. Each state must identify waters at risk and establish total daily maximum loads to protect those waters. Taxes are collected by the sewer district, and the four Westchester County sewer districts abutting the Sound face a tax increase of $235 million to upgrade sewage treatment plants. To meet federal standards in Long Island Sound, an increase of $350 per household will be necessary to pay for the upgrades.

Water quality standards are hazard-based requirements that set site-specific allowable pollutant levels for individual water bodies, and the TMDL is determined after study of the specific properties of the water body and the pollutant sources that contribute to the noncompliant status. Once the TMDL assessment is completed and the maximum pollutant loading capacity defined, an implementation plan is developed that outlines the measures needed to reduce the pollutant loading of the noncompliant water body and bring it into compliance. The TMDL target is dissolved oxygen due to bacterial metabolism of carbon compounds that doesn't cause the dissolved oxygen in the water to drop below 5 mg/L downstream of the discharge; less than 5 mg/L O_2 will kill sensitive aquatic species. More than 60,000 TMDLs are proposed or in development for U.S. waters in the next decade and a half. The CWA requires public involvement in developing TMDLs. Water quality standards are based on biocriteria, chemical levels, and antidegradation to protect the integrity of waters. Biocriteria are complex, since they include toxicant levels, temperature, dissolved oxygen, sedimentation, conditions of various aquatic communities, and so on. As of 2007, approximately half of the rivers, lakes, and bays under EPA oversight were not safe enough for fishing and swimming.

Clean Water Act Regulations

The CWA established a **National Pollutant Discharge Elimination System (NPDES)** that controls direct discharges into navigable waters. The NPDES program is administered by forty states following EPA guidelines and approval. A permit applicant must provide quantitative data identifying the types of pollutants present in the facility's effluent. The permit will then set forth the conditions and effluent limitations for discharges from a specific facility. The CWA of 1972 added the permit plus set a requirement for technology-based effluent limitations. EPA developed the standards for categories of dischargers based on the performance of pollution control technologies without regard for the conditions of a particular receiving water body. The intent of Congress was to create a level playing field by establishing a basic national discharge standard for all facilities within a category using the best available technology. More recently, NPDES permits require regulated municipalities to use best management practices to reduce pollutants to the "maximum extent practicable." Public notice of every permit must be sent out; this is the opportunity for environmental organizations or individuals to have an impact on important public policy decisions. Several state permitting agencies are willing to provide notice of permit applications long before the permit is drafted. Developing relationships with agency staff may get information on permits to the public sooner. If there are enough requests or if the permit of a discharge is controversial, there may be a public hearing in which much more detail may emerge. Following the public hearing, there may be an opportunity to appeal the decision or even go to state or federal court.

The EPA has identified 126 priority pollutants. Concentrated aquatic feeding operations are direct dischargers and require a NPDES permit. The 1987 CWA amendments required the EPA to establish a program to address storm water discharges. NDPES permits for both industrial dischargers and municipal waste treatment plants must comply with storm water considerations. The EPA enforcement of these regulations includes civil enforcement actions (including administrative penalties), criminal prosecution, and citizen suits. The CWA provides for penalties of up to $31,500 per violation per day.

Clean Water Act and Wastewater Treatment

The CWA also regulates wastewater treatment residuals referred to as sludge or **biosolids**. This rule took ten years to write, since many toxics and exposure pathways had to be considered. In spite of all the safety factors and uncertainty factors built into the process, environmental and human health risks were found to be very low.

Non-point source pollution is caused by rainfall or snowmelt moving over and through the ground; it picks up and carries away natural and human-made pollutants, finally depositing them into lakes, rivers, wetlands, coastal waters, and underground sources of drinking water. Non-point pollutants include fertilizers, herbicides, insecticides, oil, grease, toxic chemicals, sediment, salt, bacteria, and nutrients. The EPA and the states assist and encourage producers to use best management practices to reduce or prevent non-point source pollutants.

A National Estuary Program was established by the 1987 CWA amendments to maintain the integrity of whole estuaries, including chemical, physical, and biological properties. EPA promulgated regulations to address oil spill prevention in its Spill Prevention Control and Countermeasures Program, which also applies to farms and gasoline stations where there are large underground storage tanks.

Wetlands are covered by the CWA; activities covered are gravel fill for development, water resource projects (such as dams and levees), infrastructure development (such as highways and airports), and mining projects. EPA and the states are to compile a biennial report for Congress on the nation's water quality. Information from this report is used to designate "impaired waters lists." In the 1990s, numerous public interest groups across the country filed and won lawsuits against the EPA for approving lists that were demonstrably incomplete. Once a body of water is placed on the impaired waters list, it becomes one of many in line for the TDML process as required by the CWA. This process specifies problems, identifies pollution sources, determines pollution reductions needed to solve the problems, and assigns responsibilities for needed actions. Once impaired waters are placed on the list, proposals for new and increased discharges receive greater scrutiny.

Wastewater treatment is done by septic tanks in one-fourth of the nation's homes and small businesses; 10%–20% of these fail every year. The EPA has worked out a voluntary agreement with fourteen national organizations to deal with malfunctioning systems and their threat to groundwater quality.

Violations of CWA's Regulations

Since 2005, more than 23,000 manufacturing plants and other workplaces have violated the CWA more than 506,000 times.[3] The violations range from failing to report emissions to dumping toxins at concentrations regulators believe might contribute to cancer, birth defects, and other illnesses. The vast majority of these polluters have escaped punishment. State officials have repeatedly ignored obvious illegal dumping (fewer than 3% of CWA violations resulted in fines or other significant punishments), and the EPA has often declined to intervene. The number of facilities violating the CWA grew more than 16% from 2004 to 2007, the most recent year with complete data. The states' Departments of Environmental Protection have had increased workloads and dwindling resources; however, the EPA has promised to increase pressure on the states to improve their enforcement record immediately. Another problem is that some companies are pumping the polluted water into the ground, which has eventually polluted the ground water that is tapped for drinking water through artesian wells. The CWA needs to be expanded to police other types of pollution, like farm and livestock runoff, that are largely unregulated.

Protection of Wetlands under the Clean Water Act

There have been legal conflicts over the CWA application to periodic waters that may be a wetland (for example, part of the year during the rainy season a wetland may be obvious) and may or not be navigable. The CWA calls for regulatory permits, administered by the Army Corps of Engineers to be obtained before any work or construction involving wetlands can be performed. This includes real estate development where the property may include a wetland area. In *U.S. v. Riverside Bayview Homes, Inc.*, in 1985, the CWA was upheld in regulating wetlands that intermingle with navigable waters.

From 1997 to 2005 the Clinton Clean Water Action Plan called for a goal of protecting 100,000 acres of wetlands. What constitutes a wetland has been addressed by the judiciary. In *Solid Waste Agency of Northern Cook County v. U.S. Army Corps of Engineers*, the U.S. Supreme Court decided in 2001 that the United States did not have authority over "isolated" wetlands used by migratory birds. In *Rapanos v. U.S.*, in 2006, a plurality Supreme Court decision redefined the federal jurisdiction of wetlands in defining "navigable waters" and "waters of the U.S." The Court stated that the federal government needed a substantial link between navigable federal waters and wetlands and held onto a "significant nexus" test. Environmental groups considered this a major loss, repealing protection for as much as 60% of the nation's waters and 20 million acres of wetlands. More than 400 cases of suspected violation of the law—nearly half of the EPA's entire docket—were dropped or delayed since regulators did not know whether the streams and wetlands in question were covered by the law. In response, in 2007 Sen. Russ Feingold (D-WI) introduced the Clean Water Restoration Act, stating that it was Congress's intention to protect all waters. In 2010 the bill had twenty-three senator co-sponsors and 162 co-sponsors in the companion bill in the U.S. House of Representatives.

Safe Drinking Water Act

The **Safe Drinking Water Act (SDWA)** of 1974 was enacted in response to outbreaks of water-borne disease and increasing chemical contamination of public water sources. The SDWA authorizes the EPA to set **maximum contaminant levels (MCLs)** for dangerous chemicals, water-borne bacteria, and viruses in the public's drinking water. MCLs are enforceable standards and are the highest level of a contaminant that is allowed in drinking water. Each state writes a source assessment plan for each district's drinking water, requiring that the public be notified where the water comes from and levels of contaminants.

Arsenic Contamination in Water

Contamination sources of arsenic include mineral extraction and processing wastes, poultry and swine feed additives, pesticides, and highly soluble arsenic trioxide stockpiles that have caused contamination of ground waters. In 1942, the U.S. Public Health Service (USPHS) set the first drinking water arsenic standard at 50 μg/L, and in 1986, Congress directed the EPA to set a new standard by 1989. EPA estimated that 50 μg/L would result in a skin cancer risk of 1 in 400 and an internal cancer risk of 1.3 per 100 persons.[4] In 1996, Congress directed the EPA to set the new standard by 2000, and in January 2000 President Bill Clinton's EPA set a new arsenic standard of 10 parts per billion (10 μg/L).

The largest public health problems with arsenic are in the delta of the Ganges River in West Bengal, India, and Bangladesh. An estimated 36 million persons there are at risk from consuming drinking water containing elevated levels of arsenic. Arsenic poisoning leads to pigmentation changes on the upper chest and keratoses of the palms and soles of the feet (see Figure 16.1), plus cancers of the lung, bladder, and skin.

In Taiwan, 100,000 to 200,000 people have been at risk for elevated arsenic exposure for at least several decades. Epidemiological studies from Taiwan showed increased mortality from lung and bladder cancers and all sites combined in a dose–response fashion in persons drinking arsenic-contaminated water after controlling for age, sex, and cigarette smoking.[5] Bladder cancer mortality rates for those with more than 600 μg/L of arsenic in their water were more than 30–60 times the rates in the unexposed population.[6] There was a synergistic interaction ranging from 32% to 55% between cigarette smoking and arsenic exposure among 139 newly diagnosed lung cancer cases followed for 83,783 person-years in Taiwan's endemic areas.[7] Besides increasing cancer rates in Taiwan, an endemic area of "blackfoot disease" was described with artesian well water ranging from 350 to 1,100 μg/L arsenic. Blackfoot disease, found in southwestern Taiwan, is a progressive arterial occlusion resulting in gangrenous appearance of the feet in affected patients.[8] The prevalence ranged from 6.5 to 18.9 per 1,000 persons and was associated with hyperpigmentation, hyperkeratosis, and skin cancer in a dose–response fashion with arsenic exposure. Subclinical peripheral vascular disease could be demonstrated, and implementation of tap water reduced disease prevalence. The atherogenicity of arsenic could also be associated with hypercoagulability, endothelial injury, smooth muscle proliferation, and oxidative stress. Individuals with a higher arsenic exposure and a lower capacity to methylate inorganic arsenic had a higher risk of developing peripheral vascular disease in the blackfoot disease endemic

FIGURE 16.1   Keratosis from arsenic poisoning, Bangladesh

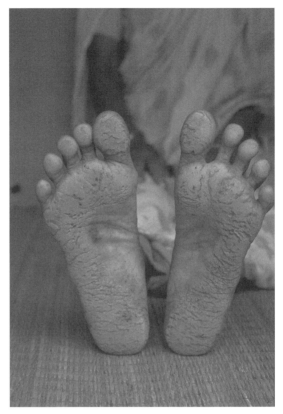

Source: Reprinted with permission from © UNICEF/NYHQ1998–0835/Shehzad Noorani.

area of Taiwan.[9] Arsenic causes gene amplification of the dihydrofolate reductase gene (sodium arsenite and sodium arsenate), but mutation has not been demonstrated.[10]

Arsenic has also affected the groundwater of Bangladesh. To create a potable water supply, about 4 million tube wells (hand pumps) were sunk into aquifers located at depths ranging from 40 to 300 feet and sometimes even deeper, assuming this water to be safe from bacterial contamination. With the primary aim of preventing cholera and other diarrheal diseases, the tube wells were installed all over the country by the government of Bangladesh and UNICEF (United Nations Children's Emergency Fund). Since the late 1960s, these wells were supposed to provide safe drinking water through simple technology at a minimum cost. Although the tube well program significantly reduced the burden of diarrheal diseases and saved millions of lives, it has resulted in a major arsenic tragedy.[11] Of sixty Bangladesh districts, 50% contained arsenic at levels above the Bangladesh safe limit of 50 μg/L, with the highest concentraton at 2,970 μg/L. In forty districts, 7,500 patients were diagnosed with arsenicosis (melanosis or hyperpigmentation on covered parts of the body and/or bilateral palmoplantar keratosis). Because arsenic crosses the placental barrier, Ahmad and colleagues studied pregnancy outcomes of ninety-six arsenic–exposed cases and ninety-six matched controls.[11] They found a significantly increased number of spontaneous abortions, stillbirths, and preterm birth rates in the arsenic-exposed group.

Water-Borne Diseases

Lack of access to clean water and basic sanitation represents a silent crisis affecting more than a third of the world's population.[12] About 1.1 billion people lack access to sand-filtered and chlorinated clean water, and 2 billion lack basic sanitation (see Figure 16.2). This contributes to water-borne diseases including cholera, hepatitis A, typhoid fever, giardia, legionella, and shigella dysentery.

FIGURE 16.2   Collecting drinking water from a polluted pond shared with livestock, Western Kenya, 2003

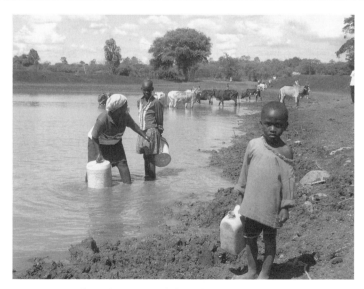

Source: © 2003 Greg S. Allgood, Courtesy of Photoshare.

In 1993 there was an outbreak of cryptosporidiosis in Milwaukee, Wisconsin, that infected 400,000 people and resulted in fifty-four deaths. This was the result of malfunctions in physicochemical drinking water purification, which has prompted interest in alternative methods to disinfect water. Milwaukee had two water treatment plants for water extracted from Lake Michigan. The southern plant had an increase in water turbidity; both cattle waste from two rivers and a sewage treatment plant entered the lake near the southern water treatment plant. Poor public health surveillance resulted in this large diarrheal outbreak. Sequential disinfection schemes, such as ultraviolet-combined chlorine and ozone-combined chlorine are being considered by many drinking water treatment plants because they are very effective in controlling *Cryptosporidium parvum* oocysts.[13] However, these new methods may still not inactivate viruses.

Water Ecosystems and Environmental and Public Health

The Klamath River Dam Removal and Water Diversion Projects

The National Wild and Scenic Rivers Act protects wild rivers, but dams, canals, roads, and other development have adversely affected rivers and swamps. Rivers that pass through several states may have segments in each state designated as wild, scenic, or recreational. For example, the 250-mile Klamath River has designations in California and Oregon and is a prime example of competing river/water interests.

In 1981, Gov. Jerry Brown of California petitioned the Secretary of the Interior to name the Klamath River a scenic river in the Klamath National Forest. This same river in Oregon was also named a scenic river managed by the Bureau of Land Management. There were four dams on the lower Klamath River whose licenses expired in 2004, allowing for an opportunity to remove these dams and create a free-flowing lower river. The Trinity River tributary was almost completely eliminated by dams and water diversions to the Sacramento Valley. The Klamath and Trinity rivers were once the spawning home to 800,000 chinook salmon, the third largest salmon fishery in the continental United States. Yurok Indians lived along its shores for 300 generations and fed themselves on its salmon. At the Klamath headwaters, the Bureau of Reclamation irrigated >100,000 acres of rich volcanic soil in the former Tule Lake Basin of the Klamath River that became the mainstay for more than 1,400 farmers. Alfalfa, grain, potatoes, and onions were grown. A downside to damming was that it created pools of warmer water that are intolerable to the fingerlings migrating downstream, and algae flourished in this warmer and phosphorus-enriched water.

In 1997, the coho salmon became so depleted that they were declared endangered; a minimum flow of water was established to protect this species under the Endangered Species Act. Additionally, in 2001, Oregon potato farmers in the upper portion of the Klamath River, suffering from a prolonged drought, demanded that the Interior Department give them water dedicated to the endangered fish.

In spring 2002, Vice President Dick Cheney and Secretary of the Interior Gale Norton personally opened the irrigation floodgates to increase the water supply to 220,000 acres of farmland. By fall 2002 poor water quality in the river led to a combination of infectious diseases, including a die-off of 30,500 adult chinook salmon due to *Ichthyophthirius multifiliis*. The fishermen were dependent on the salmon reaching their spawning grounds; the Indians needed their traditional fishing grounds; the power company controlled the water levels; and the farmers needed water for irrigation, and they had leases on federal wildlife refuges.

When all four dams' permits were up for renewal from the Federal Power Commission, negotiations began among farmers, the hydroelectric company, Native tribes, fishermen, the states, and the federal government. In 2007, low salmon populations in the Klamath led to sharply curtailed commercial fishing. In 2008, the Karuk Tribe released a report concluding that the cyanobacteria, commonly called blue-green algae, that bloom dramatically in the still summer waters behind Iron Gate Dam were releasing toxins that made fish and freshwater mussels unsafe to eat. Finally, by 2008 the Klamath Basin Restoration Agreement was concluded: four dams that provided 750,000 megawatt hours of power to 70,000 homes were to be removed through negotiation by the affected parties to allow the return of the salmon migration. Farmers switched to less water-intensive crops, pivot irrigators replaced flooding of fields, and farmers allowed fallow fields to rotate into lake and marsh in tune with the federal wildlife refuges. The four dams were to be removed by 2020, opening up 300 miles of the Klamath River.

Two major environmental groups, American Rivers and Trout Unlimited, offered immediate support for the proposal, as did representatives of the farm communities and the Indian tribes based along the river. The power company avoided expensive salmon ladders and upgrades to the old hydroelectric dams, and a surcharge to Oregon power customers plus a California bond made the business end of the deal attractive.

The Florida Everglades

The Everglades, or Grassy Waters as the Seminole Indians called it, is a fragile ecosystem that is formed by a river of fresh water 6 inches deep and 50 miles wide that flows slowly across the flat expanse of land at the southern tip of Florida. In 1947, Everglades National Park, covering 1.5 million acres, was established. More than 300 species of birds live in the park. Due to floods and limited ground to build upon, the Central and South Florida Project began in 1948 by the U.S. Army Corps of Engineers; it rerouted water for buildings and farming, severely short-changing the Everglades water ecosystem. The public perception was to drain that darned swamp! Hydrology in the Everglades was manipulated through hundreds of control gates, 720 miles of levees, 1,000 miles of canals, and dozens of pump stations. The water exits east and west, with very little reaching the Everglades. The Everglades National Park soon became starved of its own water, with the ecosystem slowly disappearing with saline water infusion. Restoration of the waterflows and the Everglades National Park soon became a political priority for the state, United States, communities, environmentalists, and the large sugar cane farming industry.

The **Comprehensive Everglades Restoration Project (CERP)** is the world's largest ecosystem restoration effort to restore the 5.7 million acre watershed and ecosystem in southern Florida. It covers sixteen counties over an 18,000 square mile area. The CERP is based on infrastructure modification and partial removal to move the ecosystem to a more natural and sustainable configuration through a forty-year, $20 billion project (1998 estimates $7.8 billion). The plan was approved in the Water Resources Development Act of 2000 and included more than sixty elements. Before 2000, there was a bipartisan agreement to restore the flow through the River of Grass from Lake Okeechobee in south-central Florida into the Everglades, including the National Park at the state's southern tip. The Department of Interior chairs the intergovernmental South Florida Ecosystem Restoration Task Force that serves as a focal point for the ongoing collaboration that is necessary to undertake the largest watershed restoration program in the world.

The plan called for new reservoirs and other storage systems to capture excess water during south Florida's rainy seasons, guaranteeing an adequate water supply for cities and farms as well as the Everglades. The cost was to be shared between the state of Florida and the federal government, but by 2008 Florida had outspent its partner 6–1, with $2 billion on sixty-eight restoration projects. This doesn't include the $1.34 billion Florida state deal to buy 180,000 acres from U.S. Sugar Corporation, which still faces uncertainty. The plan improves the quality, quantity, timing, and distribution of flows into the park.

In addition, 240 miles of canals and levees are to be removed to reestablish the natural sheetflow of water. The state of Florida purchased 207,000 acres of land—51% of what is needed for restoration. The state and U.S. Corps of Engineers have built filter marshes south of Lake Okeechobee and restored a more natural water flow in the Kissimmee River south of Orlando, which is the headwater of the Everglades ecosystem. The Kissimmee River project will recreate 52 miles of the original 103-mile river and restore 29,000 acres of wetlands. The lake receives 1.5 tons of phosphorus per day from upstream dairy farms accumulating on the bottom of the lake, accelerating the natural eutrophication process. Native species use very low levels of nutrients, so increased phosphorus and nitrogen serve to fertilize non-native species; for example, cattails drown out traditional sawgrass. Two major projects will return water flows to Everglades National Park through Shark River and Taylor Sloughs, two major channels through the River of Grass.

The U.S. Fish and Wildlife Service has a Multi-Species Recovery Plan that is a comprehensive strategy to address habitat needs of the sixty-eight endangered species in the area. Redevelopment in Miami-Dade County is looking eastward to redirect future development into the historical eastern corridor, revitalizing older urban areas. The plan replicates the natural water flow as much as possible, considering that 50% of the Everglades have been permanently lost to agriculture and urban development. Two reservoirs are to be built. The Central Lake Belt Reservoir will capture excess water and deliver this clean water to Everglades and Biscayne Bay National Parks when these natural areas need additional water flow. The Northern Lake Belt Reservoir will be designed to capture excess urban runoff that will be delivered back to the urban canal system to maintain the ground water table in the urban areas. This reservoir will serve to prevent saltwater intrusion into freshwater wells.

The South Florida Water Management District announced in 2008 that farmers had missed a phosphorus reduction target for the first time in eleven years, despite the recent construction of 45,000 acres of filter marshes to reduce contaminants in agricultural runoff. Everglades National Park was listed as a World Heritage Site in 1979, but after Hurricane Andrew and accumulated environmental threats it was listed as a World Heritage in Danger in 1993; in 2007 the World Heritage Committee removed the Everglades from the danger list after the United States had authorized $8 billion for the implementation of the Comprehensive Everglades Restoration Plan.

The Hetch Hetchy Dam Controversy

The Hetch Hetchy Valley was first visited by John Muir in 1871, prior to the protection of Yosemite National Park, granted national park status in 1890. Following the San Francisco earthquake and fire in 1906, a source of dependable water was paramount for the city. The Tuolumne River could be dammed anywhere along its course, but the cheapest point was at the entrance of the Hetch Hetchy Valley within Yosemite National Park. The city fathers fought John Muir and the Sierra Club for purchase of the lands, rights, and claims of the valley. After two denials by the Department of Interior, the City of San Francisco voted 86% in favor of approval, and the permit was approved in 1908 only to be suspended the following year. In 1913 Congress passed a bill approving the dam that was signed by President Woodrow Wilson. In 1923 the O'Shaughnessy Dam was completed. John Muir wrote in the *Yosemite* in 1912, "Dam Hetch Hetchy! As well dam for water-tanks the people's cathedrals and churches, for no holier temple has ever been consecrated by the heart of man." There is an active Restore Hetch Hetchy group aligned with the Sierra Club advocating removal of the dam and restoration of Hetch Hetchy Valley. The arguments for restoration claim that the reservoir provides only 25% of San Francisco's water and this amount could be stored in reservoirs downstream. The electric power could be made up elsewhere. Most important, restoration would take the crush of people away from Yosemite Valley and allow many others to appreciate nature's values.

Summary

The Cuyahoga River near Akron and Cleveland, Ohio, has improved from a polluted river fire in 1969 to become the home of the Cuyahoga Valley National Park nearly fifty years later because of enforcement of the Clean Water Act. The Clean Water Act has historically set levels for total suspended solids, nitrogen, and phosphorus species to limit eutrophication of U.S. rivers, bays, and lakes. The United States has seen extensive manipulation of its surface waters. Safe drinking water has been addressed by a federal law that sets levels of pollutants in waters to be met by water treatment districts. The EPA enforces the Clean and Safe Drinking Water acts. There has been considerable success in river restoration such as the Klamath River in Oregon and California, where four dams will be removed, restoring river flow to save the endangered coho salmon. The Everglades restoration projects are a collaboration of the state and federal governments to purchase sugar farms and divert water back into its historic flows.

Key Terms

Biosolids

Clean Water Act (CWA)

Comprehensive Everglades Restoration
   Project (CERP)

Maximum contaminant levels (MCLs)

National Pollutant Discharge Elimination
   System (NPDES)

Non-point source

Point source

Safe Drinking Water Act (SDWA)

Total maximum daily load (TMDL)

Water quality standards

Watershed-based strategy

Discussion Questions

1. Discuss the political and historical factors leading to the creation of the Clean Water Act.
2. What are some of the major regulations of the Clean Water Act?
3. What are some of the challenges with implementation of the Clean Water Act?
4. What are some dangers to safe drinking water?
5. How does the government seek to protect drinking water?
6. What are impediments to restoring free flows to rivers and swamps such as the Everglades?
7. Does Muir's argument that "everybody needs beauty as well as bread, places to play in and pray in, where Nature may heal and cheer and give strength to body and soul" apply to Hetch Hetchy in regard to the dam and expense of restoration?

CHAPTER 17

TOXIC CHEMICALS IN THE ENVIRONMENT

Government Regulations and Public Health

LEARNING OBJECTIVES

- To describe the chemical burden in modern humans
- To describe the Toxic Substances Control Act and its shortcomings
- To know the importance of endocrine-disrupting chemicals
- To understand the activities of the Superfund act
- To know the regulatory approaches of the Resource Conservation and Recovery Act and Federal Fungicide, Insecticide, and Rodenticide Acts

Chemical substances are pervasive in the United States, with more than 34 million metric tons of chemicals produced or imported every day.[1] Over the next quarter-century, global chemical production is projected to double, rapidly outpacing the rate of population growth. These substances ultimately enter the Earth's environment, and hundreds of chemicals can be detected in people and ecosystems worldwide. **Biomonitoring** is a growing research area that measures the types and levels of chemicals in humans. It has been used in the **National Health and Nutrition Examination Survey (NHANES),** which is a program of studies designed to assess the health and nutritional status of adults and children in the United States. The NHANES evaluated toxic chemicals, finding that 75% of people in the United States have triclosan, 100% have some type of measurable PCB (polychlorinated biphenyls), 98% have polyfluoroalkyl chemicals, and more than 90% of people have measurable levels of bisphenol A.[2] There are 80,000 chemicals in the U.S. environment regulated by EPA under the Toxic Substances Control Act (TSCA), and there are 3,000 chemicals manufactured or imported in excess of 1 million pounds each.[3]

Toxic Substances Control Act

The **Toxic Substances Control Act (TSCA)** was enacted in 1976 as a novel environmental legislation. It required the Environmental Protection Agency (EPA) to establish an inventory of chemicals manufactured or processed in the United States. Chemicals not on the inventory could not thereafter be manufactured, imported, or processed without premanufacture notification (PMN) of the EPA. TSCA operates under the default assumption that chemicals remain on the market unless or until EPA generates sufficient evidence to prove harm.

Information required in a PMN includes chemical descriptions of the material and its by-products; volume and types of uses expected; manufacturing process and locations; worker and environmental exposure; and health, safety, and environmental fate and effects test data known to the submitter or reported in the literature. The PMN is not required to demonstrate either efficacy or lack of adverse health or environmental effect. The EPA publishes a notice of its receipt of PMNs in the Federal Register. If the EPA takes no action for ninety days after the submission (or after an additional ninety-day extension that the EPA may grant itself), the chemical is added to the inventory and the submitter is free to manufacture, import, or process it. On the other hand, the EPA can prevent this by order, rule, or court action if it determines that unconditioned manufacture, processing, distribution, use, or disposal of the chemical may present an unreasonable risk of injury to health or the environment or that available data are insufficient for the EPA to determine that the chemical will not pose an unreasonable risk.

Under the Toxic Substances Control Act, EPA has broad authority to issue regulations designed to gather health and safety and exposure information on, require testing of, and control exposure to chemical substances and mixtures. The TSCA inventory is a compilation of the names of all existing chemical substances along with their respective Chemical Abstract Service (CAS) Registry numbers, production or importation volume ranges, and specific sites of production or importation. Chemicals produced in annual volumes above one million pounds are considered **high production volume (HPV) chemicals**. This subset of 3,000–4,000 HPV chemicals is the main focus of the Office of Prevention, Pesticides, and Toxic Substances' existing Chemicals Data Collection and Data Development (Testing) activities. Data on chemicals that are collected or developed are made accessible to the public and are intended to provide input for efforts to evaluate potential risk from exposures to these chemicals.

For any chemical on the inventory, the EPA is authorized to promulgate a regulation requiring manufacturers, importers, or processors of the chemical to perform testing to determine whether the chemical presents an unreasonable risk of injury to health or the environment. If it does, the EPA may also promulgate regulations to prevent the manufacture, processing, distribution, use, or disposal of a chemical from causing such an unreasonable risk. The EPA has used these authorities sparingly, but manufacturers, importers, and processors of a chemical have a continuing obligation to report to the EPA any information that comes to their attention supporting the conclusion that a chemical presents a substantial risk of injury to health or to the environment.

A special category of toxic chemicals is the **endocrine-disrupting chemicals (EDCs)**.[4] EDCs such as polychlorinated biphenyls, phthalates, and bisphenol A interfere with biological signaling mechanisms that govern the development, reproduction, or immune function in humans and wildlife.[5] Many EDCs persist in the environment and biomagnify in higher trophic levels. EDCs have been linked to population declines due to masculinization or feminization, eggshell thinning in birds and reptiles, and reduced reproductive capacity in fish, mammals, and amphibians.[6] EDCs can produce lifelong, multigenerational changes, which suggests that risk assessment should account for the timing of exposure as well as dose.[7] EDCs in combination can produce additive or synergistic effects that cannot be predicted by assessing individual chemicals in isolation.[8] Because EDCs are a new toxicological class of chemicals, they justify a policy change from assuming the safety of chemicals to producers demonstrating the safety of a chemical as a condition of its use.

CASE STUDY: POLYCHLORINATED BIPHENYLS IN THE HUDSON RIVER

Polychlorinated biphenyls (PCBs) are a group of chemicals consisting of 209 compounds used for fire prevention and insulation. PCBs are able to withstand exceptionally high temperatures in the manufacture of transformers and capacitors. PCBs can bioaccumulate in the environment, increasing in concentration as they move up the food chain from phytoplankton to zooplankton to fish. PCBs do not biodegrade in the environment. The General Electric Corporation (GE) contributed most of the PCBs to the Hudson River primarily at Hudson Falls from 1952 to 1977. These discharges were estimated at 14 kg/day or 5,000 kg/year, consisting mainly of Aroclor 1254, 1242, and 1016 with the percentage of chlorine indicated by the last two digits. GE discharged a total of 590,000 kg of PCBs, contaminating more than 200 miles of the Hudson River. More than 5 times this amount was in nearby landfills, and a similar amount was discovered in the geology beneath the two GE PCB plants. The contaminated sediments get stirred up and into the water and accumulate in fish, leading to a continued advisory from the New York State Department of Health to severely limit consumption of fish from the river. Eel, catfish, carp, shad, herring, sturgeon, and striped bass, as well as blue crab and a variety of shellfish, had been fished commercially in the Hudson River; all were found to be contaminated with PCBs exceeding Food and Drug Administration (FDA) thresholds of <2 parts per million (ppm) parts flesh. Striped bass have PCB levels of 2–6 ppm and humans average around 45 ppb. U.S. Fish and Wildlife Service studied tree swallows near the highest PCB contamination sites and found that the birds were unable to build normal nests, abandoned their eggs or had nonviable eggs, showed signs of transsexuality, and had malformations and tumors. Human health effects of PCBs have included skin changes including chloracne, suppression of immune activation, liver enzyme and microsomal enzyme increases, and neurobehavioral abnormalities in children. The EPA and the International Agency for Research on Cancer (IARC) have determined that PCBs are probably carcinogenic to humans.

The Thompson Island pool is the most heavily contaminated section of the Hudson River, and the chemical pattern there can track the PCBs to GE's particular mixtures of Aroclors. On August 1, 2002, EPA Administrator Christine Todd Whitman proposed dredging of "hot spots" of PCBs in 40 river miles of the Hudson. Approximately 2.65 million cubic yards of PCB-contaminated sediment would be removed from this Superfund site. The PCB-laden dirt and debris would be processed into a filter cake, placed inside lined railcars, taken to a disposal facility for hazardous waste near the Texas–New Mexico border, and buried in the ground surrounded by clay. The U.S. Department of Justice and the EPA have sought payment (EPA estimates are $460 million) and participation by GE in the cleanup and sampling of water and sediments for PCBs in the Hudson River. Phase 1 of the six-year project began in 2009, with 293,000 cubic yards of contaminated sediments removed. The long delay, stretching over more than three decades, demonstrates the contentious nature of the PCB pollution and the ability of the corporate polluters to deny and prolong the cleanup efforts.

European Approach to Toxic Chemicals: REACH

In 2006, the European Union (EU) leapfrogged ahead of U.S. policy with new legislation called **Registration, Evaluation, Authorization, and Restriction of Chemicals (REACH)**. The core structural difference between REACH and TSCA is the European law's requirement that chemical manufacturers and importers, not the government, provide basic information on the identity and physical properties of ~30,000 chemicals sold in volumes of more than one metric ton per year per producer.[1] More comprehensive hazard data are required for a subset of ~12,000 substances whose sales exceed 10 metric tons per year. REACH also designates some chemicals as substances of very high concern (SVHCs) based on environmental persistence and bioaccumulation or their classification as carcinogens, mutagens, or reproductive toxicants. Thus chemicals are prioritized by hazard and exposure potential, and chemicals of concern are subject to use-by-use authorization whereas TSCA has no requirements on prioritization or supply chain transparency. REACH can also regulate a chemical if it is designated as very persistent or very bioaccumulative; thus REACH put into place a precautionary approach to chemicals. REACH is estimated to save $60 billion over thirty years due to prevention of occupational diseases alone. By improving overall transparency and accountability in the chemicals market, REACH is expected to advance green chemistry innovation and may become the global standard for chemical policy.

Limitations of the TSCA

TSCA has severe limitations in implementing a rigorous chemicals control policy. For example, since 1976 the EPA has been able to apply the statute in testing only about 200 chemicals and regulating and banning only five substances. In response to this federal vacuum, some states such as Massachusetts have decided to develop their own approach to chemical regulation. Reform of TSCA has become an environmental policy imperative in the United States. One of the first tasks of President Barack Obama's administration's EPA was to enunciate "Essential Principles for Reform of Chemicals Management Legislation" in reauthorizing TSCA. These principles were

1. Chemicals should be reviewed against safety standards that are based on sound science and reflect risk-based criteria protective of human health and the environment.
2. Manufacturers should provide EPA with the necessary information to conclude that new and existing chemicals are safe and do not endanger public

health and the environment. A corollary of this is that EPA needs authority to require submission of use and exposure information to downstream processors and users of chemicals.

3. Risk management decisions should take into account sensitive subpopulations, cost, availability of substitutes and other relevant considerations.
4. Manufacturers and EPA should assess and act on priority chemicals, both existing and new, in a timely manner.
5. Green chemistry should be encouraged and provisions assuring transparency and public access to information should be strengthened.
6. EPA should be given a sustained source of funding for implementation.[9]

Sen. Frank Lautenberg (D-NJ) proposed the Safe Chemicals Act in 2010 and 2011 along these principles. Sen. Lautenberg's Subcommittee on Superfund, Toxics and Environmental Health introduced it in 2010 to the Environment and Public Works Committee after a year of hearings. There were no co-sponsors. Simultaneously, a companion bill, the Toxic Chemical Safety Act of 2010, was introduced into the House Energy and Commerce Committee by Representatives Bobby Rush (D-IL) and Henry Waxman (D-CA). Both of these bills will take years of effort to pass.

Comprehensive Environmental Response, Compensation, and Liability Act (Superfund)

The **Comprehensive Environmental Response, Compensation, and Liability Act (CERCLA)**, commonly known as **Superfund**, was enacted by Congress on December 11, 1980. CERCLA provides a federal "Superfund" to clean up uncontrolled or abandoned hazardous waste sites as well as accidents, spills, and other emergency releases of pollutants and contaminants into the environment. To pay for the Superfund, CERCLA created a tax on the chemical and petroleum industries and provided broad federal authority to respond directly to releases or threatened releases of hazardous substances that may endanger public health or the environment. The Superfund authorizes the EPA to follow one of two avenues for remediation. The first is to sue responsible parties to require them to perform the remediation work. Responsible parties include generators of the hazardous substances found at the offending site, transporters who took the substances to the site, current owners or operators of the site, and owners and operators of the site at the time the hazardous substances were disposed there. The second avenue is for the EPA to remediate the site itself and to sue the responsible parties to recover its costs. Whichever route the EPA chooses, the resulting process and remedial action are approximately the same and the responsible parties ultimately bear the cost of cleanup. There may be hundreds of responsible parties at a site. The EPA usually can handle only a limited number of these cases.

The parties the EPA identifies have the right to pursue the remaining responsible parties to recover their contribution to remedial costs. The law authorizes two kinds of response actions: short-term removals, when actions may be taken to address releases or threatened releases requiring prompt response, and long-term remedial response actions that permanently and significantly reduce the dangers associated with releases or threats of releases of hazardous substances that are serious but not immediately life threatening. These actions can be conducted only at sites listed on EPA's **National Priorities List (NPL)**, which is the list of national priorities among the known releases or threatened releases of hazardous substances, pollutants, or contaminants throughout the United States and its territories.

There are more than 30,000 sites on the EPA's **Comprehensive Environmental Response, Compensation, and Liability Information System (CERCLIS)** list for Superfund evaluation; currently some 1,300 have been placed on the NPL for Superfund action. When a site is placed on the first list, it is evaluated to determine whether any immediate action (removal of leaking drums, fencing) is necessary to prevent serious adverse effects, and a hazard evaluation is completed to determine whether the site should be placed on the NPL. Once a site is on the NPL, a remedial investigation is conducted to determine the nature and extent of contamination and the routes of exposure to people and the environment. Then a feasibility study is done to determine alternative actions and their cost. The EPA then chooses an option in a public notice and comment procedure, after which remedial action is taken. Superfund site identification, monitoring, and response activities in states are coordinated through the state environmental protection or waste management agencies.

The **Agency for Toxic Substances and Disease Registry (ATSDR)** of the Public Health Service's job is to perform a health assessment for all sites on the NPL and for sites for which physicians so petition. The assessments are to determine potential human health risk at the sites, to help decide what remedial action should be taken, and whether additional health information, including epidemiologic studies and registries of exposed persons, should be developed. In addition, ATSDR is to develop toxicologic profiles of the 100 or more most common hazardous substances found at Superfund sites. These hazardous substances are ranked based on frequency of occurrence at NPL sites, toxicity, and potential for human exposure. Toxicological profiles are developed from a priority list of 275 substances. The ATSDR toxicological profile succinctly characterizes the toxicologic and adverse health effects information for the hazardous substance described here. Each peer-reviewed profile identifies and reviews the key literature that describes a hazardous substance's toxicologic properties.

CASE STUDY: LIBBY, MONTANA, ASBESTOS EXPOSURE

In 1999, the ATSDR was asked by the Department of Health and Human Services to evaluate human health concerns related to asbestos exposure in Libby, Montana. Vermiculite mining in and near Libby began in the 1920s and was continued by W. R. Grace Company from 1963 to 1990. The vermiculite ore mined in Libby was contaminated with fibrous tremolite asbestos. In 1984, Lockey and colleagues reported on pleural disease, including pleural effusions and thickening, at an Ohio factory that processed vermiculite from Libby, Montana.[10] Mortality studies of the mine and mill workers with less than one year employment documented increased risk of lung cancer and nonmalignant respiratory disease.[11] Ambient community exposure increased risk of respiratory disease mortality among community residents and household contacts of Libby vermiculite workers.

The National Institute for Occupational Safety and Health updated the mortality of 1,672 white men hired at Libby from 1935 to 1981 and followed through 2001. Of 752 men who died, 13.2% died from lung cancer (SMR 1.7, 95% [confidence interval] CI 1.4–2.1), 2% from mesothelioma (fifteen cases), and 5.3% with asbestosis (SMR 166, 95%CI 104–251).[11] Radiographic surveys in Libby reaching 7,307 persons found 17.8% with pleural abnormalities and <1% with interstitial changes; there was an increase from 6.7% in those with no identifiable exposure pathway to 34.6% for those reporting up to twelve exposure pathways.[12] Pleural abnormalities are difficult to ascertain on a plain chest radiograph due to overlapping rib; computed tomography (CT scans) found 98 (27.8%) of 353 medical survey participants to have pleural disease when the plain chest radiograph was indeterminate.[13] Of these ninety-eight people, sixty-nine (70.4%) were either former vermiculite mine or mill workers or household contacts. Chest radiographs of former Ohio vermiculite plant workers found similar prevalences: 28.7% had pleural abnormalities and 2.9% interstitial changes.[14] A survey of more than 1,000 children from 2000 to 2001 found that respiratory symptoms of cough, shortness of breath when walking up a slight hill or hurrying on level ground, or coughing up bloody phlegm in the past year were associated with frequently handling vermiculite insulation.[15] Since vermiculite was shipped to more than seventy unique sites in twenty-three states, ATSDR evaluated mortality near these sites and found eleven sites with excess mesothelioma that could have been related to the asbestos exposure.[16]

W. R. Grace Company and its sixty-one U.S. subsidiaries filed for bankruptcy in 2001, claiming they could not afford the burden of asbestos-related lawsuits. The U.S. government filed criminal charges against W. R. Grace and several executives; the case was tried in U.S. District Court in Missoula, Montana, with the jury deciding that the U.S. government had not proven its case. The company was acquitted of eight criminal charges, including conspiracy, violation of the Clean Air Act, and obstruction of justice. EPA has designated the mill and export plant of the W. R. Grace vermiculite operation to be Superfund sites and is pursuing a cleanup plan. EPA has provided $120 million for the cleanup and another $130 million for a public health emergency to clean up homes, schools, and public buildings to remove asbestos fibers and to provide medical assistance. ATSDR has opened a respiratory clinic to treat affected workers and community residents.

CERCLA also revised the **National Contingency Plan (NCP)**, which provides the guidelines and procedures needed to respond to releases and threatened releases of hazardous substances, pollutants, or contaminants. Under the NCP and the National Response Plan, EPA emergency response personnel have worked with the Federal Emergency Management Agency (FEMA) and state and local agencies to respond to hurricanes (such as Katrina) and other natural disasters. Together, they've assessed the damage, tested health and environmental conditions, and coordinated clean-up. In emergency situations such as these, EPA serves as the lead agency for the cleanup of hazardous materials. CERCLA was amended in 1986 as the **Superfund Amendments and Reauthorization Act**, which increased the focus on human health problems posed by hazardous waste site, increased the size of the trust fund to $8.5 billion, required EPA to revise the hazard-ranking system to ensure that it accurately assessed the relative degree of risk to human health and the environment posed by uncontrolled hazardous waste sites, required cost effectiveness of cleanups in both the long term and the short term, and required cleanups to meet the Safe Drinking Water Act's recommended maximum contaminant levels (RMCLs) and the Clean Water Act's water quality criteria.

Resource Conservation and Recovery Act

The **Resource Conservation and Recovery Act (RCRA)** enacted in 1976 grafted on earlier legislation under which the EPA gave technical assistance to states on solid waste disposal and established guidelines for federal solid waste minimization and disposal programs. RCRA regulates approximately 20,000 hazardous waste generators and 280 million tons of hazardous waste; in addition, RCRA also regulates approximately 208 million tons of municipal solid waste in the United States. RCRA creates a cradle-to-grave regulatory scheme to manage storage, transport, and disposal of hazardous waste administered by the EPA or by states that have approved programs. Generators of hazardous waste must dispose of it at facilities designated for that particular waste. If the permitted disposal site is not located on the generator's facility, the generator must transport the waste to the disposal site, accompanied by an RCRA manifest to document proper disposition. Exacting standards are established in regulations for the common types of storage and disposal facilities: incinerators, landfills, and surface impoundments, among others. These requirements include prohibitions on disposal of particular wastes in specific types of facilities (for example, no liquid wastes may be disposed in landfills). Closure and postclosure requirements are also established to avoid release of the waste into the environment after the disposal facilities are closed. Permitted facilities must identify on-site pre–RCRA disposal areas and take remedial measures, if necessary, to ensure they do not release hazardous wastes into the environment. Hazardous waste generators are to certify they have taken measures to minimize the generation of hazardous waste. The high cost of disposal, however, creates an incentive for waste minimization quite apart from the requirement. It is generally thought that, as a result, hazardous waste generation has declined by some 25% since the system became effective.

Wastes covered by this system include those that are (1) corrosive; (2) ignitable; (3) reactive; (4) capable of releasing in excess of specified amounts of heavy metals, pesticides, or organic contaminants; (5) contained on a list of more than 100 specific industrial wastes; or (6) contained on a list of several hundred specific discarded commercial chemical products. These categories are broad and sweeping and contain some wastes that are not truly hazardous. The EPA's regulations contain a procedure for "delisting" such wastes to remove them from the RCRA system. Delisting, however, is an expensive and time-consuming procedure with an uncertain rate of success.

While RCRA establishes a comprehensive program for regulating hazardous waste disposal, it deals with nonhazardous waste disposal only by requiring states to bring their municipal landfills into conformity with standards established by the EPA. The EPA cannot enforce the standard against violating landfills unless it finds the state does not have a solid waste regulatory program that meets RCRA standards. As a practical matter, municipal landfills subject to these standards may be used by generators of hazardous waste who dispose of it in quantities small enough to escape hazardous waste regulation. In addition, the landfills contain the residues of household products that would be classified as hazardous wastes if they were discarded by industries in larger quantities. It is not surprising that the composition of leachates from industrial and municipal landfills is similar. There is an emerging crisis in much of the Northeast over the rapid exhaustion of existing landfill capacity coupled with the inability to locate new landfills in the face of local opposition, especially to disposal of waste generated out of state.

Recycling has emerged as a major contributor to reduction of solid waste since the 1980s. Aluminum beverage cans are the most recycled item in the United States, and because of this success, aluminum cans account for less than 1% of the total U.S. waste stream. Paper recycling is critical, since a single run of the Sunday *New York Times* consumes 75,000 trees. Americans use 85,000,000 tons of paper a year or 680 pounds per person. Each ton of recycled paper can save seventeen trees, 380 gallons of oil, 3 cubic yards of landfill space,

4,000 kilowatts of energy, and 7,000 gallons of water. This represents a 64% energy savings, a 58% water savings, and 60 pounds less of air pollution. Recycling half the world's paper would avoid the harvesting of 20 million acres of forestland. The EPA has estimated that recycling causes 35% less water pollution and 74% less air pollution than making virgin paper. The United States is the leading trash-producing country in the world at 1,609 pounds per person per year—we are 5% of the world's people and generate 40% of the world's waste. It costs approximately $30 per ton to recycle trash, $50 to send it to a landfill, and $65–$75 to incinerate it.

The Federal Hazardous and Solid Waste Amendments of 1984 to RCRA required phasing out land disposal of hazardous waste. Some of the other mandates of this strict law include increased enforcement authority for EPA, more stringent hazardous waste management standards, and a comprehensive underground storage tank program. These amendments, which provide for the management of commercial hazardous waste storage or destruction facilities, authorized ATSDR to conduct public health assessments at these sites, when requested by the EPA, states, or individuals.

The 1986 amendments to RCRA enabled EPA to address environmental problems that could result from underground tanks storing petroleum and other hazardous substances. RCRA focuses only on active and future facilities and does not address abandoned or historical sites, which are the focus of CERCLA.

Federal Insecticide, Fungicide, and Rodenticide Act

The **Federal Insecticide, Fungicide, and Rodenticide Act (FIFRA)** dates back to 1947 legislation designed to ensure the efficacy of products for agricultural customers, farmers, and other growers. In 1972 Congress substantially amended the earlier effort to focus on health and environment as well as on efficacy. The main regulatory tool of FIFRA is the registration of pesticides. The EPA must register (license) all pesticides used in the United States. Registration assures that pesticides will be properly labeled and that if in accordance with specifications will not cause unreasonable harm to the environment. To be registered for a particular use the pesticide must (1) be efficacious for that use, (2) carry a label with directions for the use, (3) perform the use without unreasonably adverse effects on health and the environment, and (4) not result in such effects when used in common practice. The EPA weighs the usefulness of pesticides against their detrimental effects. Almost by definition, pesticides have some adverse effects, but their benefits in providing an abundant food supply, preserving food from decay, or ridding premises of pests may outweigh those effects. Adverse effects may be avoided or minimized by requiring pesticide labels to give directions on how registered uses can be accomplished safely.

Some key elements of FIFRA include:

- A product licensing statute; pesticide products must obtain an EPA registration before manufacture, transport, and sale
- Registration based on a risk/benefit standard
- Strong authority to require data: authority to issue data call-ins on degradation, toxicity testing, chemical activity, and so on
- Ability to regulate pesticide use through labeling, packaging, composition, and disposal
- Emergency exemption authority: permits approval of unregistered uses of registered products on a time-limited basis
- Ability to suspend or cancel a product's registration: appeals process, adjudicatory functions, and so on

Pesticides may be registered for general or restricted use. Restricted use pesticides may be applied only by applicators who are trained and licensed by the state. Recent amendments to FIFRA require previously registered pesticides to be reregistered so that they are reviewed using contemporary data and criteria. Registration may be canceled if data developed subsequent to the registration would justify a decision not to register. Distributing an unregistered pesticide or failing to comply with the directions on the label is a violation of FIFRA.

Pesticides have both active and inert ingredients. These terms must be understood in their pesticide context. A so-called inert ingredient is not really inert; it just is not pesticidal and is used for another purpose, for instance, as a carrier. Inert ingredients in pesticides may be as harmful as active ingredients to health and the environment.

The focus of the EPA's registration activities is currently generic reregistration of each active ingredient. Under this approach, the EPA reviews the available data on each chemical used as an active ingredient, identifies data gaps that must be filled, and publishes a generic standard that sets forth the uses for which the ingredient will be authorized. These standards are interim standards, however, to be used until the data gaps are filled. The data that the EPA requires for registration include residue chemistry; environmental fate; degradation, metabolism, mobility, dissipation, and accumulation studies; acute, chronic, and subchronic effects on humans and other nontarget species; teratogenicity and mutagenicity studies; and pesticide spray drift evaluation. Moreover, pesticide registrants have a continuing obligation to provide post-registration data to the EPA whenever the registrant becomes aware of data that suggest adverse effects. This includes incomplete toxicologic studies and individual incident reports.

The EPA has a tremendous bank of information on health effects of registered pesticides. Although much of this is available to the public, the security maintained for business confidential information submitted to the EPA under FIFRA is extraordinarily tight. Indeed, a longer prison term may be imposed for disclosing business confidential FIFRA information than for violating the substantive requirements of FIFRA. This has an inhibiting effect on the EPA personnel who deal with requests for FIFRA information. Nevertheless, most of the health data are publicly available, and even confidential information may be released to doctors and others to the extent necessary to treat or prevent illness. The office to contact for such information is the Health Effects Division in the Office of Pesticide Programs in Washington, D.C.

If the pesticide is proposed for use on a food crop, EPA determines whether a safe level of pesticide residue, called a "tolerance," can be established under the Federal Food, Drug and Cosmetic Act (FFDCA). A tolerance must be established before a pesticide registration may be granted for use on food. If any registration is granted, the agency specifies the approved uses and conditions of use, including safe methods of pesticide storage and disposal, which the registrant must explain on the product label.

Summary

There are several tens of thousands chemicals in commerce that have leaked into the environment and bioaccumulated in human serum and fat. These chemicals may cause risk to humans for cancer, liver disease, cardiovascular disease, neurobehavioral effects, and altered reproduction. To avoid these adverse effects, regulatory strategies are necessary. The Toxic Substances Control Act uses the EPA as the lead agency to regulate chemicals that are found to have toxic effects. This law does not use the precautionary principle, and chemicals are not removed until hazard is demonstrated. In contrast, Europe's regulatory law demands that chemicals be proven to be safe before entering the market place. New proposals to reauthorize TSCA follow the precautionary principle. Toxic chemicals such as tremolite asbestos, PCBs, and endocrine disrupters have entered ecosystems. Superfund sites are being identified and remediated by EPA and former or current polluters. Pesticides are another chemical stream that faces EPA registration and regulation, and hazardous waste containing many toxic chemicals allows EPA to regulate chemicals from cradle to grave.

Key Terms

Agency for Toxic Substances and Disease Registry (ATSDR)

Biomonitoring

Comprehensive Environmental Response, Compensation, and Liability Act (CERCLA or Superfund)

Comprehensive Environmental Response, Compensation, and Liability Information System (CERCLIS)

Endocrine-disrupting chemicals (EDCs)

Federal Insecticide, Fungicide, and Rodenticide Act (FIFRA)

High production volume (HPV) chemicals

National Contingency Plan (NCP)

National Health and Nutrition Examination Survey (NHANES)

National Priorities List (NPL)

Registration, Evaluation, Authorization, and Restriction of Chemicals (REACH)

Resource Conservation and Recovery Act (RCRA)

Superfund Amendments and Reauthorization Act

Toxic Substances Control Act (TSCA)

Discussion Questions

1. What are the differences between the TSCA in the United States and REACH in Europe? Which act do you think is more productive?
2. Do you think the TSCA has enough power in the United States to regulate all potentially harmful chemicals? What might you do as an informed citizen to help protect our health and the environment from these potentially harmful substances?
3. In the Libby, Montana, Asbestos Exposure case study discussed in this chapter, it says that the U.S. government failed to find W. R. Grace Company at fault. Investigate the reasons for this and how the government might have taken a different approach.
4. As a consumer, how might you take remedial steps to ensure a safer environment?

Chapter 1: The Clean Air Act and the National Environmental Policy Act

1. Bulletin No. 306, Air pollution in Donora, PA, epidemiology of the unusual smog episode of October 1948 (Public Health Service).
2. Berton Roueché, The fog, New Yorker, September 30, 1950.
3. Martineau RJ, Novello DP, editors. The Clean Air Act handbook. 2nd ed. Chicago: ABA; 2004.
4. Collins J, Koplan JP. Health impact assessment: a step toward health in all policies. JAMA 2009; 302:315–317.

Chapter 2: Particulate Matter

1. Pope CA 3rd, Thun MJ, Namboodiri MM, Dockery DW, Evans JS, Speizer FE, Heath CW. Particulate air pollution as a predictor of mortality in a prospective study of U.S. adults. Am J Respir Crit Care Med 1995; 151:669–674.
2. Pope CA 3rd, Burnett RT, Thurston GD, Thun MJ, Calle EE, Krewski D, Godleski JJ. Cardiovascular mortality and long-term exposure to particulate air pollution: epidemiological evidence of general pathophysiological pathways of disease. Circulation 2004; 109:71–77.
3. Pope CA 3rd, Burnett RT, Thun MJ, Calle EE, Krewski D, Ito K, Thurston GD. Lung cancer, cardiopulmonary mortality, and long-term exposure to fine particulate air pollution. JAMA 2002; 287:1132–1141.
4. Pope CA 3rd, Ezzati M, Dockery DW. Fine-particulate air pollution and life expectancy in the United States. N Engl J Med 2009; 360:376–386.
5. Dockery DW, Pope CA 3rd, Xu X, Spengler JD, Ware JH, Fay ME, Benjamin G, Speizer FE. An association between air pollution and mortality in six U.S. cities. N Engl J Med 1993; 329:1753–1759.

6. Laden F, Schwartz J, Speizer FE, Dockery DW. Reduction in fine particulate air pollution and mortality: extended follow-up of the Harvard Six City Study. Am J Respir Crit Care Med 2006; 173:667–672.

7. Samet JM, Dominici F, Curriero FC, Coursac I, Zeger SL. Fine particulate air pollution and mortality in 20 U.S. cities, 1987–1994. N Engl J Med 2000; 343:1742–1749.

8. Dominici F, Peng RD, Bell ML, Pham L, McDermott A, Zeger SL, Samet JM. Fine particulate air pollution and hospital admission for cardiovascular and respiratory diseases. JAMA 2006; 295:1127–1134.

9. Moolgavkar SH. Air pollution and daily mortality in three U.S. counties. Environ Health Prospect 2000; 108:777–784.

10. Atkinson RW, Anderson HR, Sunyer J, Ayers J, Baccini M, Vonk JM, Boumghar A, Forastiere F, Forsberg B, Touloumi G, Schwartz J, Katsouyanni K. Acute effects of particulate air pollution on respiratory admissions. Am J Respir Crit Care Med 2001; 164:1860–1866.

11. Downs SH, Schindler C, Liu LJS, Keidel D, Bayer-Oglesby L, Brutsche MH, Gerbase MW, Keller R, Kunzli N, Leuenberger P, Probst-Hensch NM, Tschopp J-M, Zellweger J-P, Rochat T, Schwartz J, Ackermann-Liebrich U, SAPALDIA team. Reduced exposure to PM10 and attenuated age-related decline in lung function. N Engl J Med 2007; 357:2338–2347.

12. Gauderman WJ, Avol E, Gilliland F, Vora H, Thomas D, Berhane K, McConnell R, Kuenzli N, Lurmann F, Rappaport E, Margolis H, Bates D, Peters J. The effect of air pollution on lung development from 10 to 18 years of age. N Engl J Med 2004; 351:1057–1067.

13. Gauderman WJ, Vora H, McConnell R, Berhane K, Gilliland F, Thomas D, Lurmann F, Avol E, Kunzli N, Jerrett M, Peters M. Effect of exposure to traffic on lung development from 10 to 18 years of age: a cohort study. Lancet 2007; 369:571–577.

14. McConnell R, Berhane K, Yao L, Jerrett M, Lurmann F, Gilliland F, Kunzli N, Gauderman WJ, Avol E, Thomas D, Peters J. Traffic, susceptibility, and childhood asthma. Environ Health Perspect 2006; 114:766–772.

15. Avol EL, Gauderman WJ, Tan SM, London SJ, Peters JM. Respiratory effects of relocating to areas of differing pollution levels. Am J Respir Crit Care Med 2001; 164:2067–2072.

16. Hoek G, Brunekreef B, Goldbohm S, Fischer P, van den Brandt PA. Association between mortality and indicators of traffic-related air pollution in the Netherlands: a cohort study. Lancet 2002; 360:1203–1209.

17. McCreanor J, Cullinan P, Nieuwenhuijsen MJ, Stewart-Evans J, Malliarou E, Jarup L, Harrington R, Svartengren M, Han I-K, Ohman-Strickland P, Chung KF, Zhang J. Respiratory effects of exposure to diesel traffic in persons with asthma. N Engl J Med 2007; 357:2348–2358.

18. Kulkarni N, Pierse N, Rushton L, Grigg J. Carbon in airway macrophages and lung function in children. N Engl J Med 2006; 355:21–30.

19. Pope CA 3rd, Schwartz J, Ransom MR. Daily mortality and PM10 pollution in Utah Valley. Arch Environ Health 1992; 47:211–217.

20. Clancy L, Goodman P, Sinclair H, Dockery DW. Effect of air-pollution control on death rates in Dublin, Ireland: an intervention study. Lancet 2002; 360: 1210–1214.

21. Ghio AJ, Devlin RB. Inflammatory lung injury after bronchial instillation of air pollution particles. Am J Respir Crit Care Med 2001; 164:704–708.

22. Schaumann F, Borm PJA, Herbrich A, Knoch J, Pitz M, Schins RPF, Luettig B, Hohlfeld JM, Heinrich J, Krug N. Metal-rich ambient particles (Particulate Matter2.5) cause airway inflammation in healthy subjects. Am J Respir Crit Care Med 2004; 170:898–903.

23. Reibman j, Hsu Y, Chen LC, Bleck B, Gordon T. Airway epithelial cells release MIP-3α/CCL70 in response to cytokines and ambient particulate matter. Am J Respir Cell Mol Biol 2003; 28:648–654.

24. Bleck B, Tse DB, Curotto de Lafaille MA, Zhang F, Reibman J. Diesel exhaust particle-exposed human bronchial epithelial cells induce dendritic cell maturation and polarization via thymic stromal lymphopoietin. J Clin Immunol 2008; 28:147–156.

25. Seaton A, MacNee W, Donaldson K, Godden D. Particulate air pollution and acute health effects. Lancet 1995; 345:176–178.

26. Goto Y, Ishii H, Hogg JC, Shih C-H, Yatera K, Vincent R, van Eeden SF. Particulate matter air pollution stimulates monocyte release from the bone marrow. Am J Respir Crit Care Med 2004; 170:891–897.

27. Terashima T, Wiggs B, English D, Hogg JC, van Eeden SF. Phagocytosis of small carbon particles (PM10) by alveolar macrophages stimulates the release of polymorphonuclear leukocytes from bone marrow. Am J Respir Crit Care Med 1997; 155:1441–1447.

28. van Eeden SF, Yeung A, Quinlam K, Hogg JC. Systemic response to ambient particulate matter: Relevance to chronic obstructive pulmonary disease. Proc Am Thorac Soc 2005; 2:61–67.

29. Gurgueira SA, Lawrence J, Coull B, Murthy GGK, Gonzalez-Flecha B. Rapid increase in the steady-state concentration of reactive oxygen species in the lungs and heart after particulate air pollution inhalation. Environ Health Perspect 2002; 110:749–755.

30. Sun Q, Wang A, Jin X, Natanzon A, Duquaine D, Brook RD, Aguinaldo J-GS, Fayad ZA, Fuster V, Lippmann M, Chen LC, Rajagopalan S. Long-term air pollution exposure and acceleration of atherosclerosis and vascular inflammation in an animal model. JAMA 2005; 294:3003–3010.

31. Arajujo JA, Barajas B, Kleinman M, Wang X, Bennett BJ, Gong KW, Navab M, Harkema J, Sioutas C, Lusis AJ, Nel AE. Ambient particulate pollutants in the ultra fine ranges promote early atherosclerosis and systemic oxidative stress. Circ Res 2008; 102:1–8.

32. Ruckerl R, Ibald-Mulli A, Koenig W, Schneider A, Woelke G, Cyrys J, Heinrich J, Marder V, Frampton M, Wichmann HE, Peters A. Air pollution and markers of

inflammatory and coagulation in patients with coronary heart disease. Am J Respir Crit Care Med 2006; 173:432–441.

33. Peters A, von Klot S, Heier M, Trentinaglia I, Hormann A, Wichmann HE, Lowel H. Exposure to traffic and the onset of myocardial infarction. N Engl J Med 2004; 351:1721–1730.

34. Tonne C, Melly S, Mittlemann M, Coull B, Goldberg R, Schwartz J. A case-control analysis of exposure to traffic and acute myocardial infarction. Environ Health Perspect 2007; 115:53–57.

35. Chen LH, Knutsen SF, Shavlik D, Beeson WL, Petersen F, Ghamsary M, Abbey D. The association between fatal coronary heart disease and ambient particulate air pollution: Are females at greater risk? Environ Health Prospect 2005; 113:1723–1729.

36. Miller KA, Siscovick DS, Sheppard L, Shepherd K, Sullivan JH, Anderson GL, Kaufman JD. Long-term exposure to air pollution and incidence of cardiovascular events in women. N Engl J Med 2007; 356:447–458.

37. Mills NL, Tornqvist H, Gonzalez MC, Vink E, Robinson S, Soderberg S, Boon NA, Donaldson K, Sandstrom T, Blomberg A, Newby DE. Ischemic and thrombotic effects of dilute diesel-exhaust inhalation in men with coronary heart disease. N Engl J Med 2007; 357:1075–1082.

38. Kunzli N, Jerrett M, Mack WJ, Beckerman B, LaBree L, Gilliland F, Thomas D, Peters J, Hodis HN. Ambient air pollution and atherosclerosis in Los Angeles. Environ Health Perspect 2005; 113:201–206.

39. Schwartz J, Park SK, O'Neill MS, Vokona PS, Sparrow D, Weiss S, Kelsey K. Glutathione-S-transferase M1, obesity, statins, and autonomic effects of particles: gene by drug by environment interaction. Am J Respir Crit Care Med 2005; 172:1529–1533.

40. Dockery DW, Luttmann-Gibson H, Rich DQ, et al. Association of air pollution with increased incidence of ventricular tachyarrhythmias recorded by implanted cardioverter defibrillators. Environ Health Perspect 2005; 113:670–674.

41. Pereira LA, Loomis D, Conceicao GM, et al. Association between air pollution and intrauterine mortality in São Paulo, Brazil. Environ Health Perspect 1998; 106:325–329.

42. Sagiv SK, Mendola P, Loomis D, et al. A time-series analysis of air pollution and preterm birth in Pennsylvania, 1997–2001. Environ Health Perspect 2005; 113:602–606.

43. Rich DQ, Demissie K, Lu SE, Kamat L, Wartenberg D, Rhoads GG. Ambient air pollutant concentrations during pregnancy and the risk of fetal growth restriction. J Epidemiol Community Health 2009; 0:1–9.

44. Schwartz J, Norris G, Larson T, Sheppard L, Claiborne C, Koenig J. Episodes of high coarse particle concentrations are not associated with increased mortality. Environ Health Perspect 1999; 107:339–342.

45. Pope CA 3rd, Hill RW, Villegas GM. Particulate air pollution and daily mortality on Utah's Wasatch Front. Environ Health Perspect 1999; 107:567–573.

46. Vedal S, Sullivan JH. Particulate matter. In: Rom, WN, Markowitz, SB, editors. Environmental and occupational medicine. 4th ed. New York: Lippincott Williams & Wilkins; 2007. p. 1487–1506.

47. Laden F, Neas LM, Dockery DW, Schwartz J. Association of fine particulate matter from different sources with daily mortality in six U.S. cities. Environ Health Perspect 2000; 108:941–947.

48. Huang YC, Ghio AJ, Stonehuerner J, et al. The role of soluble components in ambient fine particles-induced changes in human lungs and blood. Inhal Toxicol 2003; 15:327–342.

49. Gong H Jr., Linn WS, Clark KW, Anderson KR, Geller MD, Sioutas C. Respiratory responses to exposures with fine particulates and nitrogen dioxide in the elderly with and without COPD. Inhal Toxicol 2005; 17:123–132.

50. Stenfors N, Nordenhall C, Salvi SS, et al. Different airway inflammatory responses in asthmatic and healthy humans exposed to diesel. Eur Respir J 2004; 23:82–86.

51. Nordenhall C, Pourazar J, Ledin MC, Levin JO, Sandstrom T, Adelroth E. Diesel exhaust enhances airway responsiveness in asthmatic subjects. Eur Respir J 2001; 17:909–915.

52. Svartengren M, Strand V, Bylin G, Jarup L, Pershagen G. Short-term exposure to air pollution in a road tunnel enhances the asthmatic response to allergen. Eur Respir J 2000; 15:716–724.

53. Diaz-Sanchez D, Tsien A, Fleming J, Saxon A. Combined diesel exhaust particulate and ragweed allergen challenge markedly enhances human in vivo nasal ragweed-specific IgE and skews cytokine production to a T helper cell 2-type pattern. J Immunol 1997; 158:2406–2413.

54. Heinrich J, Wichmann HE. Traffic related pollutants in Europe and their effect on allergic disease. Curr Opin Allergy Clin Immunol 2004; 4:341–348.

55. Rom WN, Samet JM. Small particles with big effects. Am J Respir Crit Care Med 2006; 173:365–369.

Chapter 3: Ozone

1. Lippmann M. Ozone. In: Rom, WN, Markowitz, SB, editors. Environmental and occupational medicine. 4th ed. New York: Lippincott Williams & Wilkins; 2007. p. 1445–1465.

2. Bates DV, Bell GM, Burnham CD, Hazucha MJ, Mantha J, Pengelly LD, Silverman F. Short-term effects of ozone on the lung. J Appl Physiol 1972; 32:176–181.

3. Mortimer KM, Neas LM, Dockery DW, et al. The effect of air pollution on inner-city children with asthma. Eur Respir J 2002; 19:699–705.

4. Folinsbee LJ, Bedi JF, Horvath SM. Respiratory responses in humans repeatedly exposed to low concentrations of ozone. Am Rev Respir Dis 1980; 121:431–439.

5. Horvath SM, Gliner JA, Folinsbee LJ. Adaptation to ozone: duration of effect. Am Rev Respir Dis 1981; 123:496–499.

6. Frank R, Liu MC, Spannhake EW, et al. Repetitive ozone exposures of young adults: evidence of persistent small airway dysfunction. Am J Respir Crit Care Med 2001; 164:1253–1260.

7. Folinsbee LJ, Horstman DH, Kehrl HR, et al. Respiratory response to repeated prolonged exposure to 0.12 ppm ozone. Am J Respir Crit Care Med 1994; 149:98–105.

8. Kinney PL, Ware JH, Spengler JD, Dockery DW, Speizer FE, Ferris BG Jr. Short-term pulmonary function change in association with ozone levels. Am Rev Respir Dis 1989; 139:56–61.

9. Thurston GD, Lippmann M, Scott MB, et al. Summertime haze air pollution and children with asthma. Am J Respir Crit Care Med 1997; 155:654–660.

10. Spektor DM, Lippmann M, Thurston GD, et al. Effects of ambient ozone on respiratory function in healthy adults exercising outdoors. Am Rev Respir Dis 1988; 138:821–828.

11. Brunekreef B, Hoek G, Brugelmans O, et al. Respiratory effects of low-level photochemical air pollution in amateur cyclists. Am J Respir Crit Care Med 1994; 150:962–966.

12. Korrick SA, Neas LM, Dockery DW, et al. Effects of ozone and other pollutants on the pulmonary function of adult hikers. Environ Health Perspect 1998; 106:93–99.

13. Brauer M, Blair J, Vedal S. Effect of ambient ozone exposure on lung function in farm workers. Am J Respir Crit Care Med 1996; 154:981–987.

14. Naeher LP, Holford TR, Beckett WS, Belanger K, Triche EW, Bracken MB, Leaderer BP. Healthy women's PEF variations with ambient summer concentrations of PM_{10}, $PM_{2.5}$, SO_4^{2-}, H^+, and O_3. Am J Respir Crit Care Med 1999; 160:117–125.

15. Chan C-C, Wu T-H. Effects of ambient ozone exposure on mail carriers' peak expiratory flow rates. Environ Health Perspect 2005; 113:735–738.

16. Folinsbee LJ, McDonnell WF, Horstman DH. Pulmonary function and symptom responses after 6.6-hour exposure to 0.12 ppm ozone with moderate exercise. JAPCA 1988; 38:28–35.

17. Horstman DH, Folinsbee LJ, Ives PJ, et al. Ozone concentration and pulmonary response relationships for 6.6-hour exposures with five hours of moderate exercise to 0.08, 0.10, and 0.12 ppm. Am Rev Respir Dis 1990; 142:1158–1163.

18. McDonnell WF, Stewart PW, Andreoni S, et al. Proportion of moderately exercising individuals responding to low-level, multi-hour ozone exposure. Am J Respir Crit Care Med 1995; 152:589–596.

19. Molfino NA, Wright SC, Katz I, Tarlo S, Silverman F, McClean PA, Szalai JP, Raizenne M, Slutsky AS, Zamel N. Effect of low concentrations of ozone on inhaled allergen responses in asthmatic subjects. Lancet 1991; 338:199–203.

20. Jorres R, Nowak D, Magnussen H, et al. The effect of ozone exposure on allergen responsiveness in subjects with asthma or rhinitis. Am J Respir Crit Care Med 1996; 153:56–64.

21. Seltzer J, Bigby BG, Stulbarg M, Holtzman MJ, Nadel JA, Ueki IF, Leikauf GD, Goetzl EJ, Boushey HA. O_3-induced change in bronchial reactivity to methacholine and airway inflammation in humans. J Appl Physiol 1986; 60:1321–1326.

22. Koren HS, Devlin RB, Graham DE, Mann R, McGee MP, Horstman DH, Kozumbo WJ, Becker S, House DE, McDonnell WF, Bromberg PA. Ozone-induced inflammation in the lower airways of human subjects. Am Rev Respir Dis 1989; 139:407–415.

23. Graham DE, Koren HS. Biomarkers of inflammation in ozone-exposed humans: Comparison of the nasal and bronchoalveolar lavage. Am Rev Respir Dis 1990; 142:152–156.

24. Devlin RB, McDonnell WF, Mann R, Becker S, House DE, Schreinemachers D, Koren HS. Exposure of humans to ambient levels of ozone for 6.6 hours causes cellular and biochemical changes in the lung. Am J Respir Cell Mol Biol 1991; 4:72–81.

25. Aris RM, Christian D, Hearne PQ, Kerr K, Finkbeiner WE, Balmes JR. Ozone-induced airway inflammation in human subjects as determined by airway lavages and biopsy. Am Rev Respir Dis 1993; 148:1363–1372.

26. Schelegle ES, Siefkin AD, McDonald RJ. Time course of ozone-induced neutrophilia in normal humans. Am Rev Respir Dis 1991; 143:1353–1358.

27. Kinney PL, Nilsen DM, Lippmann M, Brescia M, Gordon T, McGovern T, El Fawal H, Devlin RB, Rom WN. Biomarkers of lung inflammation in recreational joggers exposed to ozone. Am J Respir Crit Care Med 1996; 154:1430–1435.

28. Basha MA, Gross KB, Gwizdala CJ, Haidar AH, Popovich J Jr. Bronchoalveolar lavages neutrophilia in asthmatic and healthy volunteers after controlled exposure to ozone and filtered purified air. Chest 1994; 106:1757–1765.

29. Chen LL, Tager IB, Peden DB, Christian DL, Ferrando RE, Welch BS, Balmes JR. Effect of ozone exposures on airway responses to inhaled allergen in asthmatic subjects. Chest 2004; 125:2328–2335.

30. Mudway IS, Kelly FJ. An investigation of inhaled ozone dose and the magnitude of airway inflammation in healthy adults. Am J Respir Crit Care Med 2004; 169:1089–1095.

31. Nightingale JA, Rogers DF, Chung KF, et al. No effect of inhaled budesonide on the response to inhaled ozone in normal subjects. Am J Respir Crit Care Med 2000; 161:479–486.

32. Samet JM, Hatch GE, Horstman D, et al. Effect of antioxidant supplementation on ozone-induced lung injury in human subjects. Am J Respir Crit Care Med 2001; 164:819–825.

33. Arsalane K, Gosset P, Vanhee D, Voisin C, Hamid Q, Tonnel A-B, Wallert B. Ozone stimulates synthesis of inflammatory cytokines by alveolar macrophages in vitro. Am J Respir Cell Mol Biol 1995; 13:60–68.

34. Salmon M, Koto H, Lynch OT, Haddad E-B, Lamb NJ, Quinlan GJ, Barnes PJ, Chung KF. Proliferation of airway epithelium after ozone exposure: effect of apocynin and dexamethansone. Am J Respir Crit Care Med 1998; 157:970–977.

35. Yoon H-K, Cho H-Y, Kleeberger SR. Protective role of matrix metalloproteinase-9 in ozone-induced airway inflammation. Environ Health Perspect 2007; 115:1557–1563.

36. Cho H-Y, Morgan DL, Bauer AK, Kleeberger SR. Signal transduction pathways of tumor necrosis factor-mediated lung injury induced by ozone in mice. Am J Respir Crit Care Med 2007; 175:829–839.

37. Frischer T, Studnicka M, Gartner C, Tauber E, Horak F, Veiter A, Spengler J, Kuhr J, Urbanek R. Lung function growth and ambient ozone: a three-year population study in school children. Am J Respir Crit Care Med 1999; 160:390–396.

38. McConnell R, Berhane K, Gilliland F, London SJ, Islam T, Gauderman WJ, Avol E, Margolis HG, Peters JM. Asthma in exercising children exposed to ozone: a cohort study. Lancet 2002; 359:386–391.

39. Gilliland FD, Berhane K, Rappaport EB, Thomas DC, Avol E, Gauderman WJ, London SJ, Margolis HG, McConnell R, Islam KT, Peters JM. The effects of ambient air pollution on school absenteeism due to respiratory illnesses. Epidemiology 2001; 12:43–54.

40. Islam T, McConnell R, Gauderman WJ, Avol E, Peters JM, Gilliland FD. Ozone, oxidant defense genes, and risk of asthma during adolescence. Am J Respir Crit Care Med 2008; 177:388–395.

41. Triche EW, Gent JF, Holford TR, Belanger K, Bracken MB, Beckett WS, Naeher L, McSharry J-E, Leaderer BP. Low-level ozone exposure and respiratory symptoms in infants. Environ Health Perspect 2006; 114:911–916.

42. Mortimer KM, Tager IB, Dockery DW, Neas LM, Redline S. The effect of ozone on inner-city children with asthma. Am J Respir Crit Care Med 2000; 162:1838–1845.

43. Tolbert PE, Mulholland JA, Macintosh DL, Xu F, Daniels D, Devine OJ, Carlin BP, Klein M, Butler AJ, Nordenberg DF, Frumkin H, Ryan PB, White MC. Air quality and pediatric emergency room visits for asthma in Atlanta, Georgia. Am J Epidemiol 2000; 151:798–810.

44. Friedman MS, Powell KE, Hutwagner L, Graham LM, Teague WG. Impact of changes in transportation and commuting behaviors during the 1996 Summer Olympic Games in Atlanta on air quality and childhood asthma. JAMA 2001; 285:897–905.

45. Gent JF, Triche EW, Holford TR, Belanger K, Bracken MB, Beckett WS, Leaderer BP. Association of low-level ozone and fine particles with respiratory symptoms in children with asthma. JAMA 2003; 290:1859–1867.

46. Lewis TC, Robins TG, Dvonch T, Keeler GJ, Yip FY, Mentz GB, Lin X, Parker EA, Israel BA, Gonzalez L, Hill Y. Air pollution-associated changes in lung function among asthmatic children in Detroit. Environ Health Perspect 2005; 113:1068–1075.

47. Peel JL, Tolbert PE, Klein M, Metzger KB, Flanders WD, Todd K, Mulholland JA, Ryan PB, Frumkin H. Ambient air pollution and respiratory emergency department visits. Epidemiology 2005; 16:164–174.

48. Moore K, Neugebauer R, Lurmann F, Hall J, Brajer V, Alcorn S, Tager I. Ambient ozone concentrations cause increased hospitalizations for asthma in children: an 18-year study in southern California. Environ Health Perspect 2008; 116:1063–1070.

49. Burnett RT, Smith-Doiron M, Stieb D, Raizenne ME, Brook JR, Dales RE, Leech JA, Cakmak S, Krewski D. Association between ozone and hospitalization for acute respiratory diseases in children less than 2 years of age. Am J Epidemiol 2001; 153:444–452.

50. Dales RE, Cakmak S, Smith-Doiron M. Gaseous air pollutant and hospitalization for respiratory disease in the neonatal period. Environ Health Perspect 2006; 114:1751–1754.

51. Yang Q, Chen Y, Shi Y, et al. Association between ozone and respiratory admissions among children and the elderly in Vancouver, Canada. Inhal Toxicol 2003; 15:1297–1308.

52. Koken PJM, Piver WT, Ye F, Elixhauser A, Olsen LM, Portier CJ. Temperature, air pollution, and hospitalization for cardiovascular diseases among elderly people in Denver. Environ Health Perspect 2003; 111:1312–1317.

53. Medina-Ramon M, Zqanobetti A, Schwartz J. The effect of ozone and PM_{10} on hospital admissions for pneumonia and chronic obstructive pulmonary disease: a national multicity study. Am J Epidemiol 2006; 163:579–588.

54. Thurston GD, Ito K. Epidemiological studies of acute ozone exposure and mortality. J Expos Anal Environ Epidemiol 2001; 11:286–294.

55. Schwartz J. How sensitive is the association between ozone and daily deaths to control for temperature? Am J Respir Crit Care Med 2005; 171:627–631.

56. Bell ML, Kim JY, Dominici F. Potential confounding of particulate matter on the short-term association between ozone and mortality in multi-site time-series studies. Environ Health Perspect 2007; 115:1591–1595.

57. Bell ML, McDermott A, Zeger SL, Samet JM, Dominici F. Ozone and short-term mortality in 95 U.S. urban communities, 1987–2000. JAMA 2004; 292:2372–2378.

58. Ito K, De Leon S, Lippmann M. Associations between ozone and daily mortality: Analysis and meta-analysis. Epidemiology 2005; 16:446–457.

59. Bell ML, Dominici F, Samet JM. A meta-analysis of time-series studies of zone and mortality with comparison to the National Morbidity, Mortality, and Air Pollution Study. Epidemiology 2005; 16:436–445.

60. Levy JI, Chemerynski SM, Sarnat JA. Ozone exposure and mortality: an empiric Bayes meta-regression analysis. Epidemiology 2005; 16:458–468.

61. Gryparis A, Forsberg B, Katsouyanni K, Analitis A, Touloumi G, Schwartz J, Samoli E, Medina S, Anderson HR, Niciu EM, Wichmann HE, Kriz B, Kosnik M, Skorkovsky J, Vonk JM, Dortbudak Z. Acute effects of ozone on mortality from the "air pollution and health: a European approach" project. Am J Respir Crit Care Med 2004; 170:1080–1087.

62. Zanobetti A, Schwartz J. Mortality displacement in the association of ozone with mortality: an analysis of 48 cities in the United States. Am J Respir Crit Care Med 2008; 177:184–189.

63. Jerrett M, Burnett RT, Pope CA 3rd, Ito K, Thurston G, Krewski D, Shi Y, Calle E, Thun M. Long-term ozone exposure and mortality. N Engl J Med 2009; 360:1085–1095.

64. Schlesinger RB. Nitrogen oxides. In: Rom, WN, Markowitz, SB, editors. Environmental and occupational medicine. 4th ed. New York: Lippincott Williams & Wilkins; 2007. p. 1466–1479.

65. Frampton MW, Greaves IA. ATS Environmental Health Policy Committee. Nox-Nox: who's there? Am J Respir Crit Care Med. 2009; 179:1077–1083.

66. Barck C, Lundahl J, Hallden G, Bylin G. Brief exposure to an ambient level of NO_2 enhances asthmatic response to a nonsymptomatic allergen dose. Eur Respir J 1998; 12:6–12.

67. Lin M, Chen Y, Burnett RT, Villeneuve PJ, Krewski D. Effect of short-term exposure to gaseous pollution on asthma hospitalization in children: a bio-directional case-crossover analysis. J Epidemiol Community Health 2003; 57:50–55.

68. Strand V, Svartengren M, Rak S, Barck C, Bylin G. Repeated exposure to an ambient level of NO_2 enhances asthmatic response to a nonsymptomatic allergen dose. Eur Respir J 1998; 12:6–12.

69. National Research Council. Estimating mortality risk reduction and economic benefits from controlling ozone air pollution. Washington, DC: National Academies Press: 2008.

70. Schildcrout JS, Sheppard L, Lumley T, Slaughter JC, Koenig JQ, Shapiro GG. Ambient air pollution and asthma exacerbations in children: an eight-city analysis. Am J Epidemiol 2006; 164:505–517.

71. Adams WC. Comparison of chamber and face-mask 6.6 hour exposures to ozone on pulmonary function and symptoms responses. Inhalation Toxicol 2006; 18:127–136.

72. Adams WC. Comparison of chamber 6.6 hour exposures to 0.04–0.08 PPM ozone via square-wave and triangular profiles on pulmonary responses. Inhalation Toxicol 2006; 18:127–136.

73. Brown JS, Bateson TF, McDonnell WF. Effects of exposure to 0.06 ppm ozone on FEV_1 in humans: secondary analysis of existing data. Environ Health Perspect 2008; 116:1023–1026.

74. Schelegle ES, Morales CA, Walby WF, Allen RP. 6.6-Hour inhalation of ozone concentrations from 60 to 87 parts per billion in healthy humans. Am J Respir Crit Care Med 2009; 180:265–272.

75. Hubbell BJ, Hallberg A, McCubbin DR, Post E. Health-related benefits for attaining the 8-hr ozone standard. Environ Health Perspect 2005; 113:73–82.

Chapter 4: Sulfur Dioxide and Acid Rain

1. Frampton MW, Utell MJ. Sulfur dioxide. In: Rom, WN, Markowitz, SB, editors. Environmental and occupational medicine. 4th ed. New York: Lippincott Williams & Wilkins; 2007. p. 1480–1486.

2. Willis A, Jerrett M, Burnett RT, Krewski D. The association between sulfate air pollution and mortality at the county scale: an exploration of the impact of scale on a long-term exposure study. J Toxicol Environ Health 2003; 66:1605–1624.

3. Dominici F, McDermott A, Daniels M, Zeger SL, Samet JM. Revised analyses of the National Morbidity, Mortality, and Air Pollution Study: mortality among residents of 90 cities. J Toxicol Environ Health 2005; 68:1071–1092.

4. Lee WJ, Teschke K, Kauppinen T, et al. Mortality from lung cancer in workers exposed to sulfur dioxide in the pulp and paper industry. Environ Health Perspect 2002; 110:991–995.

5. Hedley AJ, Wong CM, Thach TQ, Ma S, Lam TH, Anderson HR. Cardiorespiratory and all-cause mortality after restrictions on sulphur content of fuel in Hong Kong: an intervention study. Lancet 2002; 360:1646–1652.

6. Burnett RT, Stieb D, Brook JR, et al. Associations between short-term changes in nitrogen dioxide and mortality in Canadian cities. Arch Environ Health 2004; 59:228–236.

7. Venners SA, Wang B, Xu Z, Schlatter Y, Wang L, Xu X. Particulate matter, sulfur dioxide, and daily mortality in Chongqing, China. Environ Health Perspect 2003; 111:562–567.

8. Sunyer J, Ballester F, Tertre AL, et al. The association of daily sulfur dioxide air pollution levels with hospital admissions for cardiovascular diseases in Europe (the Aphea-II study). Eur Heart J 2003; 24:752–760.

9. Lin M, Chen Y, Burnett RT, Villeneuve PJ, Krewski D. Effect of short-term exposure to gaseous pollution on asthma hospitalisation in children: a bi-directional case-crossover analysis. J Epidemiol Community Health 2003; 57:50–55.

10. Ware JH, Ferris BG Jr, Dockery DW, Spengler JD, Stram DO. Effects of ambient sulfur oxides and suspended particles on respiratory health of preadolescent children. Am Rev Respir Dis 1986; 133:834–842.

11. Lee BE, Ha EH, Park HS, et al. Exposure to air pollution during different gestational phases contributes to risks of low birth weight. Hum Reprod 2003; 18:638–643.

12. Lin CM, Li CY, Yang GY, Mao IF. Association between maternal exposure to elevated ambient sulfur dioxide during pregnancy and term low birth weight. Environ Res 2004; 96:41–50.

13. Frampton MW, Voter KZ, Morrow PE, Roberts NJ Jr, Culp DJ, Cox C, Utell MJ. Sulfuric acid aerosol exposure in humans assessed by bronchoalveolar lavage. Am Rev Respir Dis 1992; 146:626–632.

14. Carlisle AJ, Sharp NC. Exercise and outdoor ambient air pollution. Br J Sports Med 2001; 35:214–222.

15. Trenga CA, Koenig JQ, Williams PV. Sulphur dioxide sensitivity and plasma antioxidants in adult subjects with asthma. Occup Environ Med 1999; 56:544–547.

16. Sandstrom T, Stjernberg N, Andersson M, et al. Cell response in bronchoalveolar lavage fluid after exposure to sulfur dioxide: a time-response study. Am Rev Respir Dis 1989; 140:1828–1831.

17. Rusznak C, Devalia JL, Davies RJ. Airway response of asthmatic subjects to inhaled allergen after exposure to pollutants. Thorax 1996; 51:1105–1108.

18. Likens GE. Acid rain: the smokestack is the "smoking gun." Garden 1984; July/August:12–18.

19. Weathers KC, Likens GE, Butler TJ. Acid rain. In: Rom, WN, Markowitz, SB, editors. Environmental and occupational medicine. 4th ed. New York: Lippincott Williams & Wilkins; 2007. p. 1507–1520.

20. Likens GE, Driscoll CT, Buso DC. Long-term effects of acid rain: Response and recovery of a forest ecosystem. Science 1996; 272:244–246.

21. Dominguez G, Jackson T, Brothers L, Barnett B, Nguyen B, Thiemens MH. Discovery and measurement of an isotopically distinct source of sulfate in Earth's atmosphere. Proc Natl Acad Sci USA 2008; 105:12769–12773.

22. Corbett JJ, Winebrake JJ, Green EH, Kasibhatla P, Eyring V, Lauer A. Mortality from ship emissions: a global assessment. Environ Sci and Tech 2007; 41:8512–8518.

23. Likens GE, Bormann FH, Hedin LO, Driscoll CT, Eaton JS. Dry deposition of sulfur: a 23-yr record for the Hubbard Brook Forest ecosystem. Tellus 1990; 42B:319–329.

24. Weathers, KC, Likens, GE, Bormann, FH, et al. Cloud water chemistry from ten sites in North America. Environ Sci Tech 1988; 22:1018–1026.

25. Weathers KC, Likens GE, Bormann FH, et al. Chemical concentrations in cloud water from four sites in the eastern United States. In: Unsworth MH, Fowler D, editors. Acid deposition at high elevation sites. Norwell (MA): Kluwer Academic, 1988. p. 345–357.

26. Weathers KC, Cadenasso ML, Pickett STA. Forest edges as nutrient and pollutant concentrators: potential synergisms between fragmentation, forest canopies, and the atmosphere. Conserv Biol 2001; 15:1506–1514.

27. Galloway JN, Likens GE, Hawley ME. Acid precipitation: natural vs. anthropogenic components. Science 1984; 226:829–831.

28. Galloway JN, Keene WC, Likens GE. Processes controlling the composition of precipitation at a remote southern hemisphere location: Torres del Paine National Park, Chile. J Geophys Res 1996; 101:6883–6897.

29. Likens GE, Keene WC, Miller JM, Galloway JN. Chemistry of precipitation from a remote, terrestrial site in Australia. J Geophys Res 1987; 92:13299–13314.

30. National Atmospheric Deposition Program (NADP). NADP/NTN annual data summary: precipitation chemistry in the United States 1994. Fort Collins (CO): National Resource Ecology Laboratory, Colorado State University; 1996.

31. Lynch JA, Bowersox VC, Grimm JW. Changes in sulfate deposition in eastern USA following implementation of Phase I of Title IV of the Clean Air Act Amendments of 1990. Atm Environ 2000; 34:1665–1680.

32. Driscoll CT, Lawrence G, Bulger A, et al. Acidic deposition in the northeastern US: Sources, inputs, ecosystem effects, and management strategies. BioScience 2001; 51:180–198.

33. Schindler DW. Effects of acid rain on freshwater ecosystems. Science 1988; 239:149–157.

34. Asbury CE, Vertucci FA, Mattson MD, Likens GE. Acidification of Adirondack lakes. Environ Sci Tech 1989; 23:362–365.

35. Irving PM, editor. Acid deposition: state of science and technology. Summary report of the U.S. National Acid Precipitation Assessment Program. Washington (DC): NAPAP, 1991.

36. Havas M, Rosseland BO. Response of zooplankton, benthos, and fish to acidification: an overview. Water Air Soil Pollut 1995; 85:51–62.

37. Baker JL, Schofield CL. Aluminum toxicity to fish in acidic waters. Water Air Soil Pollut 1982; 18:289–309.

38. DeHayes DH, Schaberg PG, Hawley GJ, et al. Acid rain impacts on calcium nutrition and forest health: alteration of membrane-associated calcium leads to membrane destabilization and foliar injury in red spruce. BioScience 1999; 49:789–800.

39. Lovett GM, Weathers KC, Sobczak W. Nitrogen saturation and retention in forested watersheds of the Catskill Mountains, NY. Ecol Appl 2000; 10:73–84.

40. Likens GE, Driscoll CT, Buso DC, et al. The biogeochemistry of calcium at Hubbard Brook. Biogeochemistry 1998; 41:89–173.

41. Horsley SB, Long RP, Bailey SW, et al. Health of eastern North American sugar maple forests and factors affecting decline. North J Appl Forest 2002; 19:34–44.

42. Likens GE, Lambert KF. The importance of long-term data in addressing regional environmental issues. Northeast Natural 1998; 5:127–136.

Chapter 5: Environmental Tobacco Smoke

1. Doll R, Hill AB. Smoking and carcinoma of the lung. Br Med J 1950; 2(4681):739–748.

2. Pearl R. Tobacco smoking and longevity. Science 1938; 87(2253): 216–217.

3. Levin ML, Goldstein H, Gerhardt PR. Cancer and tobacco smoking: a preliminary report. JAMA 1950; 143:336–338.

4. Wynder EL, Graham EA. Tobacco smoking as a possible etiologic factor in bronchiogenic carcinoma: a study of six hundred and eighty-four proved cases. JAMA 1950; 143:329–336.

5. Dawber TR. The Framingham Study: the epidemiology of atherosclerotic disease. Cambridge (MA): Harvard University Press; 1980.

6. Doll R, Hill AB. The mortality of doctors in relation to their smoking habits: a preliminary report. Br Med J 1954; 1:1451–1455.

7. US Department of Health and Human Services (USDHHS), Public Health Service, National Cancer Institute (NCI). Changes in cigarette-related disease risks and their implication for prevention and control. Burns DM, Garfinkel L, Samet JM, editors. 1997. Bethesda (MD): US GPO. NIH Publication No. 97–4213. Smoking and Tobacco Control Monograph.

8. Royal College of Physicians of London. Smoking and health: summary of a report of the Royal College of Physicians of London on smoking in relation to cancer of the lung and other diseases. S2–70. London: Pitman Medical; 1962.

9. US Department of Health Education and Welfare (DHEW). Smoking and health: report of the Advisory Committee to the Surgeon General. Washington (DC): US GPO; 1964. DHEW Publication No. [PHS] 1103.

10. US Department of Health and Human Services (USDHHS). Reducing the health consequences of smoking—25 years of progress: a report of the surgeon general. Washington (DC): US GPO; 1989.

11. Willett WC, Green A, Stampfer MJ, Speizer FE, Colditz GA, Rosner B, et al. Relative and absolute excess risks of coronary heart disease among women who smoke cigarettes. N Engl J Med 1987; 317:1303–1309.

12. US Department of Health and Human Services (USDHHS). The health benefits of smoking cessation: a report of the surgeon general. Washington (DC): US GPO; 1990. DHHS Publication Number 90–8416.

13. US Department of Health and Human Services (USDHHS). Women and smoking: a report of the Surgeon General. Rockville (MD): USDHHS; 2001.

14. Evans HJ, Fletcher J, Torrance M, Hargreave TB. Sperm abnormalities and cigarette smoking. Lancet 1981; 1:627–629.

15. US Department of Health and Human Services (USDHHS). The health consequences of smoking—cardiovascular disease: a report of the surgeon general. Washington (DC): US GPO; 1983.

16. US Department of Health and Human Services (USDHHS). The health consequences of smoking—chronic obstructive lung disease: a report of the surgeon general. Washington (DC): US GPO; 1984.

17. Fletcher C, Peto R. The natural history of chronic airflow obstruction. Br Med J 1977; 1:1645–1648.

18. Samet JM, Wang SS. Environmental tobacco smoke. In: Lippmann M, editor. Environmental toxicants: human exposures and their health effects. New York: Van Nostrand Reinhold; 2000. p. 319–375.

19. US Department of Health and Human Services (USDHHS). The health consequences of involuntary smoking: a report of the surgeon general. Washington (DC): US GPO; 1986. DHHS Publication No. (CDC) 87–8398.

20. US Department of Health Education and Welfare (DHEW). The health consequences of smoking. a report of the surgeon general. Atlanta (GA): US GPO; 1972.

21. Hirayama T. Non-smoking wives of heavy smokers have a higher risk of lung cancer: a study from Japan. Bri Med J 1981; 282:183–185.

22. Trichopoulous D, Kalandidi A, Sparros L. Lung cancer and passive smoking: conclusion of Greek study. Lancet 1983; 677–678.

23. Fielding JE, Phenow KJ. Health effects of involuntary smoking. N Engl J Med 1988; 319:1452–1460.

24. National Research Council (NRC), Committee on Passive Smoking. Environmental tobacco smoke: measuring exposures and assessing health effects. Washington (DC): National Academy Press; 1986.

25. International Agency for Research on Cancer (IARC). IARC Monographs on the evaluation of the carcinogenic risk of chemicals to humans: tobacco smoking. Lyon (France): World Health Organization, IARC; 1986. Monograph 38.

26. Wald NJ, Nanchahal K, Thompson SG, Cuckle HS. Does breathing other people's tobacco smoke cause lung cancer? BMJ 1986; 293:1217–1222.

27. California Environmental Protection Agency (Cal/EPA), Office of Environmental Health Hazard Assessment. Health effects of exposure to environmental tobacco smoke. Sacramento (CA): Cal/EPA; 1997.

28. Scientific Committee on Tobacco and Health, HSMO. Report of the Scientific Committee on Tobacco and Health. Various (England): Stationary Office; 1998. 011322124x. 2–5.

29. World Health Organization (WHO). International consultation on environmental tobacco smoke (ETS) and child health: consultation report. Geneva (Switzerland): WHO; 1999.

30. International Agency for Research on Cancer (IARC). Tobacco smoke and involuntary smoking. Lyon (France): IARC; 2004. Monograph 83.

31. Peterson JE, Stewart RD. Absorption and elimination of carbon monoxide by inactive young men. Arch Environ Health 1970; 21:165–171.

32. Yolton K, Dietrich K, Auinger P, Lanphear BP, Hornung R. Exposure to environmental tobacco smoke and cognitive abilities among US children and adolescents. Environ Health Perspect 2005; 113:98–103.

33. Corbo GM, Agabiti N, Forastiere F, Dell'orco V, Pistelli R, et al. Lung functon in children and adolescents with occasional exposure to environmental tobacco smoke. Am J Respir Crit Care Med 1996; 154:695–700.

34. Tager IB, Weiss ST, Munoz A, Rosner B, Speizer FE. Longitudinal study of the effects of maternal smoking on pulmonary function in children. N Engl J Med 1983; 309:699–703.

35. Glantz SA, Parmley WW. Passive smoking and heart disease: mechanisms and risk. JAMA 1995; 273:1047–1053.

36. Taylor AE, Johnson DC, Kazemi H. Environmental tobacco smoke and cardiovascular disease: a position paper from the council on cardiopulmonary and critical care, American Heart Association. Circulation 1992; 86:1–4.

37. Law MR, Morris JK, Wald NJ. Environmental tobacco smoke exposure and ischaemic heart disease: an evaluation of the evidence. Br Med J 1997; 315 (7114):973–980.

38. Pell JP, Haw S, Cobbe S, Newby DE, Pell ACH, Fischbacher C, et al. Smoke-free legislation and hospitalizations for acute coronary syndrome. N Engl J Med 2008; 359:482–491.

39. Yanbaeva DG, Dentener MA, Creutzberg EC, Wesseling G, Wouters EFM. Systemic effects of smoking. Chest 2007; 131:1557–1566.

40. Enstrom JE, Kabat GC. Environmental tobacco smoke and tobacco related mortality in a prospective study of Californians, 1960–98. BMJ 2003; 326:1057.

41. Leuenberger P, Schwartz J, Ackermann-Liebrich U, Blaser K, Bolognini G, Gongard JP, et al. Passive smoking exposure in adults and chronic respiratory symptoms (SAPALDIA Study). Am J Respir Crit Care Med 1994; 150:1221–1228.

42. Jindal SK, Gupta D, Singh A. Indices of morbitity and control of asthma in adult patients exposed to environmental tobacco smoke. Chest 1994; 106:746–749.

43. Lam TH, Ho LM, Hedley AJ, Adab P, Fielding R, McGhee SM, et al. Environmental tobacco smoke exposure among police officers in Hong Kong. JAMA 2002; 284:756–763.

44. Eisner MD, Smith AK, Blanc PD. Bartenders' respiratory health after establishment of smoke-free bars and taverns. JAMA 1998; 280:1909–1914.

45. Goodman P, Agnew M, McCaffrey M, Paul G, Clancy L. Effects of the Irish smoking ban on respiratory health of bar workers and air quality in Dublin pubs. Am J Respir Crit Care Med 2007; 175:840–845.

46. Bouzigon E, Corda E, Aschard H, Dizier M-H, Boland A, Bousquet J, et al. Effect of 17q21 variants on smoking exposure in early-onset asthma. N Engl J Med 2008; 359:1985–1994.

47. Janerich DT, Thompson WD, Varela LR, Greenwald P, Chorost S, Tucci C, et al. Lung cancer and exposure to tobacco smoke in the household. N Engl J Med 1990; 323:632–636.

48. US Environmental Protection Agency (EPA). Respiratory health effects of passive smoking: lung cancer and other disorders. Washington (DC): US GPO; 1992. EPA/600/006F.

49. Phillips DH. Fifty years of benzo(a)pyrene. Nature 1983; 303:468–472. Review.

50. International Agency for Research on Cancer (IARC). Polynuclear aromatic compounds, Part 1, chemical, environmental, and experimental data. 33–91. Lyon (France): IARC; 1983. Monographs on the Evaluation of the Carcinogenic Risk of Chemicals to Humans 32.

51. Denissenko MF, Pao A, Tang M, Pfeifer GP. Preferential formation of benzo[a]pyrene adducts at lung cancer mutational hotspots in p53. Science 1996; 274:430–432.

52. Yoon JH, Smith LE, Feng Z, Tang M, Lee CS, Pfeifer GP. Methylated CpG dinucleotides are the preferential targets for G-to-T transversion mutations induced by benzo[a]pyrene diol epoxide in mammalian cells: similarities with the p53 mutation spectrum in smoking-associated lung cancers. Cancer Res 2001; 61:7110–7117.

53. Hecht SS. Tobacco smoke carcinogens and lung cancer. J Natl Cancer Inst 1999; 91:1194–1210.

54. Pfeifer GP, Denissenko MF, Olivier M, Tretyakova N, Hecht SS, Hainaut P. Tobacco smoke carcinogens, DNA damage and p53 mutations in smoking-associated cancers. Oncogene 2002; 21:7435–7451.

55. Christakis NA, Fowler JH. The collective dynamics of smoking in a large social network. N Engl J Med 2008; 358:2249–2258.

56. Anthonisen NR, Skeans MA, Wise RA, Manfreda J, Kanner RE, Connett JE. The effects of a smoking cessation intervention on a 14.5-year mortality. Ann Intern Med 2005; 142:233–239.

57. Anthonisen NR, Connett JE, Kiley JP, Altose MD, Bailey WC, Buist AS, et al. Effects of smoking intervention and the use of an inhaled anticholinergic broncho-dilator on the rate of decline of FEV$_1$: the Lung Health Study. JAMA 1994; 272:1497–1505.

58. Ranney L, Mlevin C, Lux L, McClain E, Lohr KN. Systematic review: smoking cessation intervention strategies for adults and adults in special populations. Ann Intern Med 2006; 145:845–856.

59. Hays JT, Ebbert JO. Varenicline for tobacco dependence. N Engl J Med 2008; 359:2018–2024.

60. Brandt AM. The cigarette century. New York: Basic Books; 2007.

61. Schroeder SA. Tobacco control in the wake of the 1998 master settlement agreement. N Engl J Med 2004; 350:293–301.

62. Jones WJ, Silvestri GA. The Master Settlement Agreement and its impact on tobacco use 10 years later. Chest 2010; 137:692–700.

63. Chang C, Leighton J, Mostashari F, McCord C, Frieden TR. The New York City Smoke-Free Air Act: second-hand smoke as a worker health and safety issue. Am J Ind Med 2004; 46:188–195.

64. Kessler DA, Witt AM, Barnett PS, Zeller MR, Natanblut SL, Wilenfeld JP, et al. The Food and Drug Administration's regulation of tobacco products. N Engl J Med 1996; 335:988–994.

65. Brandt AM. FDA regulation of tobacco: pitfalls and possibilities. N Engl J Med 2008; 395:445–448.

66. Ruling August 17, 2006 by Judge Gladys Kessler of U.S. District Court from New York in *U.S. et al. v. Philip Morris et al.*

67. Slama K. Current challenges in tobacco control. Int J Tuberc Lung Dis 2005; 1160–1171.

Chapter 6: Children's Environmental Health: Mercury and Lead

1. Thomas HM, Blackfan KD. Recurrent meningitis, due to lead, in a child of five years. Arch Pediatr Adolesc Med 1914; 8:377–380.

2. Gibson JL. A plea for painted railings and painted walls of rooms as the source of lead poisoning amongst Queensland children. Public Health Rep 2005; 120:301–304.

3. Laraque D, Trasande L. Lead poisoning: successes and 21st century challenges. Pediatr Rev 2005; 26:435–443.

4. Akinbami LJ. The state of childhood asthma, United States, 1980–2005: advance data from vital and health statistics. Hyattsville (MD): National Center for Health Statistics; 2006. p. 381.

5. Di Tanna GL, Rosano A, Mastroiacovo P. Prevalence of gastroschisis at birth: retrospective study. BMJ 2002; 325:1389–1390.

6. Williams LJ, Kucik JE, Alverson CJ, Olney RS, Correa A. Epidemiology of gastroschisis in metropolitan Atlanta, 1968 through 2000. Birth Defects Research Part A: Clinical and Molecular Teratology 2005; 73:177–183.

7. Rice C. Prevalence of autism spectrum disorders: autism and developmental disabilities monitoring network, six sites, United States, 2000. MMWR Surveill Sum 2007; 56:1–11.

8. Schechter CB. Re: Brain and other central nervous system cancers: recent trends in incidence and mortality. J Natl Cancer Inst 1999; 91:2050–2051.

9. Robison LL, Buckley JD, Bunin G. Assessment of environmental and genetic factors in the etiology of childhood cancers: the Children's Cancer Group epidemiology program. Environ Health Perspect 1995; 103:111–116.

10. Devesa SS, Blot WJ, Stone BJ, Miller BA, Tarone RE, Fraumeni JF. Recent cancer trends in the United States. JNCI 2003; 87:175–182.

11. US Environmental Protection Agency (EPA). Chemicals-in-commerce information system (Chemical Update System Database). Washington (DC): US GPO; 1998.

12. US Environmental Protection Agency (EPA). Chemical hazard data availability study: what do we really know about the safety of high production volume chemicals? Washington (DC): US GPO; 1998.

13. Centers for Disease Control and Prevention. Third national report on human exposure to environmental chemicals. Atlanta (GA): Centers for Disease Control and Prevention; 2005.

14. Gruchalla RS, Pongracic J, Plaut M, et al. Inner City Asthma Study: relationships among sensitivity, allergen exposure, and asthma morbidity. J Allergy Clin Immunol 2005; 115:478–485.

15. O'Connor GT, Walter M, Mitchell H, et al. Airborne fungi in the homes of children with asthma in low-income urban communities: the Inner-City Asthma Study. J Allergy Clin Immunol 2004; 114:599–606.

16. Trasande L, Thurston GD. The role of air pollution in asthma and other pediatric morbidities. J Allergy Clin Immunol 2005; 115:689–699.

17. Daniels JL, Olshan AF, Teschke K, et al. Residential pesticide exposure and neuroblastoma. Epidemiology 2001; 12:20–27.

18. Lee WJ, Cantor KP, Berzofsky JA, Zahm SH, Blair A. Non-Hodgkin's lymphoma among asthmatics exposed to pesticides. Int J Cancer 2004; 111:298–302.

19. National Academy of Sciences Committee on Developmental Toxicology. Scientific frontiers in developmental toxicology and risk assessment. Washington (DC): US GPO; 2000.

20. Goldman L, Falk H, Landrigan PJ, Balk SJ, Reigart JR, Etzel RA. Environmental pediatrics and its impact on government health policy. Pediatrics 2004; 113:1146.

21. Grosse SD, Matte TD, Schwartz J, Jackson RJ. Economic gains resulting from the reduction in children's exposure to lead in the United States. Environ Health Perspect 2002; 110:563–569.

22. Friedman MS, Powell KE, Hutwagner L, Graham LRM, Teague WG. Impact of changes in transportation and commuting behaviors during the 1996 Summer

Olympic Games in Atlanta on air quality and childhood asthma. JAMA 2001; 285:897–905.

23. Harada Y. Congenital (or fetal) Minamata disease. In: Study Group of Minamata Disease, editors. Minamata disease. Kumamato (Japan): Kumamato University; 1968. p. 93–118.

24. Amin-Zaki L, Elhassani S, Majeed MA, et al. Perinatal methylmercury poisoning in Iraq. Arch Pediatr Adolesc Med 1976; 130:1070–1076.

25. Kjellstrom T, Kennedy P, Wallis S, Mantell C. Physical and mental development of children with prenatal exposure to mercury from fish. Stage I: preliminary tests at age 4. Solna (Sweden): National Swedish Environmental Protection Board; 1986. Report 3080.

26. Kjellstrom T, Kennedy P, Wallis S, Stewart A, Friberg L, Lind B, et al. Physical and mental development of children with prenatal exposure to mercury from fish. Stage II: interviews and psychological tests at age 6. Solna (Sweden): National Swedish Environmental Protection Board; 1989. Report 3642.

27. Grandjean P, Budtz-Jorgensen E, White RF, et al. Methylmercury exposure biomarkers as indicators of neurotoxicity in children aged 7 years. Vol 150: © 1999 by The Johns Hopkins University, School of Hygiene and Public Health; 2003. p. 301–305.

28. Grandjean P, Weihe P, White RF, et al. Cognitive deficit in 7-year-old children with prenatal exposure to methylmercury. Neurotoxicol Teratol 1997; 19:417–428.

29. Myers GJ, Davidson PW, Cox C, Shamlaye CF, Palumbo D, Cernichiari E, et al. Prenatal methylmercury exposure from the ocean fish consumption in the Seychelles child development study. Lancet 2003; 361:1686–1692.

30. National Research Council. Toxicological effects of methylmercury. Washington (DC): National Academy Press, 2000.

31. Oken E, Wright RO, Kleinman KP, et al. Maternal fish consumption, hair mercury, and infant cognition in a US cohort. Environ Health Perspect 2005; 113:1376–1380.

32. US Environmental Protection Agency (EPA). Clean Air Act; 2008b. Available at http://www.epa.gov.

33. US Environmental Protection Agency (EPA). EPA proposes options for significantly reducing mercury emissions from electric utilities. Available at http://www.epa.gov.

34. US Environmental Protection Agency (EPA). Section B: Human and environmental benefits. 2002 technical support package for Clear Skies. Available at http://www.epa.gov.

35. Trasande L, Landrigan PJ, Schechter C. Public health and economic consequences of methyl mercury toxicity to the developing brain. Environ Health Perspect 2005; 113:590–596.

36. Trasande L, Schechter CB, Haynes KA, Landrigan PJ. Mental retardation and pre-natal methylmercury toxicity. Am J Ind Med 2006; 49:153–158.

37. Kuehn BM. Medical groups sue EPA over mercury rule. JAMA 2005; 294:415–416.

38. Jacobs DE, Clickner RP, Zhou JY, et al. The prevalence of lead-based paint hazards in US housing. Environ Health Perspect 2002; 110:A599.

39. US Dept. of Health and Human Services (USDHHS). Healthy people 2010. Washington (DC): USDHHS; 2000.

40. President's Task Force on Environmental Health Risks and Safety Risks to Children. Eliminating childhood lead poisoning: a federal strategy targeting lead paint hazards; February 2000.

41. US Congress. US Consolidated Appropriations Resolution; 2003. Available at http://thomas.loc.gov.

42. Lanphear BP, Dietrich K, Auinger P, Cox C. Cognitive deficits associated with blood lead concentrations <10 microg/dL in US children and adolescents. Public Health Reports 2000; 115:521–529.

43. Canfield RL, Henderson Jr CR, Cory-Slechta DA, Cox C, Jusko TA, Lanphear BP. Intellectual impairment in children with blood lead concentrations below 10 (micro) g per deciliter. New Eng J Med 2003; 348:1517–1526.

44. Jusko TA, Henderson Jr CR, Lanphear BP, Cory-Slechta DA, Parsons PJ, Canfield RL. Blood lead concentrations <10 μg/dL and child intelligence at 6 years of age. Environ Health Perspect 2008; 116:243–248.

45. Brown MJ, Rhoads GG. Responding to blood lead levels <10 μg/dL. Environ Health Perspect 2008; 116:A60. Guest editorial.

46. Steinbrook R. Science, politics, and federal advisory committees. N Engl J Med 2004; 350:1454–1460.

47. Gent JF, Triche EW, Holford TR, et al. Association of low-level ozone and fine particles with respiratory symptoms in children with asthma. JAMA 2003; 290:1859–1867.

48. Gent JF, Ren P, Belanger K, et al. Levels of household mold associated with respiratory symptoms in the first year of life in a cohort at risk for asthma. Environ Health Perspect 2002; 110:A781.

49. Thurston GD, Lippmann M, Scott MB, Fine JM. Summertime haze air pollution and children with asthma. Am J Respir Crit Care Med 1997; 155:654–660.

50. Committee on Environmental H. Ambient air pollution: health hazards to children. Pediatrics 2004; 114:1699–1707.

51. epa.gov/cleanschoolbus/antiidling.htm

52. Zajac L, Sprecher E, Landrigan PJ, Trasande L. A systematic review of US state environmental legislation and regulation with regards to the prevention of neurodevelopmental disabilities and asthma. Environ Health 2009; 8:9. PMID: 19323818.

53. US Congress. Children's Health Act of 2000. Public Law 2000:106–310.

54. US Environmental Protection Agency (EPA). Summary of the Toxic Substances Control Act. Available at http://www.epa.gov.

55. US Environmental Protection Agency (EPA). Food Quality Protection Act (FQPA) of 1996. Available at http://www.epa.gov.

56. Whyatt RM, Rauh V, Barr DB, et al. Prenatal insecticide exposures and birth weight and length among an urban minority cohort. Environ Health Perspect 2004; 112:1125–1132.

57. US Environmental Protection Agency (EPA). President's Task Force on Environmental Health Risks and Safety Risks to Children. Available at http://yosemite.epa.gov.

58. Landrigan PJ, Trasande L, Thorpe LE, et al. The National Children's Study: a 21-year prospective study of 100,000 American children. Pediatrics 2006; 118: 2173–2186.

Chapter 7: The Role of Community Advocacy Groups in Environmental Protection: Example of September 11, 2001

1. EPA's response to the world trade center collapse: challenges, successes, and areas for improvement. Office of Inspector General; August 21, 2003. Report No. 2003-P-00012.

2. ABC News, Fouled air? 9/13/01; from Comments on the EPA Office of Inspector General's 1/27/03 interim report: EPA's response to the world trade center towers collapse—a documentary basis for litigation. Prepared by Cate Jenkins, July 4, 2003.

3. Newman, DM. Disaster response and grassroots environmental advocacy: the example of the world trade center community labor coalition. New Solut 2008; 18:23–56.

4. Kim ET, Fong J. The Beyond Ground Zero Network: A model for grassroots public health response following an urban environmental disaster. Advancing climate justice: transforming the economy, public health and our environment. WE ACT for Environmental Justice Conference; January 29–30, 2009, New York.

5. Survey of air quality information related to the World Trade Center collapse. Office of Inspector General; September 26, 2003. Report No. 2003-P-00014.

6. Appendix B: Environmental analysis framework and performance commitments. LMDC letter dated October 31, 2003 from LMDC to Federal Transit Administration. Available at http://www.renewnyc.com.

7. Kunkel T, Held K. Particulate monitoring and control in Lower Manhattan during large urban redevelopment. Presented at Air & Waste Management Association Annual Meeting; June 2007, Charleston, SC.

8. Technical Working Group. Gold standard for remediation of WTC contaminations. New Solut 2004; 14:199–217.

9. EPA response to September 11th. Available at http://www.epa.gov.

10. September 11: Health effects in the aftermath of the World Trade Center attack; September 8, 2008. GAO Report 2004–1068T. Available at http://www.gao.gov.

11. Friedman S, Cone J, Eros-Sarnyai M. Clinical guidelines for adults exposed to the World Trade Center disaster. City Health Information 2008; 27(6):41–54.

12. Government Accountability Office. Preliminary observations of the EPA's second program to address indoor contamination. Testimony before the Subcommittee on Superfund and Environmental Health, Committee on Environment and Public Works, US Senate; June 20, 2007.

13. Government Accountability Office. EPA's more recent test and clean program raises concerns that need to be addressed to better prepare for indoor contamination following disasters. Report to Congressional Requesters; September 2007.

14. Thomas PA, Brackbill R, Thalji L, DiGrande L, Campolucci S, Thorpe L, Henning K. Respiratory and other health effects reported in children exposed to the World Trade Center disaster of 11 September 2001. Environ Health Perspect 2008; 116:1383–90.

15. Website covering information on asthma to 9/11 environmental health. Available at http://www.asthmamoms.com.

Chapter 8: The Medical Response to an Environmental Disaster: Lessons from the World Trade Center Attacks

1. Whitman C. Whitman details ongoing agency efforts to monitor disaster sites, contribute to cleanup efforts. US Environmental Protection Agency; September 18, 2001. Press release.

2. Environmental Protection Agency. Region 2, New York City response and recovery operations. World Trade Center Residential Dust Cleanup Program; March 2004. Draft final report.

3. Nordgen GE, Izeman MA. The environmental impacts of the World Trade Center attacks: a preliminary assessment. Natural Resources Defense Council; February 2002.

4. Lioy PJ, Weisel CP, Millette JR, Eisenreich S, Vallero D, Offenberg J, Buckley B, Turpin B, Zhong M, Cohen MD, Prophete C, Yang I, Stiles R, Chee G, Johnson W, Porcja R, Alimokhtari S, Hale RC, Weschler C, Chen L.C. Characterization of the dust/smoke aerosol that settled east of the World Trade Center (WTC) in lower Manhattan after the collapse of the WTC 11 September 2001. Environ Health Perspect 2002; 110(7):703–714.

5. Lioy PJ, Gochfeld M. Lessons learned on environmental, occupational, and residential exposures from the attack on the World Trade Center. Am J Ind Med 2002; 42 (6):560–565.

6. Landrigan PJ, Lioy PJ, Thurston G, Berkowitz G, Chen LC, Chillrud SN, Gavett SH, Georgopoulos PG, Geyh AS, Levin S, Perera F, Rappaport SM, Small C. NIEHS World Trade Center Working Group. Health and environmental consequences of the World Trade Center disaster. Environ Health Perspect 2004; 112(6):731–739.

7. Samet JM, Geyh AS, Utell MJ. The legacy of World Trade Center dust. N Engl J Med 2007; 356(22):2233–2236.

8. Rom WN, Weiden M, Garcia R, Yie TA, Vathesatogkit P, Tse DB, McGuinness G, Roggli V, Prezant D. Acute eosinophilic pneumonia in a New York City firefighter exposed to World Trade Center dust. Am J Respir Crit Care Med 2002; 166(6): 797–800.

9. Lorber M, Gibb H, Grant L, Pinto J, Pleil J, Cleverly D. Assessment of inhalation exposures and potential health risks to the general population that resulted from the collapse of the World Trade Center towers. Risk Anal 2007; 27(5):1203–1221.

10. McGee JK, Chen LC, Cohen MD, Chee GR, Prophete CM, Haykal-Coates N, Wasson SJ, Conner TL, Costa DL, Gavett SH. Chemical analysis of World Trade Center fine particulate matter for use in toxicologic assessment. Environ Health Perspect 2003; 111(7):972–980.

11. Gavett SH, Haykal-Coates N, Highfill JW, Ledbetter AD, Chen LC, Cohen MD, Harkema JR, Wagner J.G, Costa D.L. World Trade Center fine particulate matter causes respiratory tract hyperresponsiveness in mice. Environ Health Perspect 2003; 111(7):981–991.

12. Offenberg JH, Eisenreich SJ, Chen LC, Cohen MD, Chee G, Prophete C, Weisel C, Lioy PJ. Persistent organic pollutants in the dusts that settled across lower Manhattan after September 11, 2001. Environ Sci Technol 2003; 37(3):502–508.

13. Yiin LM, Millette JR, Vette A, Ilacqua V, Quan C, Gorczynski J, Kendall M, Chen LC, Weisel CP, Buckley B, Yang I, Lioy PJ. Comparisons of the dust/smoke particulate that settled inside the surrounding buildings and outside on the streets of southern New York City after the collapse of the World Trade Center, September 11, 2001. J Air Waste Manag Assoc 2004; 54(5):515–528.

14. Offenberg JH, Eisenreich SJ, Gigliotti CL, Chen LC, Xiong JQ, Quan C, Lou X, Zhong M, Gorczynski J, Yiin LM, Illacqua V, Lioy PJ. Persistent organic pollutants in dusts that settled indoors in lower Manhattan after September 11, 2001. J Expo Anal Environ Epidemiol 2004; 14(2):164–172.

15. Pleil JD, Vette AF, Johnson BA, Rappaport SM. Air levels of carcinogenic polycyclic aromatic hydrocarbons after the World Trade Center disaster. Proc Natl Acad Sci USA 2004; 101(32):11685–11688.

16. Banauch G, McLaughlin M, Hirschhorn R, Corrigan M, Kelly K, Prezant D. Injuries and illnesses among New York City Fire Department rescue workers after responding to the World Trade Center attacks. MMWR 2002; 51:6–8.

17. Banauch GI, Dhala A, Prezant DJ. Pulmonary disease in rescue workers at the World Trade Center site. Curr Opin Pulm Med 2005; 11(2):160–168.

18. Prezant DJ, Weiden M, Banauch GI, McGuinness G, Rom WN, Aldrich TK, Kelly KJ. Cough and bronchial responsiveness in firefighters at the World Trade Center site. N Engl J Med 2002; 347(11):806–815.

19. Fireman EM, Lerman Y, Ganor E, Greif J, Fireman-Shoresh S, Lioy PJ, Banauch GI, Weiden M, Kelly KJ, Prezant DJ. Induced sputum assessment in New York City firefighters exposed to World Trade Center dust. Environ Health Perspect 2004; 112 (15):1564–1569.

20. Feldman DM, Baron SL, Bernard BP, Lushniak BD, Banauch G, Arcentales N, Kelly KJ, Prezant DJ. Symptoms, respirator use, and pulmonary function changes among New York City firefighters responding to the World Trade Center disaster. Chest 2004; 125(4):1256–1264.

21. Banauch GI, Alleyne D, Sanchez R, Olender K, Cohen HW, Weiden M, Kelly KJ, Prezant DJ. Persistent hyperreactivity and reactive airway dysfunction in firefighters at the World Trade Center. Am J Respir Crit Care Med 2003; 168(1):54–62.

22. Banauch GI, Hall C, Weiden M, Cohen HW, Aldrich TK, Christodoulou V, Arcentales N, Kelly KJ, Prezant, D J. Pulmonary function after exposure to the World Trade Center collapse in the New York City Fire Department. Am J Respir Crit Care Med 2006; 174(3):312–319.

23. Izbicki G, Chavko R, Banauch GI, Weiden MD, Berger KI, Aldrich TK, Hall C, Kelly KJ, Prezant DJ. World Trade Center "sarcoid-like" granulomatous pulmonary disease in New York City Fire Department rescue workers. Chest 2007; 131 (5):1414–1423.

24. Levin S, Herbert R, Skloot G, Szeinuk J, Teirstein A, Fischler D, Milek D, Piligian G, Wilk-Rivard E, Moline J. Health effects of World Trade Center site workers. Am J Ind Med 2002; 42(6):545–547.

25. Herbert R, Moline J, Skloot G, Metzger K, Baron S, Luft B, Markowitz S, Udasin I, Harrison D, Stein D, Todd A, Enright P, Stellman JM, Landrigan PJ, Levin SM. The World Trade Center disaster and the health of workers: five-year assessment of a unique medical screening program. Environ Health Perspect 2006; 114(12):1853–1858.

26. Moline JM, Herbert R, Levin S, Stein D, Luft BJ, Udasin IG, Landrigan PJ. WTC medical monitoring and treatment program: comprehensive health care response in aftermath of disaster. Mt Sinai J Med 2008; 75(2):67–75.

27. Savitz DA, Oxman RT, Metzger KB, Wallenstein S, Stein D, Moline JM, Herbert R. Epidemiologic research on man-made disasters: strategies and implications of cohort definition for World Trade Center worker and volunteer surveillance program. Mt Sinai J Med 2008; 75(2):77–87.

28. Skloot GS, Schechter CB, Herbert R, et al. Longitudinal assessment of spirometry in the World Trade Center medical monitoring program. Chest 2009; 135(2):492–498.

29. Mendelson DS, Roggeveen M, Levin SM, Herbert R, de la Hoz RE. Air trapping detected on end-expiratory high-resolution computed tomography in symptomatic World Trade Center rescue and recovery workers. J Occup Environ Med 2007; 49 (8): 840–845.

30. De la Hoz RE, Christie J, Teamer JA, Bienenfeld LA, Afilaka AA, Crane M, Levin, SM, Herbert R. Reflux symptoms and disorders and pulmonary disease in former World Trade Center rescue and recovery workers and volunteers. J Occup Environ Med 2008; 50(12):1351–1354.

31. Stellman JM, Smith RP, Katz CL, Sharma V, Charney DS, Herbert R, Moline J, Luft BJ, Markowitz S, Udasin I, Harrison D, Baron S, Landrigan PJ, Levin SM, Southwick S. Enduring mental health morbidity and social function impairment in World Trade Center rescue, recovery, and cleanup workers: the psychological dimension of an environmental health disaster. Environ Health Perspect 2008; 116(9):1248–1253.

32. Agency, U.E.P., Office of Inspector General. EPA's response to the World Trade Center collapse: challenges, successes, and areas for improvement; 2003. EPA 2003-P-00012.

33. NYC Department of Health and Mental Health. Response to the World Trade Center disaster: recommendations for people re-occupying commercial buildings and residents re-entering their homes; 2001.

34. Brackbill RM, Thorpe LE, DiGrande L, Perrin M, Sapp JH 2nd, Wu D, Campolucci S, Walker DJ, Cone J, Pulliam P, Thalji L, Farfel MR, Thomas P. Surveillance for World Trade Center disaster health effects among survivors of collapsed and damaged buildings. MMWR Surveill Summ 2006; 55(2):1–18.

35. Newman DM. 9/11 environmental health: disaster and response. New Solut 2008; 18(1):3–22.

36. Group TW. "Gold standard" for remediation of WTC contamination. New Solut 2004; 13, No. 3.

37. Reibman J, Lin S, Hwang SA, Gulati M, Bowers JA, Rogers L, Berger KI, Hoerning A, Gomez M, Fitzgerald EF. The World Trade Center residents' respiratory health study: new-onset respiratory symptoms and pulmonary function. Environ Health Perspect 2005; 113(4):406–411.

38. Lin S, Reibman J, Bowers JA, Hwang SA, Hoerning, A, Gomez MI, Fitzgerald EF. Upper respiratory symptoms and other health effects among residents living near the World Trade Center site after September 11, 2001. Am J Epidemiol 2005; 162 (6):499–507.

39. Lin S, Jones R, Reibman J, Bowers J, Fitzgerald EF, Hwang SA. Reported respiratory symptoms and adverse home conditions after 9/11 among residents living near the World Trade Center. J Asthma 2007; 44(4):325–332.

40. Fagan J, Galea S, Ahern J, Bonner S, Vlahov D. Self-reported increase in asthma severity after the September 11 attacks on the World Trade Center—Manhattan, New York, 2001. MMWR Morb Mortal Wkly Rep 2002; 51(35):781–784.

41. Szema AM, Khedkar M, Maloney PF, Takach PA, Nickels MS, PatelH, Modugno F, Tso AY, Lin DH. Clinical deterioration in pediatric asthmatic patients after September 11, 2001. J Allergy Clin Immunol 2004; 113(3):420–426.

42. Berkowitz GS, Wolff MS, Janevic TM, Holzman IR, Yehuda R, Landrigan PJ. The World Trade Center disaster and intrauterine growth restriction. JAMA 2003; 290 (5):595–596.

43. Wolff MS, Teitelbaum SL, Lioy PJ, Santella RM, Wang RY, Jones RL, Caldwell KL, Sjodin A, Turner WE, Li W, Georgopoulos P, Berkowitz GS. Exposures among pregnant women near the World Trade Center site on 11 September 2001. Environ Health Perspect 2005; 113(6):739–748.

44. Lederman SA, Rauh V, Weiss L, Stein JL, Hoepner LA, Becker M, Perera FP. The effects of the World Trade Center event on birth outcomes among term deliveries at three lower Manhattan hospitals. Environ Health Perspect 2004; 112(17):1772–1778.

45. Perera FP, Tang D, Rauh V, Lester K, Tsai WY, Tu YH, Weiss L, Hoepner L, King J, Del Priore G, Lederman SA. Relationships among polycyclic aromatic hydrocarbon-DNA adducts, proximity to the World Trade Center, and effects on fetal growth. Environ Health Perspect 2005; 113(8):1062–1067.

46. Lederman SA, Rauh V, Weiss L, Stein JL, Hoepner LA, Becker M, Perera FP. Relation between cord blood mercury levels and early child development in a World Trade Center cohort. Environ Health Perspect 2008; 116(8):1085–1091.

47. Perera FP, Tang D, Rauh V, Tu YH, Tsai WY, Becker M, Stein JL, King J, Del Priore G, Lederman SA. Relationship between polycyclic aromatic hydrocarbon-DNA adducts, environmental tobacco smoke, and child development in the World Trade Center cohort. Environ Health Perspect 2007; 115(10): 1497–1502.

48. Reibman J, Liu M, Cheng Q, Liautaud S, Rogers L, Lau S, Berger KI, Goldring RM, Marmor M, Fernandez-Beros ME, Tonorezos ES, Caplan-Shaw CE, Gonzalez J, Filner J, Walter D, Kyng K, Rom WN. Characteristics of a residential and working community with diverse exposure to World Trade Center dust, gas, and fumes. J Occup Environ Med 2009; 51(5):534–541.

49. Galea S, Ahern J, Resnick H, Kilpatrick D, Bucuvalas M, Gold J, Vlahov D. Psychological sequelae of the September 11 terrorist attacks in New York City. N Engl J Med 2002; 346(13):982–987.

50. DeLisi LE, Maurizio A, Yost M, Papparozzi C, Fulchino C, Katz CL, Altesman J, Biel M, Lee J, Stevens P. A survey of New Yorkers after the September 11, 2001, terrorist attacks. Am J Psychiatry 2003; 160(4):1019.

51. Farfel M, Digrande L, Brackbill R, Prann A, Cone J, Friedman S, Walker DJ, Pezeshki G, Thomas P, Galea S, Williamson D, Frieden TR, Thorpe L. An overview of 9/11 experiences and respiratory and mental health conditions among World Trade Center Health Registry enrollees. J Urban Health 2008; 85(6): 880–909.

52. Thomas PA, Brackbill R, Thalji L, DiGrande L, Campolucci S, Thorpe L, Henning K. Respiratory and other health effects reported in children exposed to the World Trade Center disaster of 11 September 2001. Environ Health Perspect 2008; 116 (10):1383–1390.

53. Wheeler K, McKelvey W, Thorpe L, Perrin M, Cone J, Kass D, Farfel M, Thomas P, Brackbill R. Asthma diagnosed after 11 September 2001 among rescue and recovery workers: findings from the World Trade Center Health Registry. Environ Health Perspect 2007; 115(11):1584–1590.

54. Perrin MA, DiGrande L, Wheeler K, Thorpe L, Farfel M. Brackbill R. Differences in PTSD prevalence and associated risk factors among World Trade Center disaster rescue and recovery workers. Am J Psychiatry 2007; 164(9):1385–1394.

55. DiGrande L, Perrin MA, Thorpe LE, Thalji L, Murphy J, Wu D, Farfel M, Brackbill RM. Posttraumatic stress symptoms, PTSD, and risk factors among lower Manhattan residents 2–3 years after the September 11, 2001 terrorist attacks. J Trauma Stress 2008; 21(3):264–273.

56. Lioy PJ, Pellizzari E, Prezant D. The World Trade Center aftermath and its effects on health: understanding and learning through human-exposure science. Environ Sci Technol 2006; 40(22):6876–6885.

Chapter 9: Chlorofluorocarbons and the Development of the Ozone Hole

1. Molina MJ, Rowland FS. Stratospheric sink for chlorofluoromethanes: chlorine-atom catalyzed destruction of ozone. Nature 1974; 249:810–812.
2. Molina MJ, Molina LT. Chlorofluorocarbons and destruction of the ozone layer. In: Rom, WN, Markowitz, SB, editors. Environmental and occupational medicine. 4th ed. New York: Lippincott Williams & Wilkins; 2007. p. 1605–1615.
3. Midgley T. From the periodic table to production. Ind Engr Chem 1937; 29: 241–244.
4. Rowland FS, Molina MJ. Chlorofluoromethanes in the environment. Rev Geophys Space Phys 1975; 13:1–35.
5. Chapman S. A theory of upper atmospheric ozone. Mem R Meteorol Soc 1930; 3:103.
6. Crutzen PJ. The influence of nitrogen oxides on atmosphere ozone content. Q J R Meteorol Soc 1970; 96:320–325.
7. Lovelock JE, Maggs RJ, Wade RJ. Halogenated hydrocarbons in and over the Atlantic. Nature 1973; 241:194–196.
8. Toumi R, Jones RL, Pyle JA. Stratospheric ozone depletion by $ClONO_2$ photolysis. Nature 1993; 365:37–39.
9. Minton TK, Nelson CM, Moore TA, Okumura M. Direct observation of ClO from chlorine nitrate photolysis. Science 1992; 258:1342–1345.
10. Cicerone RJ. Changes in stratospheric ozone. Science 1987; 237:35–42.
11. World Meteorological Organization (WHO). Scientific assessment of ozone depletion: 1998. Geneva (Switzerland): WMO; 1999. WMO Global Ozone Research and Monitoring Project, Report no. 44.
12. Ravishankara AR, Turnipseed AA, Jensen NR, Barone S, Mills, M, Howard CJ, Solomon S. Do hydrofluorocarbons destroy stratospheric ozone? Science 1994; 263:71–75.
13. Solomon S, Garcia RR, Rowland FS, Wuebbles DJ. On the depletion of Antarctic ozone. Nature 1986; 321:755–758.
14. Molina LT, Molina MJ, Stachnick RA, Tom RD. An upper limit to the rate of the $HCl + ClONO_2$ reaction. J Phys Chem 1985; 89:3779–3781.
15. Abbatt JPD, Beyer KD, Fucaloro AF, et al. Interaction of HCl vapor with water-ice: implications for the stratosphere. J Geophys Res 1992; 97:15819–15826.
16. Gertner BJ, Hynes JT. Molecular dynamics simulation of hydrochloric acid ionization at the surface of stratospheric ice. Science 1996; 271:1563–1566.
17. Molina LT, Molina MJ. Production of Cl_2O_2 from the self-reaction of the ClO radical. J Phys Chem 1987; 91:433–436.
18. Farman JC, Gardiner BG, Shanklin JD. Large losses of total ozone in Antarctica reveal seasonal ClO_x/NO_x interactions. Nature 1985; 315:207–210.

19. Russell JM III, Luo M, Cicerone RJ, Deaver LE. Satellite confirmation of the dominance of chlorofluorocarbons in the global stratospheric chlorine budget. Nature 1996; 379:526–529.

20. Stolarski RS, Bloomfield P, McPeters RD, Herman JR. Total ozone trends deduced from Nimbus 7 TOMS data. Geophys Res Lett 1991; 18:1015–1018.

21. Proffitt MH, Aikin K, Margitan JJ, Loewenstein M, Podolske JR, Weaver A, Chan KR, Fast H, Elkins JW. Ozone loss inside the northern polar vortex during the 1991–1992 winter. Science 1993; 261:1150–1158.

22. Anderson JG, Toohey DW, Brune WH. Free radicals within the Antarctic Vortex: the role of CFCs in Antarctic ozone loss. Science 1991; 251:39–46.

23. Proffitt MH, Steinkamp MJ, Powell JA, et al. In situ ozone measurements within the 1987 Antarctic ozone hole from a high-altitude ER-2 aircraft. J Geophys Res 1989; 94(16):547–555.

24. Turco R, Plumb A, Condon E. The Airborne Arctic Stratospheric Expedition: prologue. Geophys Res Lett 1990; 17:313–316.

25. Madronich S, McKenzie RL, Caldwell MM, Bjärn LO. Changes in ultraviolet radiation reaching the Earth's surface. Ambio 1995; 24:143–152.

26. Longstreth JD, de Grujil FR, Kripke ML, Takizawa Y, van der Leun JC. Effects of solar radiation on human health. Ambio 1995; 24:153–165.

27. van der Leun J, Tang X, Tevini M. Environmental effects of ozone depletion: 1994 assessment. Ambio 1995; 24:138.

28. Biggs RH, Joyner MEB, editors. Stratospheric ozone depletion/UV-B radiation in the biosphere. New York: Springer-Verlag; 1994.

29. Shore RE. Overview of radiation-induced skin cancer in humans. Int J Radiat Biol 1990; 57:809–827.

30. Henriksen T, Dahlback A, Larsen SHH, Moan J. Ultraviolet-radiation and skin cancer: effect of an ozone layer depletion. Photochem Photobiol 1990; 51:579–582.

31. Abarca JF, Casiccia CC. Skin cancer and ultraviolet-B radiation under the Antarctic ozone hole: southern Chile, 1987–2000. Photodermatol Photoimmunol Photomed 2002; 18:294–302.

32. Brash DE, Rudolph JA, Simon JA, et al. A role for sunlight in skin cancer: UV-induced p53 mutations in squamous cell carcinoma. Proc Natl Acad Sci USA 1991; 88(10): 124–128.

33. Caldwell MM, Teramura AH, Tevini M, Bomman JF, Björn LO, Kulandaivelu G. Effects of increased solar ultraviolet radiation on terrestrial plants. Ambio 1995; 24:166–173.

34. Smith RC, Prezelin BB, Baker KS, Bidigare RR, Boucher NP, Coley T, et al. Ozone depletion: ultraviolet radiation and phytoplankton biology in Antarctic waters. Science 1992; 255:952–959.

35. National Research Council. Halocarbon: environmental effects of chlorofluoromethane release. Halocarbons: effects on stratospheric ozone. Washington (DC): National Academy of Sciences; 1976.

36. Montzka SA, Butler JH, Myers RC, et al. Decline in the tropospheric abundance of halogen from halocarbons: implications for stratospheric ozone depletion. Science 1996; 272:1318–1322.
37. Austin J, Butchart N, Shine KP. Possibility of an Arctic ozone hole in a doubled-CO_2 climate. Nature 1992: 360:221–225.
38. Ravishankara AR, Daniel JS, Portmann RW. Nitrous oxide (N_2O): the dominant ozone-depleting substance emitted in the 21st century. Science 2009; 326:123–125.

Chapter 10: Global Warming Science and Consequences

1. Intergovernmental Panel on Climate Change website: htpp://www.ipcc.ch/about/ipcc-bureau-tfb.htm.
2. Oppenheimer M, O'Neill BC, Webster M, Agrawala S. The limits of consensus. Science 2007; 317:1505–1506.
3. Hansen J, Sato M, Kharecha P, Russell G, Lea DW, Siddall M. Climate change and trace gases. Phil Trans R Soc A 2007; 365:1925–1954.
4. Sitch S, Cox PM, Collins WJ, Huntingford C. Indirect radiative forcing of climate change through ozone effects on the land-carbon sink. Nature 2007; 448:791–794.
5. Keppler F, Hamilton JTG, Braß M, Röckmann T. Methane emissions from terrestrial plants under aerobic conditions. Nature 2006; 439:187–191.
6. Hansen J, Nazarenko L, Ruedy R, Sato M, Willis J, Del Genio A, et al. Earth's energy imbalance: confirmation and implications. Science 2005; 308:1431–1435.
7. Hansen J, Sato M. Greenhouse gas growth rates. Proc Nat Acad Sci 2004; 101:16109–16114.
8. Keeling CD, Whorf TP. Atmospheric CO_2 concentrations derived from flask air samples at sites in the SIO network. In Trends: a compendium of data on global change. Oak Ridge (TN): Carbon Dioxide Information Analysis Center, Oak Ridge National Laboratory, US Department of Energy; 2004. Available at http://cdiac.ornl.gov.
9. Brook EJ. Tiny bubbles tell all. Science 2005; 310:1285–1287.
10. Siegenthaler U, Stocker TF, Monnin E, Luthi D, Schwander J, Stauffer B, et al. Stable carbon cycle-climate relationship during the late Pleistocene. Science 2005; 310:1313–1317.
11. Luthi D, Le Floch M, Bereiter B, Blunier T, Barnola JM, Siegenthaler U, et al. High-resolution carbon dioxide concentration record 650,000–800,000 years before present. Nature 2008; 453:379–382.
12. Rosenzweig C, Karoly D, Vicarelli M, Neofotis P, Wu Q, Casassa G, et al. Attributing physical and biological impacts to anthropogenic climate change. Nature 2008; 453:353–357.
13. Ramanathan V, Carmichael G. Global and regional climate changes due to black carbon. Nat Geo 2008; 1:221–227.

14. Ramanathan V, Ramana MV, Roberts G, Kim D, Corrigan C, Chung C, et al. Warming trends in Asia amplified by brown cloud solar absorption. Nature 2007; 448:575–578.

15. McConnell JR, Edwards R, Kok GL, Flanner MG, Zender CS, Saltzman ES, et al. 20th-century industrial black carbon emissions altered Arctic climate forcing. Science 2007; 317:1381–1384.

16. Serreze MC, Holland MM, Stroeve J. Perspectives on the Arctic's shrinking sea-ice cover. Science 2007; 315:1533–1536.

17. Steffen K, Nghiem SV, Huff R, Neumann G. The melt anomaly of 2002 on the Greenland ice sheet from active and passive microwave satellite observations. Geophys Res Lett 2004; 31:L20402.

18. Lenton TM, Held H, Kriegler E, Hall JW, Lucht W, Rahmstorf S, et al. Tipping elements in the Earth's climate system. Proc Nat Acad Sci 2008; 105:1786–1793.

19. Smith LC, MacDonald GM, Velichko AA, Beilman DW, Borisova OK, Frey KE, et al. Siberian peatlands a net carbon sink and global methane source since the early Holocene. Science 2004; 303:353–356.

20. Rignot E, Bamber JL, Van Den Broeke MR, Davis C, Li Y, Van De Berg WJ, et al. Recent Antarctic ice mass loss from radar interferometry and regional climate modeling. Nat Geo 2008:106–110.

21. Steig EJ, Schneider DP, Rutherford SD, Mann ME, Comiso JC, Shindell DT. Warming of the Antarctic ice-sheet surface since the 1957 International Geophysical Year. Nature 2009; 457:459–462.

22. Jenouvrier S, Caswell H, Barbraud C, Holland M, Stroeve J, Weimerskirch H. Demographic models and IPCC climate projections predict the decline of an emperor penguin population. Proc Natl Acad Sci 2009; 106(6):1844–1847.

23. Pfeffer WT. The opening of a new landscape: Columbia Glacier at mid-retreat. Washington, DC: American Geophysical Union; 2007.

24. Pfeffer WT, Harper JT, O'Neel S. Kinematic constraints on glacier contributions to 21st-century sea-level rise. Science 2008; 321:1340–1343.

25. Pounds JA, Bustamante MR, Coloma LA, Consuegra JA, Fogden MPL, Foster PN, et al. Widespread amphibian extinctions from epidemic disease driven by global warming. Nature 2006; 439:161–167.

26. Thomas CD, Cameron A, Green RE, Bakkenes M, Beaumont LJ, Collingham YC, et al. Extinction risk from climate change. Nature 2004; 427:145–148.

27. Burns CE, Johnston KM, Schmitz OJ. Global climate change and mammalian species diversity in U.S. national parks. Proc Nat Acad Sci 2003; 100:11474–11477.

28. McMenamin SK, Hadly EA, Wright CK. Climatic change and wetland desiccation cause amphibian decline in Yellowstone National Park. Proc Nat Acad Sci 2008; 105:16988–16993.

29. Moritz C, Patton JL, Conroy CJ, Parra JL, White GC, Beissinger SR. Impact of a century of climate change on small-mammal communities in Yosemite National Park, USA. Science 2008; 322:261–264.

30. Kausrud KL, Mysterud A, Steen H, Vik JO, Ostbye E, Cazelles B, et al. Linking climate change to lemming cycles. Nature 2008; 456:93–96.

31. Le Bohec C, Durant JM, Gauthier-Clerc M, Stenseth NC, Park Y-H, Pradel R, et al. King penguin population threatened by southern ocean warming. Proc Nat Acad Sci 2008; 105:2493–2497.

32. Willis CG, Ruhfel B, Primack RB, Miller-Rushing AJ, Davis CC. Phylogenetic patterns of species loss in Thoreau's woods are driven by climate change. Proc Nat Acad Sci 2008; 105:17029–17033.

33. World Commission on Environment and Development. Our common future. Oxford (England): Oxford University Press; 1987.

34. Hoegh-Guldberg O, Mumby PJ, Hooten AJ, Steneck RS, Greenfield P, Gomez E, et al. Coral reefs under rapid climate change and ocean acidification. Science 2007; 318:1737–1742.

35. Anthony KRN, Kline DI, Diaz-Pulido G, Dove S, Hoegh-Guldberg O. Ocean acidification causes bleaching and productivity loss in coral reef builders. Proc Nat Acad Sci 2008; 105:17442–17446.

36. Carpenter KE, Abrar M, Aeby G, Aronson RB, Banks S, Bruckner A, et al. One-third of reef-building corals face elevated extinction risk from climate change and local impacts. Science 2008; 321:560–563.

37. De'ath G, Lough JM, Fabricius KE. Declining coral calcification on the Great Barrier Reef. Science 2009; 323:116–119.

38. Webster PJ, Holland GJ, Curry JA, Chang H-R. Changes in tropical cyclone number, duration, and intensity in a warming environment. Science 2005; 309:1844–1846.

39. Emanuel K. Increasing destructiveness of tropical cyclones over the past 30 years. Nature 2005; 436:686–688.

40. Karl TR, Knight RW, Plummer N. Trends in high-frequency climate variability in the twentieth century. Nature 1995; 377:217–220.

41. Epstein PR. Climate change and human health. N Engl J Med 2005; 353:1433–1436.

42. Broecker WS. Thermohaline circulation, the Achilles heel of our climate system: will man-made CO_2 upset the current balance? Science 1997; 278:1582–1588.

43. Bryden HL, Longworth HR, Cunningham SA. Slowing of the Atlantic meridional overturning circulation at 25N. Nature 2005; 438:655–7.

44. Epstein, PR, Leaf A. Biological and medical implications of global warming. In: Rom, WN, Markowitz, SB, editors. Environmental and occupational medicine. 4th ed. New York: Lippincott Williams & Wilkins; 2007. p. 1590–1604.

45. Hansen J, Nazarenko L, Ruedy R, Tausnev N, et al. Earth's energy imbalance: confirmation and implications. Science 2005; 308:1431–1435.

46. McMichael AJ, Woodruff RE, Hales S. Climate change and human health: present and future risks. Lancet 2006; 367:859–869.

47. Rom WN, Pinkerton KE, Martin WJ, Forastiere F. Global warming: a challenge to all American Thoracic Society members. Am J Respir Crit Care Med 2008; 177:1053–1057.

48. Patz JA, Campbell-Lendrum D, Holloway T, Foley JA. Impact of regional climate change on human health. Nature 2005; 438:310–317.

49. Dematte JE, O'Mara K, Buescher J, Whitney CG, Forsythe S, McNamee T, et al. Near-fatal heat stroke during the 1995 heat wave in Chicago. Ann Intern Med 1998; 129:173–181.

50. Filleul L, Cassadou S, Medina S, Fabres P, Lefranc A, Eilstein D, et al. The relation between temperature, ozone and mortality in nine French cities during the heat wave of 2003. Environ Health Perspect 2006; 114:1344–1347.

51. Dhainaut JF, Claessens Y-E, Ginsberg C, Riou B. Unprecedented heat-related deaths during the 2003 heat wave in Paris: consequences on emergency departments. Crit Care 2004; 8:1–2.

52. Schar C, Vidale PL, Luthi D, et al. The role of increasing temperature variability in European summer heatwaves. Nature 2004; 427:332–335.

53. Stoot PA, Stone DA, Allen MR. Human contribution to the European heatwave of 2003. Nature 2004; 432:610–614.

54. Stafoggia M, Forastiere F, Berti G, Bisanti L, Cadum E, Caranci N, et al. Factors associated with heat-related in-hospital mortality: a multicity case-crossover analysis. Epidemiology 2006; 17:S163–S164.

55. Stafoggia M, Forastiere F, Agostini D, Caranci N, De'Donato F, Demaria M, et al. Factors affecting in-hospital heat-related mortality: a multi-city case-crossover analysis. J Epidemiol Community Health 2008; 62:209–215.

56. Argaud L, Ferry T, Le Q-H, Marfisi A, Ciorba D, Achache P, et al. Short- and long-term outcomes of heatstroke following the 2003 heat wave in Lyon, France. Arch Intern Med 2007; 167:2177–2183.

57. Cado E, Rodwin VG, Spira A. In the heat of the summer: lessons from the heat waves in Paris. J Urban Health 2007; 84:466–468.

58. Schar C, Vidale PL, Luthi D, et al. The role of increasing temperature variability in European summer heatwaves. Nature 2004; 427:332–335.

59. Karl TR, Jones PD, Knight RW, et al. A new perspective on recent global warming: asymmetric trends of daily maximum and minimum temperature. Bull Am Meteorol Soc 1993; 74:1007–1023.

60. Fouillet A, Rey G, Laurent F, Pavillon G, Bellec S, Guihenneuc-Jouyaux C, et al. Excess mortality related to the August 2003 heat wave in France. Int Arch Occup Environ Health 2006; 80:16–24.

61. Medina-Ramon M, Zanobetti A, Cavanagh DP, Schwartz J. Extreme temperatures and mortality: assessing effect modification by personal characteristics and specific cause of death in a multi-city case-only analysis. Environ Health Perspect 2006; 114:1331–1336.

62. Luber G, McGeehin M. Climate change and extreme heat events. Am J Prev Med 2008; 35:429–435.

63. Gaffen DJ, Ross RJ. Increased summertime heat stress in the US. Nature 1998; 396:529–530.

64. Ren C, Williams GM, Morawska L, Mengersen K, Tong S. Ozone modifies associations between temperature and cardiovascular mortality: analysis of the NMMAPS data. Occup Environ Med 2008; 65:255–260.

65. Schwartz J, Samet JM, Patz JA. Hospital admissions for heart disease: the effects of temperature and humidity. Epidemiol 2004; 15:755–761.

66. Qian Z, He Q, Lin HM, Kong L, Bentley CM, Liu W, et al. High temperatures enhanced acute mortality effects of ambient particle pollution in the "oven" city of Wuhan, China. Environ Health Perspect 2008; 116:1172–1178.

67. Hansen A, Bi P, Nitschke M, Ryan P, Pisaniello D, Tucker G. The effect of heat waves on mental health in a temperate Australian City. Environ Health Perspect 2008; 116:1369–1375.

68. Yoganathan D, Rom WN. Medical aspects of global warming. Am J Indust Med 2001; 40:199–210.

69. Beggs PJ, Bambrick HJ. Is the global rise of asthma an early impact of anthropogenic climate change? Environ Health Perspect 2005; 113:915–919.

70. Wayne P, Forster S, Connelly J, Bazzaz FA, Epstein PR. Production of allergenic pollen by ragweed (*Ambrosia artemisiifolia* L.) is increased in CO_2 enriched atmospheres. Ann Allergy Asthma Immunol 2002; 88:279–282.

71. Singer BD, Ziska LH, Frenz DA, Gebhard DE, Straka JG. Increasing Amb a 1 content in common ragweed (*Ambrosia artemisiifolia*) pollen as a function of rising atmospheric CO_2 concentration. Functional Plant Biology 2005; 32:667–670.

72. Wolf, J, O'Neill NR, Rogers CA, Muilenberg ML, Ziska LH. Elevated atmospheric carbon dioxide concentrations amplify *Alternaria alternata* sporulation and total antigen production. Environ Health Perspect 2010; 118: 1223–1228.

73. Beggs PJ. Impacts of climate change on aeroallergens: past and future. Clin Exp Allergy 2004; 34:1507–1513.

74. Gold JA, Jagirdar J, Hay JG, Addrizzo-Harris D, Naidich DP, Rom WN. Hut lung: a domestically acquired particulate lung disease. Medicine 2000; 79:310–317.

75. Jiang R, Bell ML. A comparison of particulate matter from biomass-burning rural and non-biomass-burning urban households in northeast china. Environ Health Perspect 2008; 116:907–914.

76. Torres-Duque C, Maldonado D, Perez-Padilla R, Ezzati M, Viegi G. Biomass fuels and respiratory diseases: A review of the evidence. Proc Am Thorac Soc 2008; 5:557–590.

77. Gage KL, Burkot TR, Eisen RJ, Hayes EB. Climate and vectorborne diseases. Am J Prev Med 2008; 35:436–450.

78. Pascual M, Ahumada JA, Chaves LF, Rodo X, Bouma M. Malaria resurgence in the East African highlands: temperature trends revisited. Proc Nat Acad Sci 2006; 103:5829–5834.

79. Patz JA, Olson SH. Malaria risk and temperature: influences from global climate change and local land use practices. Proc Nat Acad Sci 2006; 103:5635–5636.

80. Milly PCD, Wetherhald RT, Dunne KA, Delworth TL. Increasing risk of great floods in a changing climate. Nature 2001; 415:514–517.

81. Alonso D, Bouma MJ, Pascual M. Epidemic malaria and warmer temperatures in recent decades in an East African highland. Proceedings of the Royal Society B 2010; doi:10.1098/rspb.2010.2020.

82. Hales S, de Wet N, Maindonald J, Woodward A. Potential effect of population and climate changes on global distribution of dengue fever: an empirical model. Lancet 2002; 360:830–834.

83. Haines A, Patz JA. Health effects of climate change. JAMA 2004; 291 99–103.

84. Ebi KL, Mills DM, Smith JB, Grambsch A. Climate change and human health impacts in the United States: an update on the results of the U.S. National Assessment. Environ Health Perspect 2006; 114:1318–1324.

85. Ramanathan V, Feng Y. On avoiding dangerous anthropogenic interference with the climate system: formidable challenges ahead. Proc Nat Acad Sci 2008; 105:14245–14250.

Chapter 11: National Green Energy Plan

1. Frumkin H, Hess J, Vindigni S. Peak petroleum and public health. JAMA 2007; 298:1688–1690.

2. Goldstein BD, Osofsky HJ, Lichtveld MY. The Gulf oil spill. N Engl J Med 2011; 364:1334–1348.

3. Warnecke F, Luginbuhl P, Ivanova N, Ghassemian M, Richardson TH, Stege JT, et al. Metagenomic and functional analysis of hindgut microbiota of a wood-feeding higher termite. Nature 2007; 450:560–564.

4. Atsumi S, Hanai T, Liao JC. Non-fermentative pathways for synthesis of branched-chain higher alcohols as biofuels. Nature 2008; 451:86–89.

5. Fargione J, Hill J, Tilman D, Polasky S, Hawthorne P. Land clearing and the biofuel carbon debt. Science 2008; 319:1235–1238.

6. Hill J, Nelson E, Tilman D, Polasky S, Tiffany D. Environmental, economic, and energetic costs and benefits of biodiesel and other ethanol biofuels. Proc Nat Acad Sci 2006; 103:11206–11210.

7. Righelato R, Spracklen DV. Carbon mitigation by biofuels or by saving and restoring forests? Science 2007; 317:902.

8. Searchinger T, Heimlich R, Haughton RA, Dong F, Elobeid A, Fabiosa J, et al. Use of U.S. croplands for biofuels increases greenhouse gases through emissions from land use change. Science 2008; 319:1238–1240.

9. Gold JA, Jagirdar J, Hay JG, Addrizzo-Harris D, Naidich DP, Rom WN. Hut lung: a domestically acquired particulate lung disease. Medicine 2000; 79:310–317.

Chapter 12 Climate Change Policy Options

1. Anderegg WRL, Prall JW, Harold J, Schneider SH. Expert credibility in climate change. Proc Natl Acad Sci USA 2010; 107:12107–12109.
2. O'Neill BC, Oppenheimer M. Dangerous climate impacts and the Kyoto Protocol. Science 2002; 296:1971–1972.
3. Hasselmann K, Latif M, Hooss G, Azar C, Eedenhofer O, Jaeger CC, et al. The challenge of long-term climate change. Science 2003; 302:1923–1925.
4. Manne A, Richels R. U.S. rejection of the Kyoto Protocol: the impact on compliance costs and CO_2 emissions. Energy Policy 2004; 32:447–454.
5. Reilly J, Prinn R, Harnisch J, Fitzmaurice J, Jacoby H, Kicklighter D, et al. Multi-gas assessment of the Kyoto Protocol. Nature 1999; 401:549–555.
6. Campbell-Lendrum D, Corvalan C. Climate change and developing-country cities: implications for environmental health and equity. J Urban Health 2007; 84:109–117.
7. Victor DG, House JC, Joy S. Climate. A Madisonian approach to climate policy. Science 2005; 309:1820–1821.
8. Pacala S, Socolow R. Stabilization wedges: solving the climate problem for the next 50 years with current technologies. Science 2004; 305:968–971.

Chapter 13: Environmental Policy and the Land: Wilderness Preservation

1. Fuller RA, Irvine KN, Devine-Wright P, Warren PH, Gaston KJ. Psychological benefits of greenspace increase with biodiversity. Biol Lett 2007; 3(4):390–394.
2. Leopold, A. Wilderness as a form of land use. The Journal of Land & Public Utility Economics 1925; 1: 400–401.
3. Leopold, A. A Sand County Almanac. New York: Oxford University Press, 1966.
4. Marshall, R. The problem of the wilderness. Scientific Monthly 1930; 30: 145–148.
5. Marshall R. Alaska Wilderness. Berkeley, CA: University of California Press, Second Edition, 1956.
6. Udall S. testimony, Senate Committee on Interior and Insular Affairs, National Wilderness Preservation Act: Hearings before the Committee on Interior and Insular Affairs, 88th Cong., 1st sess., Feb. 28-Mar. 1 1963, 16.
7. Scott D. The Enduring Wilderness: Protecting Our Natural Heritage Through the Wilderness Act. Golden, Colorado: Fulcrum, 2004.
8. Olson SF. The Singing Wilderness. New York: Alfred A. Knopf, 1956.
9. Taylor MFJ, Suckling KF, Rachlinski JJ. The effectiveness of the Endangered Species Act: A quantitative analysis. Bioscience 2005; 55: 360–367.

Chapter 14: Environmental Policy and Advocacy Groups: The Wilderness Society: A Case Study

1. Stegner, W. Wilderness letter; 1960. Available at http://wilderness.org/content/wilderness-letter.

Chapter 15: Alaska: America's Wilderness Frontier: A Case Study

1. Waterman, J. Where mountains are nameless. New York: WW Norton; 2005.
2. Marshall, R. Alaska wilderness. Berkeley (CA): University of California Press; 1973.
3. US Dept. of Interior, Geological Survey. The oil and gas potential of the Arctic National Wildlife Refuge 1002 Area, Alaska. USGS Open File Report 98–34. Washington (DC): [PUBLISHER]; 1999.
4. National Academies of Science. Cumulative environmental effects of oil and gas activities on Alaska's north slope (March 2003). 452 pp.

Chapter 16: The Clean Water Act and Water Ecosystems

1. Clean Water Act-Full text with amendments through 2006–01–11. (http://www.waterboards.ca.gov/water_laws/docs/fedwaterpollutioncontolact.pdf). Maintained by California Water Resources Control Board.
2. Schindler DW, Hecky RE, Findlay DL, Stainton MP, Parker BR, Paterson MJ, Beaty KG, Lyng M, Kasian SE. Eutrophication of lakes cannot be controlled by reducing nitrogen input: results of a 37-year whole-ecosystem experiment. Proc Natl Acad Sci 2008; 105:11039–11040.
3. Duhig C. Clean Water Laws Are Neglected, at a Cost in Suffering. http://www.nytimes.com/2009/09/13/us/13water.html.
4. Smith AH, Lopipero PA, Bates MN, Steinmaus CM. Public health: arsenic epidemiology and drinking water standards. Science 2002; 296:2145–2146.
5. Chiu HY, Hsueh YM, Liaw KF, Horng SF, Chiang MH, Pu YS, Lin JSN, Huang CH, Chen CJ. Incidence of internal cancers and ingested inorganic arsenic: a seven-year follow-up study in Taiwan. Cancer Res 1995; 55:1296–1300.
6. Chen CH, Chiou HY, Hsueh YM, Chen CJ, Yu HJ, Pu YS. Clinicopathological characteristics and survival outcome of arsenic related bladder cancer in Taiwan. J Urol 2009; 181:547–553.
7. Chen CL, Hsu LI, Chiou HY, Hsueh YM, Chen SY, Wu MM, Chen CJ. Blackfoot Disease study group. JAMA 2004; 292:2984–2990.

8. Tseng CH. An overview on peripheral vascular disease in blackfoot disease-hyper-endemic villages in Taiwan. Angiology 2002; 53:529–537.

9. Tseng CH, Huang YK, Huang YL, Chung CJ, Yang MH, Chen CJ, Hsueh YM. Arsenic exposure, urinary arsenic speciation, and peripheral vascular disease in blackfoot disease-hyperendemic villages in Taiwan. Toxicol Appl Pharmacol 2005; 206:299–308.

10. Lee TC, Tanaka N, Lamb PW, Gilmer TM, Barrett JC. Induction of gene amplification by arsenic. Science 1988; 241:79–81.

11. Ahmad SA, Sayed MHS, Barua S, Khan MH, Faruquee MH, Jalil A, Hadi SA, Talukder HK. Arsenic in drinking water and pregnancy outcomes. Environ Health Perspect 2001; 109:629–631.

12. Barry M, Hughes JM. Talking dirty: the politics of clean water and sanitation. N Engl J Med 2008; 359:784–787.

13. Shanon MA, Bohn PW, Elimelech M, Georgiadis JG, Marinas BJ, Mayes AM. Science and technology for water purification in the coming decades. Nature 2008; 452:301–310.

Chapter 17: Toxic Chemicals in the Environment: Government Regulations and Public Health

1. Schwarzman MR, Wilson MP. New science for chemicals policy. Science 2009; 326:1065–1066.

2. CDC, Fourth National Report on Human Exposure to Environmental Chemicals. 2009, Centers for Disease Control and Prevention, National Center for Environmental Health: Atlanta, GA.

3. USEPA. What is the TSCA Chemical Substance Inventory? 2006 (cited April 4, 2007) Available from http://www.epa.gov.

4. Gee D. Late lessons from early warnings: toward realism and precaution with endocrine-disrupting substances. Environ Health Perspect 2006; 114:152–160.

5. National Toxicology Program, Center for the Evaluation of Risks to Human Reproduction, Reproductive and Developmental Effects of Bisphenol A. September 2008 NIH Publication No. 08–5994. Available at http://cerhr.niehs.nih.gov.

6. Li, D, Zhou Z. Occupational exposure to bisphenol-A (BPA) and the risk of self-reported male sexual dysfunction. Hum Reprod 2010; 25:519–527.

7. Woodruff TJ, Zeise L, Axelrod DA, et al. Moving upstream: evaluating adverse upstream end points for improved risk assessment and decision-making. Environ Health Perspect 2008; 116:1568–1575. Meeting report.

8. Carpenter DO, Arcaro K, Spink DC. Understanding the human health effects of chemical mixtures. Environ Health Perspect 2002; 110:25–42.

9. http://www.epa.gov/oppt/existingchemicals/pubs/principles.pdf.

10. Lockey JE, Brooks SM, Jarabek AM, Khoury PR, McKay RT, Carson A, et al. Pulmonary changes after exposure to vermiculite contaminated with fibrous tremolite. Am Rev Respir Dis 1984; 129:952–958.

11. Sullivan PA. Vermiculite, respiratory disease and asbestos exposure in Libby, Montana: update of a cohort mortality study. Environ Health Perspect 2007; 115: 579–585.

12. Peipins LA, Lewin M, Campolucci S, et al. Radiographic abnormalities and exposure to asbestos-contaminated vermiculite in the community of Libby, Montana, USA. Environ Health Perspect 2003; 111:1753–1759.

13. Muravov OI, Kaye WE, Lewin M, et al. The usefulness of computed tomography in detecting asbestos-related pleural abnormalities in people who had indeterminate chest radiographs: the Libby, MT, experience. Int J Hyg Environ Health 2009; 208:87–99.

14. Rohs AM, Lockey JE, Dunning KK, et al. Low-level fiber-induced radiographic changes caused by Libby vermiculite. Am J Respir Crit Care Med 2008; 177: 630–637.

15. Vinikoor LC, Larson TC, Bateson TF, Birnbaum L. Exposure to asbestos-containing vermiculite ore and respiratory symptoms among individuals who were children while the mine was active in Libby, Montana. Environ Health Perspect 2010; 118:1033–1038.

16. Horton DK, Bove F, Kapil V. Select mortality and cancer incidence among residents in various U.S. communities that received asbestos-contaminated vermiculite ore from Libby, Montana. Inhalation Toxicology 2008; 20:767–775.

Page references followed by *fig* indicate an illustrated figure; followed by *t* indicate a table.